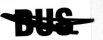
Asthma

ASTHMA

THE COMPLETE GUIDE
TO INTEGRATIVE THERAPIES

Jonathan Brostoff, M.D.
Linda Gamlin

Healing Arts Press
Rochester, Vermont

Healing Arts Press
One Park Street
Rochester, Vermont 05767
www.InnerTraditions.com

Healing Arts Press is a division of Inner Traditions International

Copyright © 1999, 2000 by Dr. Jonathan Brostoff and Linda Gamlin
Originally published in London by Bloomsbury

First U.S. edition published by Healing Arts Press

*Note to the reader: This book is intended as an informational guide. The remedies,
approaches, and techniques described herein are meant to supplement, and not to be
a substitute for, professional medical care or treatment. They should not be used to
treat a serious ailment without prior consultation with a qualified health care
professional.*

Library of Congress Cataloging-in-Publication Data

Brostoff, Jonathan.
    Asthma : the complete guide to integrative therapies / Jonathan Brostoff
and Linda Gamlin.—1st U.S. ed.
        p. cm.
    Originally Published: London : Bloomsbury, 1999.
    Includes index.
    ISBN 0-89281-932-4 (alk. paper)
        1. Asthma—Popular works. 2. Asthma—Alternative treatment.
        I. Gamlin, Linda. II. Title.

RC591 .B77 2000
616.2'38—dc21

00-040844

Printed and bound in the United States

10 9 8 7 6 5 4 3 2 1

This book was typeset in Berling Agency

Acknowledgements

This book would not have been possible without the work of thousands of different doctors, medical researchers and other health professionals, in many parts of the world. We cannot possibly mention all those whose work we have drawn on from scientific journals and textbooks, but we would like to thank those who have taken time to talk to us, allowed us to quote their opinions on asthma, or checked certain sections of the book: Dr Raymond Agius and all those at the Department of Public Health Sciences at Edinburgh University, Professor Jon Ayres, Dr Neil G. M. Beattie, Liz Bell, Dr Sybil Birtwhistle, Peter Blackaby, Dr Simon Bowler, Sue Clarke, Dr Joe Collier, Dr Adnan Custovic, John Green, Professor Claire Infante-Rivard, Dr Richard Lawson, Huy Le, Pat MacDonald, Sally Magnusson, Dr John Maunder, Dr Robin Monro, Ilana Nevill, Professor Tom Platts-Mills, David Reading, Robin Shepherd, Dr Veronica Spooner, Dr Martin Stern, Owen Tudor, Dr Erika von Mutius, Jessica Ward and Des Whitrow.

We are also grateful to the many asthma sufferers, and parents of asthmatics, who have shared their experiences with us: Helen Adam, Barny Allan, Chris Allan, Helen Arnold, Rollo Arnold, Peter Barnes, Ella Blamble, Catherine Bligh, Chrissie Bligh, Tom Bragg, Gerry Day, Ken Day, Dee Gill, Gerry Gill, Penny Gillam, Stephen Gordon-Saker, Sarah Hughes, Christer Nordlund, Jill Olney, Louise Pirouet, Donna Price, Henry Stobart, Maurice Teulan, Arthur Wainwright, Mo Wakeman, Lucy Wendover and Jean Wilkins. They have helped us realise, among other things, how varied the experiences of asthmatics are, and how often they differ from the standard medical picture of asthma. We hope that this book reflects that great diversity and individuality of experience, and will therefore be of help to other asthmatics.

Finally, we would like to thank Philippa Porter, Lisa Cummings, and Polly Heffer for their considerable help with the final hectic stages of this book.

A Note to American Readers:

The brand names of prescription and over-the-counter drugs sometimes vary from country to country, and American readers should refer to the list of generic drug names that begins on p. 370 if they do not recognize a particular drug name. The generic name should be listed in small type somewhere on the package or insert. If you have any questions, your pharmacist should be able to answer them.

Likewise, laws relevant to those with occupational asthma are different in the USA, and readers will want to consult with their local trade union, the state department of health, or a private attorney to determine their legal rights and options.

Linda Gamlin's Web site offers information of interest to readers around the globe and can be reached at www.allergy-intolerance.com.

Contents

1 **How this book can help you**
Feel better and get more out of life   2
Twenty things every asthmatic should know (before it's too late)   7
Children with asthma – how to help   11

2 **Basic information**
What is asthma – and why does it develop?   20
Technical words used about asthma – what they mean   31
Is asthma 'all in the mind'?   34
Does asthma get worse in time? Or does it go away?   42

3 **Asthma attacks – what to do**
Recognizing an asthma attack   45
Coping with an asthma attack   50
After an attack: the next steps are crucial   59

4 **Understanding your symptoms**
Why do asthma symptoms vary so much?   65
Why does exercise trigger asthma attacks?   68
Why is asthma worse at night?   74

5 **The asthma epidemic – and how to beat it**
Why is asthma on the increase?   79
Can parents prevent their children from getting asthma?   87
Can a good diet protect against asthma?   96
What does the future hold for asthma treatment?   105

6 **Allergies**
Asthma and allergies – what's the connection?   110
How to tell if allergies are at the root of your asthma   113
Avoiding house dust mites   127
Avoiding pollen, cats, moulds and other allergens   156
Is it true that food allergies can affect asthma?   179
Tackling the cause of allergies: desensitization treatments   197

7 **The air we breathe**
Air pollution   204
Cigarette smoking – the link with asthma   216
Indoor air pollution and how to prevent it in your home   221
Why does the weather affect asthma?   227
Can asthma attacks be brought on by smells?   232

8 **Diseases and drugs that make asthma worse**
Colds, flu and chest infections   237
Sinusitis   240
Athlete's foot, ringworm, *Candida* and other fungal infections   246
Other medical problems that can make asthma worse   253
Aspirin and aspirin-like drugs   257
Other drugs that can affect asthma   262

9 **Special situations**
Work and asthma – which jobs are risky?   268
Pregnancy, birth and breast-feeding   287
Sport and asthma   293

10 **Getting medical help**
Doctors, asthma nurses and specialists   298
Medical tests used for asthma   303
Can the doctor be sure it's asthma?   306
Peak-flow meters: an early-warning system for asthma   315

11 **Drug treatment**
Are all these drugs really necessary? And are they safe?   319
What are the different drugs supposed to do?   334
Side-effects: which ones are worth worrying about?   350
Identify your drugs   370
How to use inhalers, spacers and nebulizers   376
Decisions about drugs: what to take, how much and when   388

12 **Alternative medicine**
What can alternative medicine offer?   394
Yoga and yoga therapy   397
Osteopaths and chiropractors   400
Alexander Technique and Feldenkrais Method   403
Herbal remedies, homeopathy and aromatherapy   407
Acupuncture and shiatsu   410
Breathing exercises and the Buteyko Method   414
Methods that promote calmness and relaxation   446

Appendix 1 **Useful addresses**   452
Appendix 2 **Allergen particles – the range of sizes**   462
Appendix 3 **Products for those with asthma**   465
Index   483

1

How this book can help you

'Now I feel I've really got on top of it . . .'

Jenny is 23 and has had asthma ever since she can remember. 'At one time I was a real Ventolin junkie – once someone stole my bag and I was in a total panic because I hadn't got my inhaler – I didn't care about my credit cards or money. I got an attack just like that, because the inhaler wasn't there.

'My asthma was pretty bad all the time, and it just dominated my life, it stopped me doing so many things. I felt I really couldn't go on like that. It wasn't any sort of life.

'Now I feel I've really got on top of it, and I hardly ever get asthma attacks. I'm much more careful about avoiding dust and cats, which makes a big difference. Last year I started doing yoga classes, and I'm a lot more chilled out about things now. When I have an attack I don't get panicky like I used to.

'I don't hang around with people who smoke any more. I think, "If they want to kill themselves that's okay but they're not taking me with them." Now my asthma is better I can go running and I swim quite a lot, a couple of times a week. I just feel so much healthier now. I haven't needed my inhaler for months.'

FEEL BETTER AND GET MORE OUT OF LIFE

Most asthmatics could feel substantially better, need fewer drugs, and enjoy life more – it is just a question of tackling asthma from several different angles, rather than relying solely on drugs. This section summarizes the steps you can take to deal with your asthma, and guides you to different parts of the book which give more detailed advice.

Identify allergies and avoid allergens

Few doctors or asthma nurses have time to talk to their asthmatic patients about allergies, and they often know very little about avoidance measures. This is unfortunate because allergies are a very common cause (or contributing factor) in asthma, particularly in children – more than 80 per cent of asthmatic children are allergic to something. Their allergies are a fundamental cause of the asthma (not just a trigger for attacks), and reducing exposure to the allergen can make a huge difference.

There is far more that can be done to avoid allergens than most people (including doctors) realize. Don't believe anyone who says 'You can't get rid of house dust mites,' or 'Pollen is unavoidable.'

You can begin working out what you or your child are allergic to, if you don't already know, by using the checklists on pp. 115–25. Remember that workplace allergens are also a possible cause of asthma (see pp. 280–3). Avoidance measures for house dust mite are described on pp. 127–155 and for other airborne allergens on pp. 156–178. For allergens that really are unavoidable, desensitization treatments (see pp. 197–202) may be helpful.

Identify your major triggers and avoid them

There are many potential triggers for asthma attacks. These include some apparently harmless things such as breathing cold air or taking exercise, and some genuinely harmful things such as cigarette smoke or other irritants in the air. Triggers only produce this effect if the airways are already inflamed and 'twitchy': they are not a basic cause of asthma, but they can bring on attacks and make asthma worse. Someone who has asthma only in the pollen season, for example, will be sensitive to triggers at that time, but not during the winter. (Note that a trigger is not the same thing as an allergen.)

If you can get your asthma under control you may find that triggers no longer affect you. Until then, avoiding triggers is a useful way of reducing the number of asthma attacks.

The list below gives all the common potential triggers for asthma attacks: you may well be sensitive to quite a few of them. The page references can be followed up for more information about each trigger, and for tips on avoidance.

These are the common triggers for asthma:
- cold or very dry air (see p. 227)
- exercise – but this is definitely *not* something you should avoid and you can exercise safely if you take the right precautions (see p. 70)
- colds and chest infections (see p. 237)
- emotional upsets or stressful situations (see p. 34)
- excitement (see p. 34)
- industrial pollution (see pp. 207 and 211–3)
- traffic pollution (see pp. 204–11) – note that some forms of pollution, such as ozone, are not detectable and may occur in areas with apparently light traffic
- irritants in the air at home or in public places, such as cigarette smoke, fly spray, air freshener or other aerosols (see pp. 221–6)
- irritants in the air at work (see pp. 283–5)
- strong smells – even pleasant ones such as the scent of flowers (see p. 232)
- sulphur dioxide given off by foods and drinks (see p. 180)
- aspirin and aspirin-like drugs (see pp. 257–61): note that these can affect you even if you have taken them without ill-effects before
- thunderstorms (see p. 229)

Treat hayfever and other nasal allergies
By getting any allergic symptoms in the nose under control, you may greatly reduce your asthma symptoms (see p. 253).

Learn to breathe well
It is easy to get into unhealthy patterns of breathing – this can happen to anyone, but asthmatics are especially vulnerable. Hyperventilation (see p. 419) is a particular problem and can make asthma symptoms much worse, or even mimic asthma. You need to find someone – a

physiotherapist or alternative practitioner – who can help you retrain your breathing and learn healthier patterns (see pp. 422–8). Both children and adults can benefit from breathing retraining.

Strengthen your breathing muscles
Several independent lines of research have shown that, by strengthening their breathing muscles, asthmatics can improve their condition. Exercises that are of proven benefit – tested by doctors in Canada and never previously published – are described on pp. 321–45.

Practise a relaxation exercise, or take up yoga or a martial art
Staying calm during asthma attacks, and feeling in control of your breathing, will help enormously. There are many different ways to do this, but relaxation exercises (see p. 447), hypnotherapy (see p. 450), biofeedback (see p. 449), autogenic training (see p. 447), yoga (see p. 397) and martial arts such as aikido or tai chi (see p. 429) are particularly recommended.

Look into food sensitivity
Only a minority of asthmatics have food intolerance, but for those who do, identifying the culprit food and avoiding it (see p. 181) can lead to a major improvement in their asthma symptoms.

Treat heartburn and chronic infections (sinusitis, athlete's foot etc.)
A number of lingering infections, including athlete's foot and sinusitis can be a major contributing factor in asthma. Treating these infections may improve asthma symptoms enormously (see pp. 240–52).

Heartburn (gastro-oesophageal reflux) can also make asthma worse – or even mimic asthma (see pp. 254 and 312).

Check you are not taking drugs that make asthma worse
Several different drugs, prescribed for conditions such as glaucoma, high blood pressure, angina, prevention of heart attacks, migraine, diabetes and thyroid problems, can aggravate asthma. So can the contraceptive pill and HRT (hormone replacement therapy). See pp. 262–6 for more details. Aspirin and related drugs, some of which are prescribed for arthritis or sports injuries, can make asthma worse in susceptible people (see p. 257).

Avoid chest infections

For many asthmatics, colds and chest infections are a major trigger for worsening asthma. Although it is not easy to avoid these infections, there are some steps you can take (see pp. 237–9). And you can safely use preventer drugs to reduce the impact of infections on your asthma (see p. 238).

Protect yourself from pollution

Some of the worst air pollution occurs in our houses. This can aggravate existing asthma, and make children more likely to develop asthma. Measures to combat indoor pollution are described on pp. 221–6.

You can minimize the effects of outdoor pollution in a variety of ways, from simple avoidance to wearing a pollution mask. New research shows that vitamin supplements can also protect you from the effects of pollution (see p. 213).

Consider whether your workplace is bad for your asthma

Irritants and allergens inhaled at work are a significant cause of asthma. If your workplace could be the culprit, it is important to take prompt action (see pp. 268–77). Chemicals encountered both in the workplace and at home, such as formaldehyde, can also cause asthma, or make it worse (see pp. 223–6). Because you are exposed to them at home as well as at work, the link may not be obvious.

Use a peak-flow meter

Peak-flow meters put asthma sufferers in touch with their airways, and give an early warning of asthma attacks. They can greatly improve the control of asthma symptoms (see pp. 315–7).

Review your drugs, and your inhaler devices

Many people go on taking drugs at the same dosage for months or years, when the dosage needs to be increased, or could be reduced (see pp. 390–1). Other asthmatics are taking obsolete drugs or using outdated inhaler devices, when far better drugs and inhalers are now available. If you have not seen your doctor or asthma nurse for some time, make an appointment and ask to review your treatment. Some of the new drugs available for asthma could make a big difference to your life (see pp. 340–1).

Work out a management plan with your doctor

Research shows that people get their asthma under control far more successfully if they have a management plan, worked out with their doctor or asthma nurse (see pp. 391–2). The number of emergency visits to hospital is substantially reduced and asthma no longer disrupts everyday life. Management plans are particularly useful for the parents of asthmatic children.

Have an osteopathy treatment

Asthma takes its toll on the ribcage and shoulders, because of the over-inflation of the lungs that occurs during an asthma attack. The bones and cartilage can become fixed in unnatural positions, making it more difficult for asthmatics to adopt healthy breathing patterns. An osteopath will sort out these problems and can teach you or your child useful breathing exercises (see pp. 400–2).

Take more strenuous exercise and get fit

Vigorous exercise keeps the airways elastic, and by improving your fitness you will have fewer problems with exercise-induced asthma (see pp. 68–9). It is well worth using extra doses of asthma drugs that will allow you to take exercise – in the long term, once you are fitter, you will probably need fewer drugs to control your asthma.

Lose weight

Several studies have shown that children and adults who are over-weight are more likely to develop asthma. No one yet knows if losing weight will improve asthma, once it is established, but this seems likely because the extra poundage makes breathing much harder work (see p. 255). If you improve your diet (see below) and take more exercise, losing weight will probably come fairly easily.

Improve your diet

There is good evidence now that a typical Western diet, with its high intake of salt and fat and low intake of fruit and vegetables, is part of the reason for our epidemic rates of asthma (see pp. 96–104). It is possible that improving your diet will help to alleviate asthma symptoms.

Consider chemical sensitivity

Sensitivity to everyday chemicals such as petrol fumes, cleaning fluids, perfumes and newspaper ink is a contributing factor for some asthmatics (see p. 225).

TWENTY THINGS EVERY ASTHMATIC SHOULD KNOW (BEFORE IT'S TOO LATE)

Many of the following items of information are not well publicized. There are asthmatics who would still be alive today, or in much better health, if they had known these facts.

1. Fatal asthma attacks often come on very quickly. One study found that half those who died did so within two hours of starting their asthma attack. A quarter died within 30 minutes. So don't delay seeking help if your asthma starts to get much worse (see p. 51). Knowing how to recognize a severe asthma attack (see p. 45) and what to do about it (see pp. 50–7) could be a lifesaver.

2. The air pollution in a kitchen is often worse than on a city street. Kitchens with gas cookers and no ventilation hoods frequently have levels of nitrogen dioxide that exceed WHO safety limits. A child exposed to this air is more likely to develop asthma (see p. 208). Asthmatic parents need to be aware of such risks because their children are already more likely to develop asthma (see p. 87), and exposing them to other risk factors will further increase the chance of their becoming asthmatic. The good news is that there are many things parents can do to reduce the chance of a child developing asthma (see pp. 87–95).

3. Coughing is a major symptom of asthma for many people, including children. Doctors sometimes forget this (see p. 308), so you need to be aware of it. Some asthmatics – including some with severe life-threatening asthma – have coughing as their main symptom.

4. If you have nocturnal asthma every night, this is regarded by doctors as severe asthma. Research has shown that more than half of those with regular nocturnal asthma think their asthma is 'mild' or moderate', which worries doctors because these people have greatly under-estimated the risk that their asthma poses. Most asthma deaths occur at night, or follow on from asthma attacks that began during the night. It is important to treat nocturnal asthma and get the inflammation in the airways under control (see p. 74).

5. As many as one in ten asthmatics eventually becomes sensitive to aspirin. If you have harmless growths in your nose called nasal polyps, and a constant runny or blocked nose – chronic rhinitis – this indicates that you may be sensitive to aspirin (see p. 257) or are likely to develop this sensitivity in the future. Aspirin sensitivity can come on quite suddenly, even though you have taken aspirin safely in the past. And it can produce a serious asthma attack, or collapse, which could land you in hospital. Such attacks can be fatal. Asthmatics should be cautious about taking aspirin or any related drug (see p. 258).

6. Surgical operations on the nose can make asthma much worse, or bring back asthma in someone who has outgrown it. Some doctors advise asthmatics against having operations on the nose unless absolutely essential, because it could leave them with much more serious asthma symptoms – permanently. But other doctors are unaware of this risk. Think hard before you have such an operation, and ask your doctor if it is really necessary.

7. Bathing babies and young children every day, and regular hand-washing, substantially increases the risk of asthma (see p. 93).

8. Of those who die each year from a true allergy to food or insect stings (see p. 111), the vast majority are asthmatic. Anyone with asthma and an allergy which causes anaphylaxis (see p. 48) should be seen promptly by a specialist and given proper treatment, including injectable adrenaline to carry with them.

9. Certain household cleaning products give off concentrated sulphur dioxide gas which can cause fatal asthma attacks (see p. 223). Products that release chlorine are also dangerous, and so are some DIY kits for painting cars (see p. 225). It pays to read labels when buying any new product – but the label may not always tell you about the asthma risk.

10. Some of the advice commonly given for reducing house dust mite infestation is wrong, and can actually make asthma symptoms *worse* by increasing the amount of mite allergen that you or your asthmatic child inhale (see p. 143).

11. Those who die during a severe asthma attack have often been exposed to very large doses of their allergen in the previous 24 hours. This is particularly true of those allergic to animals, house dust and *Alternaria* mould (see p. 165). The risk of a fatal asthma attack is particularly high in someone who has been taking a long course of steroid tablets, and has stopped or reduced the dose in the previous year – this is a time to be especially vigilant about allergens.

12. Although certain drugs should be avoided in pregnancy, uncontrolled asthma in a pregnant woman poses a far higher risk to the baby than the use of asthma drugs (see p. 287).

13. People with asthma and allergies are at risk of developing new allergies if they throw themselves into activities that involve heavy exposure to allergens (see pp. 110–1).

14. Antibiotics, if given to babies in the first two years of life, double the risk of asthma developing. Some antibiotics are worse than others (see p. 92). Doctors sometimes prescribe antibiotics for chest infections that are actually caused by viruses – so the antibiotic is of no value anyway.

15. Asthmatic children have died in British schools because their inhalers were kept locked away and a teacher refused access to the inhaler when an asthma attack began. Parents of asthmatic children can help schools to develop better strategies for coping with asthma (see p. 15).

16. If you develop asthma at your workplace, you should leave the job (or get a transfer) as soon as possible. People who develop asthma from something encountered at work often have it for ever – and it can be disabling (see p. 280). If you leave your job (or get transferred to another part of the same workplace, where there is no exposure to the offending substance), you have a much better chance of recovering (see p. 268). It may not be obvious that your asthma is due to your work (see p. 270).

17. Asthma may not always be asthma – misdiagnosis does occur. There are many different medical conditions – from stomach acid reflux to low-level carbon monoxide poisoning – that can be mistaken for asthma by doctors (see p. 309).

18. Steroid tablets have damaging and sometimes dangerous side-effects, whereas inhaled steroids are far safer. It makes sense to use inhaled steroids regularly and keep asthma under control, rather than let asthma get out of control and need steroid tablets (see p. 326).

19. Many asthmatics use reliever inhalers (such as Ventolin) far too often, and this can lead to severe, sometimes fatal, asthma attacks (see p. 322). Some doctors are still not giving their patients the correct advice about over-using these drugs.

20. Ignoring exercise-induced asthma, and continuing to exercise regardless, is dangerous because the lungs are over-inflated and the oxygen levels in the blood are low. Fatal asthma attacks have occurred in these circumstances (see p. 70).

Did you know?

Some of the products sold in high-street shops, and labelled as being useful for allergies or asthma, are completely ineffective. These include sprays for pets (see p. 164), pesticide sprays for bedding and mattresses which will have no effect on the main source of trouble – dust mites or their allergens inside the mattress (see p. 150), and air ionizers, which can actually make asthma symptoms worse. Room vaporizers, described as being useful for allergy sufferers, will also tend to make matters worse for anyone allergic to house dust mite by increasing humidity in the room (see p. 140).

CHILDREN WITH ASTHMA – HOW TO HELP

Helping a child during an asthma attack

All the basic information on recognizing and coping with asthma attacks (see pp. 45–58) applies to children as much as to adults. It helps to be familiar with all this in advance, and to visualize the situation and what you would do. Visualize doing the right things and *keeping calm* at the same time – that is the only way you can help the child to stay calm. If you tend to be nervy and over-anxious, consider learning some special relaxation skills (see p. 446). Remember that it is very rare for a child to die during an asthma attack. Those who do suffer fatal attacks have generally been neglecting their preventer medication, missing out on regular asthma check-ups, and failing to notice worsening asthma.

A child may be very scared by the attack, and holding hands can be reassuring, but don't put your arm around the child's shoulders as this makes it more difficult to take a breath. So does lying down – make sure that all the child's carers know this, and teach the child the best positions to adopt during an attack (see p. 54). Loosen any tight clothing.

If you don't already have a spacer, consider getting one in case of severe attacks, when inhalers can become difficult to use. Prime the spacer ready for use (see pp. 382–3).

When a child does have to go into hospital with an asthma attack, one parent should try to go too, stay in sight of the child during treatment, and remain there overnight if possible. Being left in hospital without any familiar faces close at hand is very frightening for a child.

Children and asthma drugs

With the help of modern preventer drugs, almost every child with asthma should be able to lead a normal life and do most of the things that other children do. If your child cannot play or run around without getting breathless, or if you feel as though you live on a roller-coaster, lurching from one asthma crisis to another, then your child is probably being under-treated (see pp. 390–1).

Basically, drug treatment for children is much the same as for adults (see pp. 334–49). However, children may have difficulty in using inhalers, especially when very young. Spacers (see p. 380) overcome this problem.

The B-2 reliever drugs are available as tablets or syrup, and may be much easier for children to take. However, they take longer to work and are much more likely to cause side-effects, because a larger dose is required. For this reason, children should be encouraged to inhale the drugs, if they possibly can: this gives the maximum benefit with the minimum of side-effects.

The new drugs called leukotriene antagonists (see p. 340) are taken once a day in tablet form, and may be useful for children who have serious difficulty with inhaling their asthma drugs.

Most children with asthma have allergies, and the cromoglycate-type drugs are excellent preventers which can stop allergic reactions before they start. They are used for children over one year old and are extremely safe (see p. 338). If you have not been offered these, ask your doctor about them.

With children suffering from severe asthma who are taking steroid tablets, keep an eye on their growth (see p. 355). Make sure they don't come into contact with other children suffering from chicken-pox, measles or shingles, and see the doctor urgently if there is any contact (see p. 360).

At the end of a long course of steroid tablets (anything more than three weeks), or when the dose of tablets is reduced, be extra careful about allergens and asthma triggers. A child is more vulnerable to severe asthma attacks for as much as a year after long-term steroid tablets are stopped or the dosage reduced.

There have been reports that theophylline-type drugs may produce behavioural problems and learning difficulties in children. Recent research in the USA suggests that this is not true for children aged six and over, but theophylline might affect younger children. Inhaled steroids were also studied by these researchers and found to have no effects on behaviour in children over six.

Parents often worry a great deal about all the drugs an asthmatic child takes. Generally speaking, these drugs are very safe and only children with severe asthma are at risk of serious side-effects (see pp. 350–69). Obviously, if you can reduce the need for drugs by taking steps to reduce allergen exposure (see pp. 127–78) and avoid asthma triggers (see pp. 2–3) you should do so, but if the child still need drugs it is far better to accept them than to struggle with all the limitations and problems that asthma imposes on a child's life (see p. 333).

If you are still concerned about drugs after reading pp. 319–33, talk to your doctor about your fears. Where there are doubts and dis-agreements about drugs within the family, try not to air these in front of the asthmatic child. Sort out an agreed policy on asthma drugs with your partner and present a united front to the child.

Getting children to take asthma drugs

Babies and toddlers may object strongly to being dosed with asthma drugs. There are various ways of getting them used to the spacer (see p. 382), and it helps to make the whole thing seem like a game. If this doesn't work, don't get into a battle of wills – it is best to leave it a while, reassure the child, and try again later. But if you have repeated difficulty, and doses are being missed, talk to your doctor about the problem.

Children usually become more cooperative as they get older, especially if you take the time to talk to them about their asthma and explain why they need the medicines. As soon as the child can understand, explain the difference between preventers and relievers. The important message to get across is that using preventers regularly will keep asthma under control and mean that there are fewer embarrassing attacks and less need to use the reliever inhaler in public.

It will help to talk about asthma to your child's schoolfriends, when you get the chance, so that it is easier for him or her when an attack does happen. By welcoming the child's friends into your home, and building up good relationships with them, you will be helping to smooth the difficult transition into independence that occurs later.

Six-year-olds will still need to be reminded to take their drugs and check their peak flow, but by the time they are seven or eight most children can remember for themselves. Encourage them to take as much responsibility as possible for their own medication, while keep-ing a careful eye on how they are doing. By taking a more 'hands-off' approach at this stage you will build up their own sense of indepen-dence and maturity. This will pay dividends later, when they get into their teens, because taking their asthma drugs will already be a self-directed habit, not something they identify with being nagged about or fussed over. With luck, their teenage rebelliousness will then be directed elsewhere, not at their asthma treatment.

Adolescence may bring a new spate of problems and worries. This is a time when the need to be exactly like the peer group and free from parental direction is overwhelming, and when emotional problems are common. Some asthmatic teenagers neglect their medication, or start smoking cigarettes, or both. Getting into a confrontational situation is likely to make matters worse, so be as tactful and diplomatic as possible. If you have already established a good relationship with your child's friends this will help a lot, as their attitudes to issues such as smoking can be crucial. Your child needs not only to refuse cigarettes but also to say, 'I can't go to that club, it's too smoky,' or 'Let's sit near the door and get some air' without being jeered at.

The Asthma and Allergy Foundation of America and other national support organizations (see Useful Addresses) offer some well-designed educational material specifically aimed at teenagers which can be helpful.

Although this is *extremely rare*, asthmatic teenagers (or their friends) may begin abusing inhaled short-acting B-2 relievers, or become addicted to the propellants used (see pp. 330–1). You should be alert to such problems but not worry unduly.

Growing up with asthma

The most useful thing you can do for an asthmatic child, especially when he or she first starts school, is to build up self-esteem and boost confidence. The problems of having asthma can easily make children feel 'not good enough' or 'different'. They may be very anxious and fearful, but feel that they have to protect their parents by never admitting this. Young children can even think that they have developed asthma because of something they have done wrong, but they may not tell you this unless you spend some quiet, unhurried time talking to them about their asthma.

If the asthma is severe, and limits physical activity, try to find other interests and hobbies that the child can do well. Focus on the positive things all the time:

- the steps you can both take to keep the asthma under control
- the successful way you have both dealt with some asthma attacks in the past
- the difficulties that he or she has already overcome
- the fact that he or she is good at many things despite having asthma
- the idea that coping with a challenge like asthma makes you a stronger and more determined person in the end

Make sure that friends or schoolteachers are not undermining your efforts by giving out negative messages.

Wanting to protect your child from asthma triggers can slip into being over-protective, and you should avoid this trap (see p. 38). Let your child live as normal a life as possible, and try not to say 'No' automatically to risky activities such as going out to play when it's cold. Think about it each time, take small risks, and don't always make the decision yourself – the child will gain a lot from being given the responsibility, even if the decision is sometimes the wrong one.

Tempting though it is to be extra nice to a child with asthma, you must be careful not to link asthma attacks to special treats or privileges. There should be no 'secondary gain' from asthma, no advantages to having an attack. Where there are other non-asthmatic children in the family, it is particularly important to treat them all just the same. Never let a child use asthma as a way of getting out of things or winning battles with brothers and sisters (see p. 39).

Should your child have to miss school because of asthma, ask the teacher to supply work that can be done at home, and make sure that it is done, so that your child does not fall behind in class. Encourage schoolfriends to visit, to relieve the isolation.

Taking care of yourself is also essential. The strain that severe asthma puts on a family is enormous. Research in the USA shows that divorce is more common in families where a child suffers from severe asthma. Don't add to the inevitable stress by feeling guilty about the fact that your child has asthma. It probably couldn't have been avoided, and even if it could, there is absolutely no point in blaming yourself or anyone else – a lot of the information about what causes asthma has only become known very recently.

If the stress of having an asthmatic child is getting too much, don't be afraid to admit it and ask for help. Your doctor may be able to arrange for counselling for you, or indeed for the whole family, if that seems appropriate.

Asthma and schools

Before your child starts a new school (or if asthma begins when the child is already at the school), don't hesitate to arrange a meeting with the class teacher to talk about asthma. Ask if the school has an asthma policy, if teachers are trained to deal with asthma attacks, and what arrangements are made for inhalers.

Ideally, children who can take responsibility for their own treatment (and most seven- to eight-year-olds can) should keep their inhalers with them, in their pocket or in a belt-pouch. For younger children, the inhaler should be in the classroom in a place that is immediately accessible (not locked in a cupboard or desk) and should be taken along at playtime and mealtimes, so that the child is always within easy reach of the inhaler. It is not acceptable to keep the inhaler in another room or with the school nurse – a slight delay in getting to the inhaler when an attack begins can have serious consequences.

Be diplomatic but persevere – children have died because teachers refused to let them use an inhaler at a crucial moment. Reassure staff that there is little danger of an asthmatic child over-dosing (though as a parent you should be keeping an eye on how quickly inhalers are used up – see p. 379) and if other children borrow the inhaler and have a few puffs they will suffer no ill-effects.

Check that the teacher realizes that cold air and exercise can bring on attacks, and that the child might need a reminder to take an extra puff of the reliever before games. You may want to talk to the games teacher or sports coach, and the playground attendants as well. It is important that games teachers are encouraging and supportive with asthmatic children, and never tell them to continue exercising if they are feeling breathless (see p. 70).

Would the teacher be able to recognize when an attack is not under control, and know what to do? (You could supply a photocopy of pp. 45–58.) Will the teacher keep an eye on your child and check that he or she is not embarrassed about using the inhaler in front of classmates? Teasing or bullying can be a problem for asthmatic children.

If the teacher seems to be saddled with the out-dated idea that asthma is a psychological problem, or that children are 'putting it on', go and talk to the principal. Suggest that a local asthma nurse or doctor come in and talk to the school about asthma – this can be useful to educate other children, as well as the teachers.

You might also consider directing your child's principal, teacher, or school nurse to information available from a national educational organization such as the Asthma and Allergy Foundation of America (see Useful Addresses).

Allergens in schools

These days schools often have carpets and soft furnishings to make them more homely. These may well be old and riddled with dust mites. If your child is allergic to mites, and if attacks are frequent at school, have a look around the classroom to see if this might be the explanation. Before talking to the head teacher, or the class teacher, about removing the offending items, make sure you know all the facts about dust mites (see pp. 127–55) so that you can assess whether proposed solutions to the problem would actually work. The teacher may suggest, for example, shampooing the carpet and furnishings, but this would not help at all (see p. 140).

Pets such as hamsters and mice are also common in classrooms these days. Some children may be allergic to these animals (see p. 119). Moulds can flourish if there is a damp problem in any of the school buildings, and these will affect children with mould allergy (see pp. 117–8).

In addition to allergens, there may be irritants in the air, such as the fumes produced during science lessons. Make sure the science teacher is aware that there are asthmatics in the class, and that any experiment producing fumes (e.g. sulphur dioxide or nitrogen dioxide) should be done in a fume cupboard. Bear in mind that strong-smelling substances such as glue, paint, felt-tip pens or air fresheners may also trigger attacks.

Children with true allergies to food or insect stings

True allergies to foods or insect stings can lead to anaphylaxis (see p. 111), which can be life-threatening, especially for those with asthma. It is very important that anyone looking after a child with such an allergy should know how to recognize anaphylactic shock and be aware of exactly what must be done in an emergency (see p. 55). Adrenaline (epinephrine) injector kits and inhalers must be within easy reach, never locked away in a cupboard. Check that the child's class teacher and others at the school know how to deal with anaphylaxis, and that a review of the procedures occurs at the beginning of each new school year, and before school trips. During a severe reaction, a child may find it difficult to self-inject, and may need adult help, so the teacher should have been shown how the injector kit works. Sports teachers and coaches, lifeguards, school bus drivers, club leaders, babysitters, childminders, best friends and grandparents should all be briefed on emergency procedures.

If you live in the USA or Canada, you may be asked to sign a waiver by the school. *Do* sign a waiver allowing the school to inject epinephrine (adrenaline) when necessary, but *don't* sign a waiver absolving them from responsibility if epinephrine was not used.

'I'm meant to be taking Flixotide . . .'

Tim is 15 and his asthma started when he was six. Tim's mother says 'He used to cough and cough and cough until he made himself sick. And there were a couple of times when he couldn't get his breath at all. Once in particular we had to rush him to the surgery in the middle of the night.'

Tim describes how it is now: 'When I wake up in the mornings, I just wheeze like anything. It gets better during the daytime, but when I play football at lunchtime I can't run around too much, because then I'll wheeze and it'll hurt. So I just stand around and wait for the ball to come by.

'I'm meant to be taking Flixotide – what did they say? – twice a day? Morning and evening, I think. The asthma nurse tries to get me to take the Flixotide. But the thing is, I get up in the morning and I'm in a rush and I just forget it.

'I do smoke sometimes. I know it's not a good idea really.'

Whenever Tim's asthma is discussed, the conversation degenerates into an argument. His parents blame Tim for the problem – because he doesn't use his Flixotide preventer, because he smokes occasionally, because his room is so untidy that it's impossible to clean it, and so on.

They talk to Tim about it in a way that makes him feel angry and uncooperative, for example, describing how the asthma nurse 'tells him off' for not taking his preventer. In fact the asthma nurse tries to talk to Tim as if he were a responsible adult, but his parents, by presenting the situation in this way, undermine her efforts and make Tim feel like a resentful child.

2

Basic information

'Patients have to make a lot of the decisions for themselves . . .'

Janey is an asthma nurse at a busy general practice. 'I think education about asthma is so important. We really need to get the message across. You just can't rely on the doctor and nurse all the time if you're asthmatic. Patients have to make a lot of the decisions for themselves, and if they knew more about asthma and really understood how the treatments work, as well as how to avoid things that make asthma worse, it would help them so much.

'Asthma is very worrying too, and people always think that maybe it will get worse as they get older. A lot of my job is about reassuring them that this probably won't happen.'

WHAT IS ASTHMA – AND WHY DOES IT DEVELOP?

How the lungs work

To understand asthma, it is important to know about the structure of the healthy lung. Diagrams of the lungs show them as two balloon-like objects in the chest. When we breathe in and the chest expands, it is easy to imagine the lungs expanding like two balloons being inflated. But in fact the lungs are not really like this – they are much more complex inside than a balloon.

To picture the structure of a lung, imagine a tree turned upside down, with millions of miniature balloons instead of leaves. These little balloons are called alveoli or air sacs. They are all packed together over the surface of the tree, with their sides touching, so you cannot normally see the twigs and branches of the tree.

The twigs and branches of the tree are all hollow tubes – these are the airways of the lung. When you breathe in, air rushes through the tree trunk (the trachea), along each branch (the bronchi), along each twig (the bronchioles), and into each air sac. When you breathe out, old stale air runs out of each air sac and along the twigs and branches to flow out again through the trunk.

What happens during an asthma attack?

During an asthma attack the airways (the twigs and branches of the tree) become narrower. The air sacs are not affected, just the tubes leading to them.

What are the consequences of airway-narrowing? Notice that the airways are not a 'dual carriageway' – they are a single-lane road. Air has to go in and come out along the same route, and it can't go in both directions at once.

Normally, the airways are organized rather like a road with roadworks, where temporary traffic lights are put up, allowing cars to go in one direction for a while (breathing in), then in the other direction (breathing out). When our breathing pattern is healthy we don't experience this as a problem. But during an asthma attack, when the airways narrow, the system breaks down: it takes so long for the out-breath to get out that you need a new in-breath before the out-breath is complete. As a result there is a 'traffic jam': it is as if cars from both directions are trying to get through the narrow gap at once. Stale air trying to escape gets in the way of fresh air trying to come in.

The asthmatic feels as if there isn't enough air coming in, and tries hard to inhale, when in fact what he or she needs to do is to breathe *out* more, in order to clear a path for the incoming air. It can be useful to remember this during an asthma attack: many sufferers find it helpful to focus their attention on breathing out.

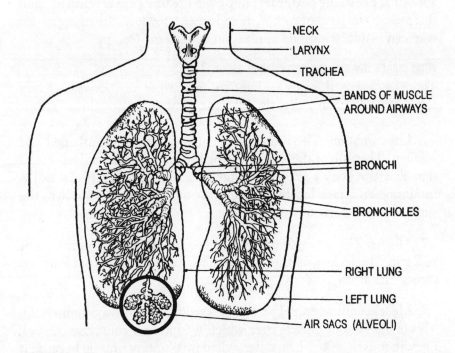

Why we breathe

Air is necessary because it contains oxygen, without which we suffocate. When fresh new air reaches the air sacs of our lungs, the oxygen gas is extracted from it by our blood. Oxygen can get into the blood because the blood flows all around the air sacs in a network of tiny blood vessels known as capillaries. As oxygen moves from the air sacs into the blood, another gas, carbon dioxide, moves in the opposite direction. Carbon dioxide is a waste gas which is produced in all parts of the body and disposed of via the blood.

The blood flows away from the lungs, carrying its precious load of oxygen which it takes to every part of the body. At the same time, the air sacs empty and the stale air, loaded with carbon dioxide, is breathed out.

The purpose of breathing is to get oxygen into the blood, and carbon dioxide out. But it is wrong to think of oxygen as wholly good and carbon dioxide as wholly bad. Each of these gases has a correct level in the blood, and there should not be too little or too much of either. In an effort to deal with their attacks, some asthmatics develop abnormal breathing patterns. They over-breathe (hyperventilate) and this pushes the level of carbon dioxide down too low. Breathing in this way can produce various unpleasant symptoms (see pp. 419–20).

What makes the airways narrower in asthma?

Three different things can happen to narrow the airways. Every asthmatic will have a slightly different combination of these factors:

1. **Inflammation**: The lining of the airways becomes inflamed and swollen. This is like the swelling which occurs around a deep cut: a sign that the body's immune system (its defence against disease) is mounting an attack locally. Because the airway lining is swollen, the tube becomes narrower inside.

2. **Mucus**: The airway lining produces a lot of thick sticky mucus or phlegm, which clogs up the airways. This mucus is white or clear, and sometimes frothy.

3. **Muscle contraction**: The muscles around the airways tighten up. This is the kind of muscle over which we have no conscious control, like the muscle of the heart. It is called involuntary muscle because it contracts or relaxes without our having much say in the matter. (Asthmatics may, with training, gain some degree of control over these muscles – see p. 449). When the muscles of the airways (bronchial muscles) contract during an asthma attack, they do so very sharply, and this is known as bronchospasm.

The reactions that occur in asthma are just exaggerated versions of normal, healthy reactions that our lungs use to defend themselves:

1. **Inflammation** is a reaction by the immune defences which is normally used to fend off bacteria, viruses and other infectious microbes (germs).

2. Mucus is produced to 'mop up' irritating dust particles, so that they can be ejected from the airways by coughing.

3. The muscles around the airways can tighten temporarily to reduce the inflow of air when it is thick with smoke or other irritants.

All three are basically healthy reactions, but in asthma they become unhealthy over-reactions.

Once asthma is established, the muscles around the airways will tighten in response to many different triggers (see pp. 2–3). The problem is that the airways are over-sensitive or hyper-reactive: in other words, they narrow at the smallest provocation. Doctors sometimes describe these airways as 'twitchy'. One of the aims of asthma treatment is to calm down the airways so that they are less sensitive.

The symptoms of asthma

There are four main symptoms of asthma. Not all asthmatics show all these symptoms: often only one or two are present.

1. **Shortness of breath**: This may not be noticeable normally, but walking upstairs, playing sport, or running to catch a bus may suddenly leave the asthmatic gasping for breath. The activity itself has not necessarily brought on the asthma (although this does happen for many asthmatics – see p. 68). It is just that the narrowed airways are no particular problem when standing, sitting, or walking slowly on level ground, because the body does not need much oxygen for these activities. When the body gets active and demands more oxygen, the narrow airways start to become a problem.

2. **Tightness in the chest**: Asthmatics often feel as if there is a tight band around their chest (or a very heavy weight on it, when they are lying down). This feeling indicates that there is stale air trapped in the chest which has not been able to escape through the narrow airways. New air is being inhaled before the out-breath is complete, and this is forced in on top of the stale air still left in the lungs, making the lungs and chest expand excessively.

3. **Coughing**: One of the lungs' most powerful weapons against unwelcome guests is the cough. It forces air and mucus out sharply, and this takes any rubbish and debris with it, pushing it upwards and out of the lungs. We cough when a crumb goes down the wrong way, or when we have phlegm in the lungs from a chest infection. In asthmatics, the cough can be a healthy and useful reaction to the mucus produced as part of the asthma, pushing it out of the lungs. But in some asthmatics the cough seems to be just a reflex reaction to the inflammation and obstruction in the airways; this sort of cough does not produce any mucus and is not particularly helpful. (However, it is *not* a good idea to treat it with cough mixtures – see p. 349.)

4. Wheezing: If the airways tighten up enough, the air forcing its way through the narrow gaps makes a whistling noise, known as wheezing. Although wheezing is firmly linked to asthma in most people's minds, the fact is that many asthmatics never wheeze. And there are other lung diseases, such as bronchitis, which can also produce wheezing (see p. 313). Babies very often develop wheezing with chest infections, but this is not necessarily asthma (see pp. 307–8). So wheezing is not the hallmark of asthma.

As well as these basic symptoms, there will often be other effects from asthma, such as tiredness and lack of energy. This is due to the poor supply of oxygen reaching the muscles and other parts of the body. Exhaustion often continues for some time after a severe attack.

Some asthmatics have other, more unusual symptoms:
- A few develop pain in the chest, because it is over-expanded. This can be quite alarming, because it can seem as if the pain is coming from the heart, but it is just the rib joints, the chest muscles and the membranes around the lung which are hurting as they become stretched. The pain in itself is nothing to worry about.
- Occasionally there is vomiting during an asthma attack, especially in children. This occurs because the over-expanded lungs put pressure on the stomach. Emptying the stomach often makes the asthmatic child feel much better, because it reduces the pressure around the lungs.
- For a tiny minority of asthmatics, narrowing occurs mainly in the trachea, the upper part of the windpipe, just below the throat. These asthmatics feel as if they are being strangled

when they have an asthma attack. This rare form of asthma responds to treatment more slowly than the common form.

'a child may not recognize the symptoms as abnormal . . .'

A survey of British schoolchildren published in 1998 found that a third of those with regular night-time wheezing had not had their asthma diagnosed and were not receiving any treatment. Dr Balvinder Kaur, one of the doctors involved, commented, 'We need to raise awareness of asthma symptoms. It is important to ask the child not the parent about symptoms, as a child may not recognize the symptoms as abnormal and not mention them to the parent.'

The different kinds of asthma

You may hear various terms being used to describe different kinds of asthma, such as chronic asthma (see p. 32) , brittle asthma (see p. 32), occupational asthma (see p. 269), cough-variant asthma (see p. 308) and exercise-induced asthma (see p. 68).

At one time, doctors separated their asthma patients into those with 'extrinsic asthma' and those with 'intrinsic asthma'. These terms are no longer used, but for an explanation of them see p. 34.

Is asthma inherited?

Asthma does run in certain families. But what is inherited is the *susceptibility* to asthma. If you have asthma, your children will not necessarily suffer from it, but they are at more risk than the average child.

A susceptibility to *allergy* – distinct from the susceptibility to asthma – can also be inherited. Families carrying genes that can lead to allergy are called atopic families. Often one member of the family will have eczema, another hayfever, and another asthma. This is because the same atopic genes can lead to different kinds of allergic reaction: the allergic tendency comes out in different ways.

In all cases, the allergy is a mistaken reaction by the body's defences (the immune system, whose real job is to fight bacteria, viruses and parasites) against a harmless substance, such as pollen, dust or particles from pets. The immune system mistakes these harmless items for dangerous parasites.

Not all asthmatics are allergic to substances in the air, but many are, especially children (see p. 110). Once the airway lining has become inflamed by the allergic reaction, it is then very sensitive to irritants, cold air, the fast breathing caused by exercise, and other triggers (see pp. 2–3).

For some people, the inherited tendency to allergy and asthma is so strong – they have so many pro-allergy and pro-asthma genes – that the environment they grow up in makes little difference. These are the sort of people who would have got asthma in the past, before the epidemic (see p. 79) began. But for the majority of those with an inborn susceptibility, this tendency is not so strong, and they will only develop asthma if exposed to particular conditions (see below).

What factors encourage allergy and asthma to develop?

Researchers are now beginning to understand some of the factors that encourage asthma and allergy to develop.

In the case of **asthma**, certain kinds of diet – particularly those rich in salt and fat but short on fruit and vegetables – seem to make the airway linings more vulnerable to inflammation (see p. 96). Infection of the baby's throat with a particular bacterium picked up from the mother during birth (see p. 88) can also make the airways more irritable and asthma-prone.

In the case of **allergy**, it is a question of things that happen to the baby's immune system as it develops, both before and after birth. The immune system is shaped and altered by the challenges it encounters in the outside world. These challenges include:

- allergens (from dust, moulds, pets, pollen, etc.) either in the mother's blood during pregnancy or in the air after birth
- natural antibodies and other factors in the mother's breast-milk
- bacteria and viruses that cause disease
- other microbes (including, possibly, some soil bacteria) that are fairly harmless and produce no obvious symptoms
- the natural bacteria in the gut (which can be altered by taking antibiotics)
- parasitic worms
- vaccinations

- the toxic products of tobacco in the mother's bloodstream if she smokes when pregnant
- irritants such as tobacco smoke and nitrogen dioxide (see p. 207) in the air the baby breathes

Some of these challenges influence the baby's immune system to behave in one way, some in another way. For example, some bacteria, including those that cause TB (tuberculosis), encourage the production of cells called Th1 cells, at the expense of others called Th2. Both are 'helper cells' which help other immune cells to produce antibodies. Th1 and Th2 cells do the same job but in different ways: Th2 cells favour the production of allergy-type antibodies (called IgE), while Th1 cells favour other antibodies.

Vaccinations for TB with the BCG vaccine may have a similar effect to TB itself, and promote Th1 cells, so reducing the chance of allergies. Some bacteria found naturally in the soil may do the same thing, which might be why grubby children are less inclined to develop allergies than well-scrubbed, squeaky-clean children (see p. 93).

On the other hand, colds and chest infections in babies often lead on to wheezing, and one type of viral infection in babies, called RSV, may increase the likelihood of asthma developing (see p. 93). These viral infections seem to favour Th2 cells rather than Th1, which is why they may promote the development of allergies and asthma.

Parasitic worms such as tapeworms, and other multicellular parasites causing tropical diseases such as sleeping sickness, are an interesting case, because the immune system uses IgE – the 'allergy antibody' – to fight these off. This is what IgE is supposed to do, in a more natural world than the one we inhabit, where parasites are just part of life. When children are infected with parasites, they gear up to producing IgE to fight them. But rather than making the children more prone to allergies, as one might expect, it seems to have the opposite effect (see p. 83).

It is almost as if the parasite-fighting cells, in our hygienic world, have no useful job to do, so they get bored and get up to mischief, causing allergic reactions. Give them something worthwhile to do and they stay out of trouble. Few people, however, would want their children infested with worms, even briefly, to prevent them developing asthma. (Fortunately, there are several other ways in which you can reduce the chances of your children having asthma – see pp. 87–95.)

Comparing life now with conditions a century ago, there has been a general reduction in bacterial and parasitic infections. This has been achieved by antibiotics, a cleaner water supply and better sanitation. At the same time, there seems to have been an increase in viral infections, probably due to rapid international travel (which carries viruses from place to place) and more indoor living (which makes it easier for viral infections to spread from one person to another). This change in the pattern of infections may have helped to shift the immune system towards a more allergy-prone condition.

Finally, one factor that is still not well understood is the diet women eat when pregnant. Suspicions that this might affect the child's immune system are based on the curious discovery that the larger a child's head at birth, the more likely it is to develop allergies later. Head size relates to brain size, and researchers believe that the balance of nutrients eaten in the last three months of pregnancy can affect both brain growth and the development of the immune system. At the moment, unfortunately, little more is known, so no specific advice about nutrition during pregnancy can be given.

'Is asthma infectious?'

Asthma itself is not infectious in any way. Some people get the wrong idea about this, given that several children in a family often have asthma, but this is because it is inherited (see above).

While asthma itself is not infectious, there are some infections which play a part in asthma, either by starting it off, or by triggering attacks. For many people, a cold or chest infection is an important asthma trigger and invariably brings on a bad asthma attack by irritating the airway lining (see p. 237).

'Why me?' 'Why my child?'

When asthma begins, a lot of people ask, 'Why me? or 'Why my child?' – 'What caused this?' In most cases there is no single cause – it is a mixture of causes, including the genes asthmatics inherit from their parents, and all sorts of events that have happened during their lifetime.

Doctors now understand, in broad terms, why some people develop asthma and others do not (see pp. 25–8). But explaining why a particular individual has developed asthma is a completely different matter. There are usually so many different factors at work – some of them in the distant past, years before the asthma began, that it is impossible to say. Few of these factors can ever be identified for certain. Except in cases of occupational asthma (see p. 269), or where someone has an unmistakable allergy to a pet and the asthma goes when the pet goes, it is very rare to be able to say for sure what has caused a person to develop asthma.

This is not to say that there is no point in trying to find out. Understanding why asthma began may help to bring it under control, although this is not always possible. However, there is no point in trying to understand why in order to feel guilty about it, as many parents of asthmatic children do (see p. 15).

Children developing asthma

A high proportion of children with asthma (80–90 per cent) have one or more allergies, and this may be an important cause of their asthma. Although sensitization to the allergen tends to occur in the first year of life, asthma does not necessarily begin then. There may be no allergic symptoms at all at first, or the child might have another type of allergic symptom, such as eczema.

The potential for an allergic reaction in the airways may be lurking there for years before it comes out. It may be that an extra-large dose of allergen finally provokes the asthma, or exposure to irritants in the air, or even stress.

For example, moving into a 'big bed', with an old mattress full of dust mites, is sometimes the start of asthma for toddlers, although the sensitivity to dust mites was probably there already. Moving to a different house or a new area with more mould or pollen allergens in the outdoor air, or changes to the heating or ventilation at home, which allow a build-up of dust mites, can also be the starting points for asthma. In the case of a completely new allergen, such as that from a pet, it may take a year or two for the sensitivity to develop, so the child may be fine at first.

Adults developing asthma for the first time

When people develop asthma in adulthood, allergies are not always involved, but there can be an allergic factor, especially in young adults. In trying to understand the cause, think about any major changes that occurred in the year or two before the asthma began.

Changing jobs, or starting a different type of job within the same workplace, can be the cause (see p. 270). Have any fans or extractor equipment broken down at work over the past year or two, which could have caused the escape of asthma-causing substances into the air?

Pets, changes to the heating or ventilation, moving house and moving to a new area are also possibilities, as with children (see above). Staying temporarily in dusty lodgings can bring on asthma in young adults, or a spate of home improvements could have caused exposure to irritant chemicals (see p. 223). A new hobby that involves soldering can lead to asthma (see p. 284), working in cellars or basements may result in mould allergy (see pp. 117–8) and so may intensive gardening or farming work in damp conditions.

Not everyone can pinpoint a reason for their asthma, and the older you are when your asthma begins the more unlikely it is that there is some simple removable cause.

'I didn't see it as frightening then . . .'

Helen is in her thirties, and has mild asthma. 'I started to get asthma when I was about ten. I always got it when I was doing exercise in the sunshine, whenever I got "hot and bothered" – that was what triggered the attacks. It was worst when I was about 13 or 14.

'I was never given any treatment by a doctor, and it got better eventually. Now I only have it if I get an allergic reaction to a cat or a dog. The worst asthma I'd had in years was recently when I stayed in a house with a dog. That reminded me what it had been like when I was a teenager, which was quite frightening. But I didn't see it as frightening then, in my teens, it was just something that happened every day.'

TECHNICAL WORDS USED ABOUT ASTHMA – WHAT THEY MEAN

Doctors try not to use technical words when talking to patients, but sometimes they forget. The medical terms listed here are ones that may crop up during a visit to your GP or consultant, plus a few words used in this book whose meaning might not be obvious. If the word you are looking for is not here, look in the index, or try one of the following:

For the names of **drugs** (and groups of drugs) see pp. 370–5.
For the **tests** used in the diagnosis of asthma see pp. 303–5.
For the names of **parts of the lungs and airways** see pp. 20–1.
For **other diseases** that may relate in some way to asthma see pp. 237–56 and pp. 306–14.

Commonly used terms

Acute Doctors describe diseases as either 'acute' or 'chronic'. Acute means, roughly speaking, 'short-lived', while chronic means 'long-term'. So if you have had asthma for years, this is called '*chronic asthma*', but if you then develop a very bad attack that lasts for a few days or weeks, it is called a 'severe *acute* attack of asthma'.

Airway resistance The extent to which the airways slow down the passage of air is described as airway resistance. A wide airway lets air through easily, whereas a narrow airway does not – so it has higher airway resistance. Someone with uncontrolled asthma has greater airway resistance than someone without asthma.

Airways The airways are the hollow passages that lead down into the lungs. They include the trachea, the two bronchi, and the smaller tubes known as bronchioles (see p. 21).

Allergen Any substance that can cause an allergic reaction is called an allergen. There are thousands of different allergens in the things that we eat, breathe in or touch. Some asthmatics are allergic to only one substance, others are allergic to more than one substance, but no one, fortunately, is allergic to all the known allergens.

Allergic reaction An allergic reaction is a strong reaction by the immune system to a substance that is basically harmless, such as pollen or dust or cat proteins.

Allergy See *allergic reaction* above. The diseases linked to allergy are hayfever, true food allergy, allergic asthma and allergic eczema.

Alveoli The air sacs of the lungs (see pp. 20–1).

Anaphylaxis or anaphylactic shock A severe allergic reaction which, if not treated promptly, can produce a fatal asthma attack and/or total collapse due to a sharp fall in blood pressure. Anaphylaxis is life-threatening, particularly for asthmatics, and everyone at risk should be seeing a specialist (see pp. 62–3). Recognizing the early symptoms of anaphylaxis (see p. 48), and getting emergency treatment quickly, can be a life-saver.

Atopic Families or individuals may be described as atopic: it simply means 'having allergies or likely to develop allergies'. The tendency to develop allergies is inherited.

Brittle asthma Asthma that is unstable and difficult to manage is described as brittle asthma. Despite extensive and careful treatment with drugs, it can very easily develop into a severe asthma attack.

Bronchi The bronchi are two tubes that run from the trachea into the lungs (see p. 21).

Bronchioles The smaller tubes that branch off from the bronchi.

Bronchiolitis Inflammation of the bronchioles (see p. 311).

Bronchitis Inflammation of the bronchi usually caused by an infection (acute bronchitis), or by cigarette smoking or industrial pollution (chronic bronchitis). Bronchitis causes narrowing of the airways, because the airway linings become swollen. Unlike asthma, the degree of narrowing remains the same from day to day and week to week. Some people have both asthma *and* bronchitis; this is called chronic obstructive pulmonary disease (COPD) or chronic obstructive airways disease (COAD) or chronic obstructive respiratory disease (CORD). See also pp. 308–9 and p. 313.

Bronchodilators These are drugs that open up asthmatic airways by making the muscles around the airways relax. The main bronchodilators used are B-2 reliever drugs (see pp. 341–7).

Bronchospasm Contraction of the muscles around the airways (see p. 22).

Chronic Any long-term medical condition is described as 'chronic'. See also *acute*.

Chronic obstructive pulmonary disease (COPD) Asthma combined with bronchitis or emphysema, or both. See above and p. 309.

COPD, COAD or CORD See above.

Emphysema Damage to the tiny air sacs or alveoli (see p. 20) of the lung. Cigarette smoking is almost always the cause. There is breathlessness, which gets progressively worse until the sufferer stops smoking. Some people have both asthma *and* emphysema; this is called chronic obstructive pulmonary disease (COPD). See also p. 216.

Extrinsic asthma See p. 34.

Hyper-inflated Over-inflated; this term is used to describe the lungs of asthmatics when they have too much air retained in them. The problem occurs because the narrowed airways make breathing out very difficult.

Hypersensitivity Another term for *allergy* (see above).

Immune system The defensive system of the body, whose job is to protect against infectious bacteria, viruses and parasites, and to fight off cancers. The immune system can also 'get it wrong' and mount attacks against harmless items such as pollen or foods. This is the cause of allergies.

Inflammation An effect caused by immune system activity. In the skin (e.g. around a cut or graze) inflammation can be seen as redness and swelling. It also feels sore. Similar reactions occur in the lining of the airways when asthma is uncontrolled. The swelling contributes to the narrowing of the airways.

Intrinsic asthma See p. 34.

Lower airways The trachea, bronchi and bronchioles.

Mucus The sticky, thick or watery secretions produced by the nose and airways; phlegm.

Nasal Of the nose, or to do with the nose.

Occupational asthma Asthma directly caused by substances inhaled at work. Different terms are used for asthma that is simply made worse by substances inhaled at work (see p. 269).

Peak flow The fastest speed at which air can be breathed out. It is measured with a peak-flow meter (see p. 315) or a spirometer.

Post-nasal drip Mucus from a runny nose slipping down the *back* of the nose and straight into the airways.

Rhinitis Inflammation of the nose.

Trachea The tube that leads from the throat down to the bronchi. It is the largest airway.

Upper airways The nose, the back of the mouth and the throat.

Wheezing A whistling noise made by narrow airways (see p. 24).

Wheezy bronchitis A diagnosis that is now considered out of date (see p. 308).

IS ASTHMA 'ALL IN THE MIND?'

For a long time, doctors believed that there were two kinds of asthma: 'extrinsic asthma' caused by allergies, and 'intrinsic asthma' which had no obvious external cause. It was widely assumed that 'intrinsic asthma' was psychological in origin, that it was 'all in the mind'. As a result (and for no logical reason, since psychological diseases are no more shameful than physical diseases) there was a stigma attached to having asthma. Even more illogically, the stigma was attached to any kind of asthma, 'intrinsic' or 'extrinsic'.

Since the 1960s, medical attitudes have changed. As asthma has been studied in more and more detail, doctors have come to realize that there is almost always some external factor triggering off asthma, even if it is not obvious. If not an allergy, then it may be a reaction to chest infections or to irritants such as cigarette smoke in the air, or some other factor. Of course, there is an underlying reason why asthmatics respond to these triggers with narrowed airways when other people do not, but the basic reason is not in their minds, it is in their genes (see p. 25) and their airways.

When lung transplants have been carried out using lungs from asthmatic donors, the recipients have developed asthma after the operation. This shows very clearly that asthma is primarily a problem in the airways, not in the mind.

It is now agreed that asthma is never 'all in the mind', but most asthmatics are aware that the mind *does* influence their asthma symptoms. This is partly because our breathing is so tied up with our emotions. Everyone gasps with fear or pleasure, catches their breath when alarmed, and changes to quick, shallow little breaths when anxious. For asthmatics, these situations can also make the airways tighten up. Crying or laughing may also trigger an asthma attack, just by making the breath more forceful, which then stimulates the airways to contract. For some people, any upset or excitement (even feeling happily excited about something) may bring on asthma symptoms.

These are all short-term reactions to emotional triggers, but there can also be longer-term reactions. Being under a lot of stress can lead to a gradual and sustained tightening of the airways. Asthma can sometimes come on for the first time after a traumatic event, such as the death of a close relative. In these cases, the person concerned was probably susceptible to asthma beforehand, and the severe stress simply sparked it off.

For some people, their asthma only gets worse after the stress is over: it seems to be the relief from tension that brings the asthma on. This can be explained by the action of the autonomic nervous system on the airways (see pp. 417–8).

There is often an interaction between stress and allergens. For example, someone who normally gets asthma only when the pollen count is high may find, on a stressful day, that a moderate or low pollen count will bring on an attack.

Is there an 'asthma personality'?

When asthma was thought to be a psychosomatic disease, many doctors and psychiatrists believed that there must be a typical 'asthma personality': a particular psychological make-up which predisposed a person to asthma. But research has failed to identify any such personality traits. Only in those with very severe asthma ('brittle asthma') are there more psychological problems than in the average healthy person, and these problems (such as anxiety) seem to be a consequence of asthma, not its cause. Given the unstable nature of brittle asthma, and its profound impact on all aspects of life, it is hardly surprising that it should produce psychological problems for many people.

The power of suggestion

Asthmatics, like everybody else, can be 'conditioned' to respond in particular ways to a particular stimulus. It is the same reaction that Pavlov showed with his famous dog: he rang a bell every time he fed the dog, and eventually the dog's mouth would water in anticipation whenever it heard the bell, even if there was no food on offer. In the same way, experiments show that a large number of asthmatics will develop an asthma attack in any situation that has regularly brought on an attack in the past – even if the allergic trigger in that situation has now been removed.

Suggestion works in a similar way. Laboratory tests show that many people who are allergic to grass pollen will suffer an asthma attack if told that they are inhaling grass pollen, even though they are actually inhaling something harmless. What is more, telling them that they are inhaling a reliever drug will relieve the attack, even though they are not inhaling any drug. Some people are more inclined to respond to these suggestions than others, but on the whole, asthmatics are no more or less susceptible to conditioning than non-asthmatics: almost everyone will feel some pain relief from a tablet that they believe to be a powerful painkiller, even though it contains no drug at all. This is known as the 'placebo effect'.

What does all this mean in everyday life? Firstly, if you are severely allergic to cats, simply seeing a cat in the distance or on TV may be enough to start you wheezing. If it does, there is no reason to feel embarrassed or to suspect that your asthma is 'all in the mind': conditioning is a perfectly natural reaction to repeated asthma attacks. However, it may be helpful to try out relaxation techniques (see pp. 446–51) – or other methods that may help you get these conditioned reactions under better control. Hypnotherapy (see p. 450) could be a useful approach, because people who are most susceptible to conditioning are also easily hypnotized.

Secondly, and more commonly, you may have a psychological response to your reliever inhaler, a placebo effect that boosts the actual effect of the drug. There is no harm in this, but it can develop into a problem if you are also very anxious about your asthma and become psychologically addicted to your inhaler. As one asthmatic put it 'If I didn't have my inhaler with me, that was enough to give me an asthma attack – just knowing that I hadn't got it there would start me off wheezing.' If this sounds familiar, try to sort the problem out, because you will probably be using your reliever too often, and this is potentially damaging (see p. 322). Hypnotherapy, counselling or psychotherapy (see pp. 446–51) might be helpful in this situation, or you could try yoga (see p. 397) or a martial art (see p. 429) as a way of feeling more in control of your asthma.

Hyperventilation

Hyperventilation is fast, shallow breathing, using the upper part of the chest. If you breathe in this way habitually, the chances are that you will not realize you do it – it will seem perfectly normal to you. Some asthmatics (and some non-asthmatics) get into this type of breathing pattern, which can make their asthma seem much worse. In some cases, people diagnosed with asthma are actually suffering from hyperventilation alone – one of the symptoms is breathlessness and this can be mistaken for asthma, even by doctors. Other symptoms of hyperventilation may include dizziness, tingling of the hands and feet, numbness and muscle cramps. For a full list of symptoms see p. 419.

There are often psychological effects from hyperventilation, the most common one being anxiety. And hyperventilation often begins through psychological causes such as fear and anxiety. Once hyperventilation is established, cause and effect become hard to distinguish. Fortunately, this problem is fairly easy to treat (see pp. 422–8).

Problems from the past

It is not just things happening in the here-and-now that cause us stress, but also things that occurred long ago in our childhood. Often we have forgotten the actual details of the event, but the emotional hurt remains. When something happens to remind us of that hurt, this can trigger an asthma attack.

One woman who had been mistreated by her father as a child noticed that her asthma always got worse when her father was around. Even talking to him on the phone could start her wheezing. With the help of psychotherapy she was able to come to terms with her childhood experiences, and could then cope better with her father's presence. All this helped to make her asthma less severe.

Another asthmatic believed that she was allergic to goldfish, although this is impossible because they do not produce airborne allergens. Scientific tests showed that she genuinely suffered from narrowed airways whenever she saw a goldfish, but she would also react in the same way to an empty goldfish bowl. Eventually the problem was traced back to a traumatic moment in her childhood, when her mother took her pet goldfish in its bowl and threw it into the dustbin, smashing the bowl and killing the fish. Once she became aware of the source of the problem, her 'allergy' to goldfish disappeared.

In both these cases there was real asthma as well, and skin-prick tests showed allergies to house dust mites and other allergens. The psychological component was just 'added on' to the genuine asthma symptoms. This is almost always the case: it is very rare to find an asthmatic whose attacks are triggered *solely* by psychological or emotional factors.

Can stress *cure* asthma?

There may be a sudden improvement in your asthma if you become very frightened or angry. An asthmatic doctor described a classic example of this, where he suffered an attack of asthma while at the wheel of his car. A few moments later he put the car into neutral by mistake, while going down a steep hill, and the car began to accelerate wildly. For a few seconds he felt completely out of control of the car and he was terrified there would be an accident. When he got the car under control, at the bottom of the hill, he found his asthma had completely cleared up. The explanation for this is that during those few seconds when he was racing down the hill, he was so terrified that he had a rush of adrenaline, and this opened up his airways. Adrena-line was one of the first modern drugs used for asthma, and the B-2 relievers (such as Ventolin) are modified forms of adrenalin that act on the airways in the same way.

Can sustained stress have the same effect as a sudden burst of fear? For a minority of asthmatics it clearly does: rather than their asthma getting worse when they are under stress, they find that it actually improves.

Parents and children

Children with very severe asthma often benefit from going to stay in a residential home. Such homes for asthmatic children are designed to have very low levels of allergens, and it was originally assumed that this explained the children's improvement. But doctors suspected that, for some children, being separated from their parents might also be playing a part, so they tried sending the parents away to a hotel while other people looked after the children in their own homes. For some of the children there was just as much improvement as when they themselves had gone away to a residential home.

The parents concerned were not uncaring – quite the opposite. Most of them were anxious, protective parents whose lives were completely caught up with the worry of having a severely asthmatic child. The sense of constant anxiety which they communicated to the child, intentionally or otherwise, made the child feel so tense that the asthma symptoms became much worse. What the children needed was some sense of freedom from worry – a chance to relax, run around, mess about, be silly and generally feel like other children.

In addition to this type of problem, the sort of stresses that any child might find difficult to cope with can bring on attacks for asthmatic children. The death of a parent, neglect or abuse by one or both parents, constant arguments between the father and mother, separation and divorce can all make asthma worse in a child. Bullying at school, or problems with brothers or sisters, can also affect the asthmatic child badly.

Unfortunately, just to complicate matters, a few children learn to use their asthma to manipulate difficult situations. They find they can bring on attacks by breathing in a particular way, or just by thinking about having an attack. As one asthmatic explained, 'When I was little, if I got into a fight with my sister, I could bring on an asthma attack, and that meant she'd give in and let me have what I wanted, or I could go running to my mum and she'd be nice to me.' Dealing with this type of behaviour is obviously tricky, and it needs careful handling. For a start, try to make sure that having an asthma attack is not associated with any special treats or privileges. Then give your child the benefit of the doubt until you are absolutely sure that the asthma attacks are self-induced. When you are sure, try to talk to the child gently about it, and explain why it is wrong to use an illness in this way – the story of the little boy who cried 'Wolf!' might prove useful.

Asthma and anxiety
Feeling anxious during an asthma attack is an entirely natural reaction to not being able to breathe properly. Only another asthmatic can understand just how frightening this is. But while this anxiety is natural, it can add to the problems if it gets out of hand.

A certain amount of anxiety is helpful in focusing your attention on your breathing, so that you recognize an attack before it gets too bad, and take appropriate action. (This sort of anxiety is a lot more healthy than 'denial' – pretending there's no problem and neglecting medication – which tends to land people in hospital, or worse.) Beyond a certain point, however, anxiety during an attack can lead to panic and hyperventilation (see p. 419), making the attack far worse. Some asthmatics also become so panicky and fearful that they use their reliever inhalers far too frequently, which is dangerous in the long run (see p. 322). It is a good idea to learn to control anxiety during attacks, by practising yoga or a relaxation technique for example, as you will then cope with the attacks much better.

For some asthmatics, the anxiety does not really go away when an attack ends, and they feel anxious all or most of the time. This is especially likely if the asthma is severe or unpredictable. Constant worrying about asthma can increase your general level of anxiety about life, which may undermine your ability to cope and make decisions. This in turn can sometimes make asthma worse, because making the right decisions about treatment is crucial for day-to-day asthma management. If you feel you may be caught in this type of vicious circle, it would be a good idea to get some outside help. Talking to a counsellor or therapist may be very valuable. Your GP should be able to recommend someone, or see Useful Addresses for organizations that can point you in the right direction. In Britain, more and more GP surgeries now have a counsellor on the staff, so you may not have to pay for this kind of help.

Learning to breathe correctly (see pp. 421–3) can also allay a lot of your anxieties about asthma attacks. Knowing exactly what to do in an emergency (see pp. 50–8) and how to overcome feelings of panic, is also very helpful.

Asthma and depression
Severe asthma can, quite understandably, be a very depressing experience. Patients who are depressed often find it difficult to remember to take their medication at the right times, and because they are not following the recommended treatment plan, their asthma then deteriorates. Being depressed is a significant risk factor for suffering a fatal asthma attack, which is why any asthmatic with depression should be given professional help.

Don't be afraid to talk to your family doctor: he or she will be very sympathetic and can do a lot to help. Depression is very common, and nothing to be ashamed of: it is a mistake to think that you can (or should) struggle alone with depression.

Depression makes it very hard to think straight or to see the world as it really is. So it is easy to get trapped by your problems. Simply *realizing* that you are not thinking clearly about problems (that you are seeing everything as if through a distorting mirror that makes life seem utterly worthless and bleak) is half the battle. You may need to tell yourself this repeatedly (or have a close friend tell you) to make it possible even to ask for help from your doctor. Effective treatment will put everything back in proportion so that you do not feel overwhelmed.

When asthma attacks produce depression
There is another way in which asthma is linked to depression. Some people, who are normally cheerful and well balanced, find that when they suffer an attack of asthma they also feel depressed. The depres-

sion may even come on before any noticeable asthma symptoms and therefore act as a warning sign. There is no explanation yet for this link. It seems to be the asthma that affects that mood, rather than the depressed mood producing an attack: when the asthma is successfully treated with drugs, the depression lifts. If you are affected in this way, you can use the change in your mood as a warning sign that your asthma is getting worse, and that you may need to increase the dose of preventer drugs.

Did you know?

Many asthmatics have dreams in which they are drowning or being stifled. This seems to be a natural response to the anxiety of having asthma.

'. . . when I got married the attacks got much worse . . .'

'I'd had asthma most of my life, but when I got married the attacks got much worse, especially when I went to bed at night. As soon as I got into bed I started wheezing. We bought a new mattress, because I'd heard about dust mites and I thought it might be that, but I wasn't any better. The doctor gave me different inhalers – I tried all kinds of different things, but I was just the same. This went on for over a year. It put a lot of stress on our marriage.

'Then my dad died, and just after that my sister had a breakdown. I spent a lot of time trying to help her, and she saw a psychiatrist, and slowly the whole story came out about our childhood and the things that our dad had done . . . I've found out since that it's quite common for someone to just forget everything that happened to them as children, if some of it was really bad. I always wondered why I could hardly remember a thing about when I was a kid. Now I've been seeing a therapist for a couple of years, and I understand it all a lot more, and I'm coping much better. Looking back, I can see that the reason for those attacks whenever I got into bed was just that I was terrified of my husband touching me – and if I had an asthma attack he couldn't.'

DOES ASTHMA GET WORSE IN TIME?
OR DOES IT GO AWAY?

Many people are very worried when first told that they have asthma, because they think it will inevitably get worse. This is usually not the case.

Asthma in children

The outlook is best for young children, because their asthma often goes away in time. They are said to 'grow out of it', although no one knows exactly what this means. Other childhood allergies, such as allergic eczema, also have a tendency to disappear in time: it seems as if the immune system learns to ignore the allergens.

Wheezy babies and toddlers are the ones most likely to lose their asthma. One study showed that, of children who wheezed before the age of five, 85 per cent had no sign of asthma at the age of 16. There are several things you can do to help your child become one of the 85 per cent who grow out of wheezing rather than one of the 15 per cent who develop asthma. A wheezy child who is breathing in a lot of cigarette smoke or large amounts of allergen (from house dust, pets, moulds, etc.) is going to be more inclined to develop asthma in the long term than one who is not. High levels of nitrogen dioxide in the air could also increase the chance of the wheezing turning into asthma. For detailed information on how to reduce allergens, nitrogen dioxide and other asthma risks in the home, look at p. 89 (under the heading 'Improving the baby's environment') which will direct you to the relevant sections of the book.

Many doctors believe that wheezing in young children should be treated with inhaled steroids, and that this will reduce the chance of it developing into asthma. There is some evidence from Sweden for the benefits of this approach (see pp. 327–8). Other studies show that children with persistent wheeze tend to have a steady decline in lung function over the years, whereas treatment with inhaled steroids stops this decline.

Teenagers and young adults with asthma

The more severe a child's asthma, the more likely it is to persist into teenage years and adult life. However, only 2 per cent of children who wheeze at seven years of age have asthma that never goes away again.

Many children and teenagers who have asthma lose their symptoms when they are in their late teens or twenties. It can seem as if they have grown out of their asthma for ever. For some – about a third of those who wheeze at age seven – this is the case, but for others the asthma comes back in their late twenties or thirties. *Smoking cigarettes makes it very much more likely that the asthma will come back, so it is vitally important that former asthmatics do not take up smoking.* It is no good thinking, 'Well, if the asthma comes back I'll just stop again, and it will go away.' Unfortunately, the asthma may persist even though you stop smoking.

As well as avoiding cigarettes, former asthmatics are well advised to reduce their exposure to allergens (see pp. 127–78) and indoor pollution (see pp. 221–6) as much as possible, and avoid jobs where there is a high risk of asthma developing (see pp. 268–86). They should also avoid surgical operations to the nose unless absolutely necessary (see p. 8).

If you had asthma as a child and still have it at the age of 30, you are probably going to have it for ever. It may get worse in time, and you would be well advised to avoid anything that can help to make it worse (see above).

Asthma that comes on later in life

Many people develop asthma in their middle years, or even in old age. In such cases, it is unlikely that the asthma will ever go away. But it will not necessarily get much worse, and it is unlikely to involve severe life-threatening asthma attacks.

If you get asthma later in life, try not to get the problem out of perspective, or to worry excessively. Many older people find it alarming to be told that they have asthma, because they see it as a very frightening disease. In fact, with modern drug treatment, you should find that the asthma does not affect your lifestyle very much. By using a preventer inhaler (see p. 334) you can keep the inflammation in the airways under control, and this will help to stop the asthma from getting worse.

Once again, smoking cigarettes is the sure way to make your asthma worse, especially if you have bronchitis or emphysema as well (see p. 216).

3

Asthma attacks – what to do

> '. . . *as a parent you have to trust your own judgement* . . .'

Suzie's son Barnaby has had asthma since he was a few months old. 'One thing I've learned is that as a parent you have to trust your own judgement, and don't ever be fobbed off. One time Barny had a cough that I just didn't feel right about. I was really concerned so I rang the doctors, and this young newly qualified GP came out. He was a bit patronizing and said that there was nothing wrong with him – "But of course if you're worried again do call us" – only he said it in a way that made me feel I couldn't call them again.

'Barny got worse and worse that evening, but because this doctor had made me feel a bit silly, I didn't phone, even though I felt I should. Eventually I phoned at about 11.30 p.m., in a panic. When the doctor arrived, Barny's asthma was so bad that he took one look at him and told me to drive him to the hospital. I said, "Shouldn't we call an ambulance?" And he said, "No, it would take too long, we must just get him in." That was just awful.

'Because I hadn't had an asthmatic child before, and because I'd been fobbed off earlier in the day, I was very nervous about calling them again. I think some doctors can very easily undermine your instincts as a mother.'

(Although the doctor in this case thought it better to drive to the hospital, in most areas calling an ambulance is the best policy – see p. 50).

RECOGNIZING AN ASTHMA ATTACK

Why you should read this page

You should read this page even if you (or your child) have never had a serious asthma attack. No one with asthma should think, 'It won't happen to me.' And no parent of an asthmatic child should think, 'It won't happen to my child.' Any asthmatic, even one with mild disease who has never had a serious attack before, can suddenly have the kind of attack that requires emergency treatment.

We don't wish to alarm you unnecessarily, or make you over-anxious, but it is vital that you know what to do if an attack like this happens.

You must be able to recognize when an asthma attack is getting out of control and you need to call medical help. So don't just read this page – read the next ten pages as well. It could literally be a matter of life or death.

Know what you're supposed to do, and always, *always* have your reliever inhaler (see p. 334) with you, wherever you go. If you are a parent, make sure all your child's clothes have a pocket large enough to carry the inhaler, and check that he or she never leaves home without it.

Owning a peak-flow meter and using it morning and evening (or as recommended by your doctor), will give you advance warning of asthma attacks (see p. 315). But if your peak flow seems normal, yet you feel breathless or have a tight chest, *pay attention to your symptoms* – they always matter more than the peak-flow reading.

Some asthma attacks come on fast, some come on slowly. You need to be able to recognize both types of attack, and react accordingly.

Remember that it is always better to deal with the attack sooner rather than later: the sooner you act, the fewer drugs you'll need in the long run to control the attack, and the sooner it will be over. In a crisis, most people wait too long and then under-treat their asthma. Surveys show that this 'too-little too-late' tendency is especially common among teenagers and the elderly. It can be a very dangerous mistake to make.

Not every asthma attack will follow the exact course described below, whether it is a rapid or a slow attack. Even if you do not have all the symptoms described here, you may still be having an attack, and you should take action.

There is one very simple sign that your asthma is not well controlled and an attack may be coming on: if your reliever inhaler does not work as well as usual, or if the effect wears off in less than three hours. Always increase your dose of reliever inhaler when this happens, and see your doctor as soon as possible – or follow your management plan (see p. 391) if that tells you how to deal with this situation. You will probably need to increase your dose of preventer to get the asthma back under control.

Rapid asthma attacks

Stage 1: Having been fine all day, you (or your child) suddenly start to feel very breathless and wheezy (or begin coughing badly, if coughing is the main asthma symptom).

Stage 2: Half an hour later, despite using the reliever, the breathlessness is getting worse. It is now difficult to walk across the room, or to say a complete sentence without gasping for breath.
This is a severe attack: don't delay in getting medical help.

Stage 3: Another half hour later, the breathlessness has got even worse, and it is difficult to speak at all, or to rise from a chair.
Unless you know that an ambulance or doctor is on the way, you should take steps to get to a hospital with an Accident and Emergency Department as quickly as possible.

For more detailed information on what to do at each stage, see p. 51.

Slow asthma attacks

Stage 1: You (or your child) are more breathless and wheezy than usual, for two or three days. The reliever inhaler (the 'blue one') is not working as well as usual.

Stage 2: For the next two nights, asthma disturbs sleep more often each night, and it is difficult to go back to sleep afterwards. There is much more breathlessness than usual in the early morning, and it takes longer to clear up.
This could be the beginning of a severe attack: don't delay in getting medical help.

Stage 3: About six to seven days after the attack began (Stage 1), asthma disturbs sleep regularly every night, and in the morning the breathlessness is so bad that it is difficult to speak or walk about.
See your doctor or go to the hospital now.

For more detailed information on what to do at each stage, see pp. 51–2.

Very young children with asthma: how to recognize an attack

It may be difficult to judge just how bad a child's asthma is, especially when the child is very young. The following pointers indicate a severe asthma attack:

- The child can only say one or two words between breaths.
- The tongue is blue.
- The lips are blue or grey.
- The fingernails are blue.
- The nostrils are flared.
- The child is leaning forward with shoulders held unusually high.
- The ribs are pushed out and the shoulders pushed up, because the lungs are too full of air
- There are hollows between the ribs.
- The pulse rate is high (over 100 per minute).
- You can hear wheezing (a whistling noise) in the chest.
- There has been wheezing but this stops without the child seeming better in other ways. This indicates that the attack is really bad: wheezing stops when the airways have become so narrow that no air is passing through them. Doctors call this a 'silent chest', and it needs urgent medical attention.

Make sure that everyone who normally looks after the child knows about all these signs: you could give them a photocopy of these pages.

Recognizing asthma attacks brought on by aspirin

A bad reaction to aspirin or aspirin-like drugs takes between 30 minutes and two hours to develop. If you have polyps in the nose, this reaction is a distinct possibility (see p. 257).

- At first the nose usually starts running, or is badly blocked, and the eyes get red.
- Some people feel hot, flushed and sweaty, and a rash may develop.

- There might be a feeling of tightness in the chest and a dry cough.
- A feeling of exhaustion and general ill-health is common.
- As the reaction proceeds, the airways get very narrow, producing breathlessness.
- A few people are sick or have diarrhoea.
- Some have swelling and puffiness (oedema), or a type of rash called urticaria or hives that resembles nettle stings.

You may not have all the symptoms listed here, and they may come on in a different order.

If you have any of these symptoms after taking aspirin or aspirin-like drugs, seek emergency medical help *immediately* – call an ambulance, and then read p. 55.

Recognizing anaphylactic shock

Some asthmatics have strong allergic reactions to food, insect stings or latex, which produce a reaction called anaphylactic shock (see p. 111). There can be the signs of an asthma attack but there will probably be other signs as well.

If full anaphylaxis occurs, it is a serious emergency. Do not hesitate to call an ambulance the moment you suspect anaphylactic shock. Use injectable or inhaled adrenaline (epinephrine) straight away if you are carrying it, *and call the emergency services as well.*

If you have any of these warning signs, anaphylactic shock is a possibility:
- nettle rash (hives) and swelling
- dizziness or feeling faint
- itching all over
- sneezing and a runny nose
- red or itchy eyes
- diarrhoea, stomach pains
- weakness
- skin pale or blue
- a feeling of general warmth
- a feeling of apprehension or dread
- palpitations and rapid pulse
- incontinence
- disorientation, dizziness, anxiety

- abdominal pains
- slurred speech
- general collapse

If food is the allergen, there are other signs as well:
- tingling or itching in the mouth
- swelling of the lips, tongue and throat
- nausea and vomiting
- hoarseness or a 'lump-in-the-throat' sensation

See pp. 55–7 for further advice on coping with anaphylactic shock, including serious attacks and mild 'first-time' attacks.

Get in touch with your airways

Most asthmatics could learn to recognize severe attacks earlier, and much more reliably. In one interesting experiment, researchers set out to teach asthmatics to recognize how open or obstructed their airways were, without using a peak-flow meter. The researchers asked them to breathe through a tube and the diameter of the tube was then increased or decreased by specific amounts, so that breathing became easier or more difficult: the idea was to mimic the effects of an asthma attack.

The asthmatics were asked to assess how difficult it had become to breathe, and were then told how well their assessment corresponded to reality. After going through this training procedure several times, everyone had a much better sense of how narrow the tube was. This made them more aware of how badly their breathing was obstructed by asthma, so the training was a success.

Unfortunately, this type of training is not generally available at present. But the fact that it works suggests that everyone with asthma could learn to be more aware of the state of their airways.

You can use your peak-flow meter as a do-it-yourself training device: before you take your reading, stand or sit quietly for a few minutes, with no distractions. Concentrate on your breathing and try to assess for yourself how easy it is to breathe. Now try to guess what your peak-flow reading might be. Then use your peak-flow meter and see how well your guess corresponded to the meter's measurement.

After a few days or weeks of this you should find that you are much better able to guess how tight your airways are. This gives you another powerful weapon against asthma attacks, because you can assess your own airways at any time of the day, wherever you are.

COPING WITH AN ASTHMA ATTACK

The different stages of asthma attacks are described in more detail on pp. 46–7. The instructions given here apply equally to adults or to children having an asthma attack. If you are the parent of an asthmatic child, you should make photocopies of these pages (or the child's management plan, or both) for everyone who normally takes care of the child, including teachers, grandparents, baby-sitters, child-minders, Brownie, Cub, Scout or Guide leaders, sports coaches and other club leaders. Written instructions are much more helpful than verbal ones, especially in an emergency when people tend to panic and forget what they have been told.

Severe attacks will need emergency medical help. Depending on where you live, and what the local services are like, it may be best to:

- **call an ambulance**. This is the best option for a severe attack in any area with a good ambulance service. The ambulance crew will have oxygen, and drugs such as adrenaline (epinephrine) which can stop an attack promptly.
- **call your family doctor**. If the attack is not particularly severe, or if the doctor is close by and the ambulance station a long way off, this may be a better option. Some doctors carry oxygen and adrenaline, especially in rural areas.
- **get to the nearest hospital emergency department in a car or taxi**. This is not the best option, because the attack may quickly get worse and you have nothing but the reliever inhaler to help you. But there may be times, or places, where this is the best thing to do.

It is a good idea to talk to your family doctor in advance and ask for advice about who to contact in an emergency. When staying away from home, especially somewhere remote, check in advance that you know where the nearest hospital is, and that you have the phone number of a local doctor (you may need to register as a temporary patient). Check also that the phone is working – and don't stay anywhere without one.

Coping with rapid asthma attacks
Rapid asthma attacks are those that come on in a few hours.

Stage 1: Suddenly starting to feel very breathless and wheezing or coughing badly.

Action: Use the reliever inhaler (the 'blue one' in Britain), and follow the general guidelines given on pp. 52–4. The reliever should begin to take effect within five to ten minutes.

If it does, and the asthmatic remains well for the next four hours at least, then the attack has been successfully stopped. If the attack comes back within four hours, use the reliever again and call a doctor.

If the reliever does not seem to be working at all within ten minutes, think about calling a doctor or ambulance. You should definitely call for medical help if it is difficult to talk, or if an asthmatic child seems distressed or exhausted by the attack. Use the reliever inhaler again while you call the medical services.

Stage 2: 30 minutes later, feeling so breathless that it is difficult to cross the room or say a complete sentence.

Action: Call the doctor or ambulance now, if you have not already done so. Make sure that the doctor/ambulance service knows that this is an emergency. Use the reliever inhaler again. Take another puff every five to ten minutes if needed. Alternatively, you can take up to 30 puffs all at once. Keep a count of how many puffs you've had. Use a spacer if it is difficult to inhale – this is especially important for children. If you do not have one, you can improvise a spacer from a plastic cup or a paper bag (see pp. 383–4).

Stage 3: Another 30 minutes later, it is difficult to speak at all, or to rise from a chair.

Action: Keep using the reliever inhaler, but stop when you have had a total of 30 puffs. Check that the doctor or ambulance is on the way, and how long it might be before assistance arrives.

If it is very difficult to speak, get someone else to telephone. You can explain what you want them to do by writing it down on paper.

Coping with slow asthma attacks

Slow asthma attacks are ones that build up over several days.

Stage 1: For two to three days you (or your child) are more breathless than usual. The reliever inhaler is not working as well as expected.

Action: Check the peak flow reading (see p. 315). Consult your management plan, and if the peak flow has fallen below the recommended level, double the dose of inhaled steroids now. Add any other medicines (e.g. steroid tablets) as recommended by the management plan.

If you do not have a peak-flow meter or management plan, double the dose of inhaled steroids (take twice as many puffs each time) and make an urgent appointment to see your doctor (by tomorrow at the latest).

Stage 2: Asthma disturbs sleep more often each night, and breathlessness is much worse in the early morning.
Action: Keep checking the peak-flow reading, and follow the recommendations in your management plan. If you are at all concerned, ring your doctor. Don't worry if it is at night or very early in the morning. This is often when asthma is at its worst, and your doctor knows this. He or she would much rather be disturbed than have you (or your child) deteriorate any further.

If you do not have a peak-flow meter or management plan, you must see your doctor now (unless you have already done so). A short course of steroid tablets will probably be needed to suppress the attack. These short courses of steroid tablets are very safe when taken occasionally, and you should not hesitate to take them.

Stage 3: Six to seven days after the attack began, asthma disturbs sleep regularly every night. In the morning the breathlessness is so bad that it is difficult to speak or walk about.
Action: The attack is not under control. It is crucial that you now seek urgent medical help. Do not hesitate to go to the hospital emergency department if your doctor cannot get to you quickly.

General guidelines for coping with asthma attacks
Stay calm
During an asthma attack the most important thing is to stay calm. When asthmatics begin to panic they start to breathe more quickly, using the upper part of the chest (hyperventilate) and this makes matters much worse (see p. 419). Tell yourself that you are in control of the situation, and there is no need to panic.

Parents must reassure their children and help them to stay calm. A panicky adult is the worst possible thing for an asthmatic child at this moment.

Focus on breathing out

Because you feel you cannot get enough air, it is natural to gasp for breath, but this is a mistake. Focus on breathing out, not on breathing in. Breathe out as fully as you can. Your in-breath will follow naturally. Do the same with the next out-breath: stay calm and focus on breathing out. Older children should be able to understand this if you explain it to them calmly.

Breathe slowly

You should also breathe as slowly as you can. This should help to bring the asthma attack under control. (If you have practised breathing slowly and improving your out-breath when you are relatively free of asthma, it will be much easier to bring it into play during an attack – see p. 429). Parents should gently explain to their child that breathing slowly will help.

Open a window

It may be helpful to open a window and get some fresh air, as long as it is not too cold outside.

Drink plenty of fluids

A lot of water is lost through the surface of the airways during an asthma attack, so it is important to drink plenty of water, fruit juice or other liquids. Try to eat a little when you can as this will keep your strength up.

Do not take sleeping pills

Never take anything to help you sleep, even herbal sleeping pills. When asthma gets worse during the night, it is natural and healthy to wake up so that you can get more air. Sleeping pills may make you sleep very heavily.

Get into a good position

Take up a position that makes breathing as easy as possible. The diagrams below show some possibilities.

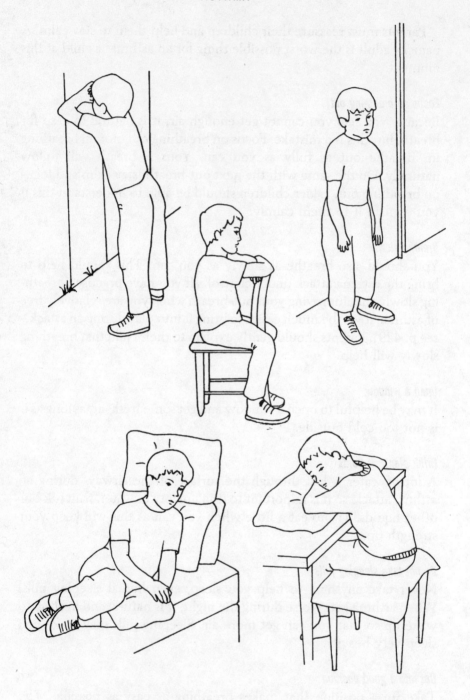

Coping with a reaction to aspirin or aspirin-like drugs

For help with recognizing this type of reaction see pp. 47–8.

Ring for an ambulance. The reaction can progress quickly to severe asthma, or to shock, collapse and unconsciousness. The ambulance crew will have drugs and resuscitation equipment on board, so this is better than driving to the hospital in almost all circumstances. Use your reliever as much as required (up to 30 puffs) until the ambulance arrives.

If you happen to have an adrenaline (epinephrine) inhaler, you can use this as well. Take up to 30 puffs or whatever maximum dose is given in the instructions with the inhaler – but be sure to tell the ambulancemen and doctors that you have done this.

Coping with anaphylactic shock

Use an adrenaline (epinephrine) injector (e.g. Epi-pen) or adrenaline inhaler as soon as you realize what the problem is, *and call the ambulance as well.* Remove the cap and inject into the outer thigh, through clothing if necessary. Do not inject it into any other part of the body.

In the USA, doctors' advice on anaphylaxis is that if you have reacted very badly in the past and know *for sure* that you have encountered your allergen (e.g. an insect sting) you can use the adrenaline injector before there are any symptoms. In Britain, the advice is to wait for symptoms. It's up to you – generally speaking, for those with no other health problems, it is better to give an unnecessary adrenaline injection than to delay giving one that was indeed necessary.

Both the injection and an adrenaline inhaler (see p. 347) can be used. You can use the inhaler first to treat symptoms in the mouth, throat and airways, and then use the injection if there are still symptoms or if new symptoms develop. This is a good approach if you have relatively mild reactions normally. Alternatively, if your reactions are often severe, use the injection first to get the reaction under control and then follow up with the inhaler if necessary. Don't worry about over-dosing by using the inhaler as well – unless you have a heart condition there is no risk of this. However, you should not exceed the maximum number of puffs recommended for the inhaler, because the propellant can be dangerous.

One shot of adrenaline is enough for most cases of anaphylaxis, but if you do not improve, a second injection can be used, 10–15 minutes after the first. Where it takes time to get to hospital, there is no medical help and the breathing is still deteriorating, another shot of adrenaline (epinephrine) can be given every 15–20 minutes, but the maximum number of shots recommended by your doctor should *never* be exceeded – this can be fatal.

If there is any difficulty in inhaling the adrenaline, improvise a spacer (see pp. 383–4). Should you not have an adrenaline inhaler, you can use your reliever inhaler (e.g. Ventolin) as well as the adrenaline injection.

Anaphylaxis is potentially life-threatening, especially in those with asthma, and *there should be absolutely no delay in calling an ambulance*. Make sure the telephone operator understands the problem. The ambulance crew should be carrying adrenaline as well as oxygen and resuscitation equipment.

During a severe reaction, if you suffer vomiting or diarrhoea and have to go to the toilet, take someone with you – do not go alone in case you collapse. Needless to say, you should already have called an ambulance before you go, or ensured that someone else is doing so.

You should be kept in hospital for six to twelve hours even when the attack seems to be under control. Repeat attacks have occurred up to eight hours later.

What to do if you do not have adrenaline

A reliever inhaler will give you some help if you do not have adrenaline. Take a puff every few minutes. Anti-histamines, such as those prescribed for hayfever, may also be of some assistance if you do not have adrenaline: take the maximum dose allowed.

First Aid for someone in anaphylactic shock

Swelling of the tongue or throat can produce suffocation in the worst cases. If there is visible swelling in the mouth and throat, the person is unconscious or turning blue and no medical help is at hand, it may be possible to keep the top of the trachea (the main airway leading from the throat) open by using the handle of a spoon. Make sure it has really smooth edges, and slide it gently over the top of the tongue and into the throat. Press down gently but firmly to open the airway.

If the person feels faint, they should lie down, but if there is swelling in the throat and difficulty in breathing they should sit up, as this will avoid making the swelling worse.

Someone who is losing consciousness should be put in the recovery position, known to all first-aiders, to minimize the chance of inhaling vomit – a definite risk after an allergic reaction to food.

The first-ever attack

There is a first time for everything, and the first bout of anaphylactic shock can be quite mild. The initial signs may be tingling or itching of the mouth. If this happens to you, stay close to the telephone for at least an hour, so that you can summon help if necessary.

Should you begin to feel an asthma attack coming on, or have any of the other symptoms listed on pp. 48–9, ring for an ambulance and use your reliever inhaler until it arrives. For many people, the tingling/ itching will wear off, and nothing further will happen. In this case, keep well away from the food that triggered the attack in future, and see your doctor.

Everyone who has suffered anaphylactic shock should also read pp. 62–3.

'. . . when you're young you tend to panic . . .'

James is 28 and has suffered from asthma since he was seven. 'I still have asthma, although I cope with it better than when I was a kid. When you're young you tend to panic if you're having an attack, but when you're older you know that's no good, and you should just keep breathing normally. Fresh air helps in those circumstances.'

After discharge from hospital

Recent studies in Britain have shown that asthmatics admitted to hospital with a severe attack are, occasionally, sent home before they are really out of danger. Some of these patients have died. If you feel at all concerned after you leave hospital, don't hesitate to call your doctor again, or call an ambulance, or go back to the hospital.

The hospital doctors should make arrangements for some kind of follow-up treatment, either with your GP or a specialist, a few days after the emergency admission. If this does not happen, make an appointment yourself to see your GP – and read the next section.

Did you know?

The rate of asthma is reaching epidemic proportions in the United States. According to the U. S. Department of Health and Human Services, the number of Americans suffering with asthma more than doubled from 1980 to 1996 to reach nearly 15 million, including 4.4 million children. Rates of asthma among children under five are increasing at an alarming rate, although the disease is still more common among school-age children. Asthma is one of the leading causes of school absenteeism, and children with asthma miss more than 10 million school days annually.

The reasons behind this rapid increase are unclear, but the Department of Health and Human Services has initiated new efforts to raise public awareness of asthma's impact and improve access to necessary health care services.

Did you know?

A study of 90 patients who died from asthma attacks found that, in 86 per cent of cases, there were potentially preventable factors contributing to the fatal attack. These factors can include depression, smoking, heavy exposure to problem allergens, inadequate treatment with preventer drugs, repeat prescriptions given without the patient seeing a doctor or asthma nurse, and delays in seeing a specialist.

AFTER AN ATTACK: THE NEXT STEPS ARE CRUCIAL

Don't expect too much of yourself in the days after a severe attack. You need more rest than usual, because the attack takes a lot out of you. Drink plenty of fluids as you may be dehydrated.

Remember to keep on taking your preventer inhaler at the increased dose – this is vitally important, as you still need to keep the inflammation damped down. Reducing the dose or forgetting your preventer inhaler now could lead to another severe attack.

Keep on taking your steroid tablets too, following your doctor's instructions or your management plan (see pp. 391–2). Again, this is vitally important in preventing another attack.

If you produce a lot of mucus when you have asthma, there may still be some left in your chest after the attack. This mucus can sometimes form solid plugs which totally block the small airways. If you do not clear these, you are storing up trouble for yourself. You should try to clear the mucus without violent coughing, which may make matters worse. There are various steps you can take:

- Treatment by a physiotherapist is often a very effective way to clear your lungs of excessive mucus. The easiest way to find a physiotherapist in your area is to ask your doctor if he or she can recommend one.

- Medicines known as expectorants can also be useful in clearing mucus, but do not take ordinary cough medicines (see p. 349). Ask your doctor or pharmacist for advice on a suitable expectorant.

- There are also some breathing exercises which can help to clear mucus, including pursed-lips breathing and huffing (see p. 429). The objective of these exercises is to bring the mucus up to the top of the airways, where it can be cleared with a small gentle cough. The mucus may not come up straight away – often the exercise takes effect some time later, usually within the next hour. Try to repeat the exercises several times each day.

- There are reports that the Heimlich manoeuvre, used to treat choking, can also be effective in freeing mucus plugs in asthmatics. The technique must be used more gently than usual on asthmatics. It is probably best if asthmatics can perform the treatment for themselves. It is *essential* that you ask your doctor before trying this, even if you have been trained in the Heimlich manoeuvre.

Ask yourself what went wrong

Asthma attacks happen for a reason. If you have had a severe attack, take the time to think over what happened just before it, and to ask yourself what went wrong:

- Were you exposed to a high dose of allergen? This is one of the most common causes of severe and sudden asthma attacks. Possible sources of allergen are listed on pp. 113–26. Ways of avoiding allergens are dealt with on pp. 127–78.
- Did you have any other symptoms such as tingling, itching or swelling of the lips, tongue or face? If so, you may have a food allergy (see p. 179). Consult your doctor about this as it is a potentially serious problem.
- Were you forgetting to take your preventer inhaler regularly? This is another very common cause of sudden asthma attacks. You should always keep taking your preventer inhaler (e.g. steroids or cromoglycate-type drugs, see p. 334) even when you feel well. If you stop taking the preventer, or frequently skip doses, the inflammation that causes asthma attacks gradually builds up to dangerous levels (see p. 22). It may be helpful to read p. 327 and pp. 388–90 if you have misgivings about taking your preventer regularly.
- Is it a long time since you had your medicines reviewed by the doctor or asthma clinic? If so, make an appointment now.
- Have you been using your peak-flow meter regularly and recording the results? If you do not have a peak-flow meter, ask your doctor for one now (see p. 315).
- Have you been using your reliever inhaler regularly, more than once a day (see p. 322)? If so, see your doctor now.
- Did you have a cold or chest infection which might have triggered the attack? Did you double your dose of preventer inhaler when the infection started (see p. 238)?
- Were you exposed to any of the triggers listed on pp. 2–3 just before the attack? How could you avoid this exposure in future?

Did you cope well with the attack?

Every attack is also a chance to learn more about coping with asthma. You may just want to forget all about it, but please don't – not just yet. It really helps to look back over events, so that you understand how the attack developed, and how you might have prevented it from getting out of hand. If you do this now, you will reduce your chance of having another severe attack in the future. You should also see your doctor after an attack, to have your treatment reviewed.

Did you recognize the attack in good time?

Read pp. 45–9 on recognizing an asthma attack. A small number of asthmatics have great difficulty recognizing when they are increasingly breathless, and they are likely to be taken by surprise when a severe attack occurs. If you think this might be your problem, talk to your doctor or asthma nurse. Using a peak-flow meter every day would help.

Did you react in the right way?

Read pp. 51–4 on coping with an asthma attack. Then try answering these questions:

1. What would you do differently if it happened again? You could try writing down some general guidelines for yourself, based on this experience.
2. Did you have everything with you that you needed? Your reliever inhaler? A spacer? (There are collapsible ones that you can carry around with you – see p. 469.) Your peak-flow meter? Your preventer inhaler and/or steroid tablets? Your management plan? Your doctor's phone number? Enough money for a taxi? A pencil and paper so that you could explain your problem when too breathless to speak (or a message written out in advance)?
3. What would help you to ensure that these things are always to hand? Have them in a bag that you always carry with you? A bigger pocket in your favourite jacket? Sometimes these small practical improvements can make all the difference. Be imaginative – if you are male and you wouldn't be seen dead with anything resembling a handbag, you could use a small camera bag or sports bag for your inhalers, or carry them in a pouch made from a sunglasses case attached to a belt.

> ### '. . . ill-judged over-confidence can kill . . .'
>
> Dr Joe Collier describes a situation that many doctors are
> familiar with: 'Inevitably, serious illness will impair judgement
> even in the most level-headed and resilient patient. One of the
> most vulnerable times for an asthmatic is just when he or she is
> beginning to recover after a serious attack. They fail to recognize
> the severity of their disability and are prone to over-exert
> themselves while neglecting vital medication. I have seen such
> ill-judged over-confidence kill patients who were released from
> hospital too soon.'

After anaphylactic shock

Any asthmatic who has suffered anaphylactic shock must be treated
properly by a specialist (see p. 301). If you are not being treated by a
hospital allergist, and have not been given a special syringe loaded
with adrenaline (epinephrine), see your doctor immediately. Some
asthmatics may also be given an adrenaline inhaler (see p. 347), and
this is useful, but not a substitute for an injector kit.

Always take your injector kit with you, and keep it close at hand at
all times: you need to be able to use it within minutes of the attack
beginning, and you may be unable to speak (and so ask someone else
to get it) quite soon after the attack begins. The day you leave your
adrenaline injector at home, in a cloakroom locker or in your desk far
away from the canteen, might be the one day when it could save your
life. Protect the kit from sunlight and excess heat – don't leave it in a
parked car on a sunny day.

If you are going off camping or hiking somewhere remote, it would
be wise to have a second injector kit, or one that can deliver multiple
injections. Make sure you know the maximum number of allowable
injections.

Wearing a Medic-Alert bracelet (see Useful Addresses) is a sensible
idea for anyone who suffers from anaphylaxis.

Carry your adrenaline inhaler at all times too. For children, a spacer
may be valuable during a bad attack (see pp. 380–4).

Drugs known as beta-blockers can make anaphylaxis worse, and adrenaline (epinephrine) less effective. Be sure never to take beta-blockers (see p. 262).

You need to be extremely careful about avoiding your offending food if you suffer from food-induced anaphylaxis. Becoming an expert on things like food-labelling regulations and cross-contamination in food factories may not seem like fun, but it could one day make the difference between life and death. The information you need can be found in *Food Allergies and Food Intolerance* by Jonathan Brostoff and Linda Gamlin, published by Healing Arts Press. Joining the Food Allergy Network (see Useful Addresses) will ensure that you remain up to date about any new and unexpected hazards, such as contaminated food.

'. . . all of a sudden they're in trouble.'

Harry is a college principal in Sydney, with many asthmatic students in his care. 'In Australia, the people who die are not those who are known to be serious asthma sufferers – those people know themselves very well, they've seen the limits, they've experienced the danger and they are very good at monitoring themselves and getting attention quickly and properly. The people who have died are the ones who've only had a bit of asthma – they may carry Ventolin, but they don't worry too much about it. They don't notice the asthma attack coming on, and all of a sudden they're in trouble.'

'We have had a number of students with life-threatening asthma attacks, and they would educate their friends and immediate house-mates in recognizing it, and treating it. It's part of first-aid training to deal with an asthma attack, but by law you're not allowed to hand out Ventolin as a first-aider. A lot of people do it though, and doctors tend to say, off the record, that you should – a lot more people die from undermedication than from overmedication.'

4

Understanding your symptoms

'That seems to me like a really hard way to learn a lesson . . .'

Dr. Veronica Spooner is a GP working in Cambridge. 'I was on emergency call the other night, and there was a girl of about 20 who is asthmatic. She's been asthmatic since she was a child, and she just stopped taking all her medication, because she decided she'd grown out of her asthma. She'd even recognized that she was getting more and more unwell over a period of three or four days, but she didn't call us. In fact she didn't call us until her peak flow was down to 60, and she could scarcely speak, which meant that she wound up in hospital with oxygen and nebulizers and drugs being given on an intravenous drip. That seems to me like a really hard way to learn a lesson. Patients do need to realize that asthma is potentially fatal, and that you can't take those sorts of chances.'

WHY DO ASTHMA SYMPTOMS VARY SO MUCH?

One of the essential features of asthma is that the symptoms vary. The inflammation in the airways flares up and then dies down again, and the muscles in the airway walls can relax as well as tighten up (see p. 22). Even when there are no obvious symptoms, the asthma is usually still there in the sense that the airways are not like those of a healthy person – if medical tests are made it is clear that these airways are asthmatic.

There is usually a reason why asthma symptoms are worse at some times than others, and trying to get to the bottom of those reasons may well help you to avoid the things that make you or your child worse.

As a first step, consider the likely triggers for asthma attacks (see pp. 2–3) and see whether any of these could explain the pattern of your asthma variations. Or could it be something encountered at work (see pp. 268–86) or at school (see p. 17). It may help to keep a symptom diary for a few weeks or months – this can help to reveal the pattern of your asthma, and relate it to your activities. The weather affects asthma symptoms for many people (see pp. 227–31), so you may want to make a note of weather conditions as well.

Reasons why asthma might be worse at certain times of the year

An allergy to pollen is often to blame for asthma getting worse at certain seasons of the year (see pp. 120–3). Your asthma may not coincide with what everyone thinks of as the 'pollen season'. In the northeastern USA this means the grass pollen season (May–July), and most people don't realize that there are other allergenic pollens which appear in spring or late summer.

Mould allergy may also produce seasonal symptoms, with asthma being worse in summer, autumn or winter, depending on the type of mould (see pp. 117–9). In places with cold winters, cockroach allergy can produce symptoms that are much worse in summer (see p.123).

In many countries a large number of asthmatics get worse during autumn and early winter. Research has shown that this autumn surge in asthma is not related to any increase in levels of outdoor pollution. There is an increase in the number of dust mites in houses from September to December, which may partially account for the generally increased levels of asthma, although cold air, and colds and chest infections also play their part. So if you get worse in the autumn, and this is not always related to having a cold or breathing cold air, consider the possibility of dust-mite allergy (see pp. 115–6). Getting worse when the central heating first comes on may well indicate problems with dust mites.

Very occasionally, seasonal symptoms are due to a food intolerance (see pp. 181–96), where the culprit food is only eaten at certain times of the year.

Why is asthma worse at certain times of the month?

About 30–40 per cent of women find that their asthma gets a little worse when they have their monthly period, or just beforehand. A small number of women get much worse at this time. This seems to be due to changes in the levels of the female hormones, oestrogen and progesterone, in the bloodstream. (When these are taken in tablet form, they can make asthma worse – see p. 263.) If your asthma gets a lot worse each month, talk to your doctor about this. You may have to increase your dose of preventer, or have some other form of treatment. Some women are helped by hormone treatment, for example high doses of progesterone. To get this type of treatment, you will probably need to be seen by a gynaecologist as well as a chest physician.

Why is asthma worse in some places than others?

The first suspect, when your asthma is worse in certain places, should be allergens. Is the place damp, either indoors or out? If so, it could be moulds (see p. 117) or dust mites (see pp. 115–6) to which you are allergic. Don't dismiss the possibility of dust-mite allergy just because you are sometimes well in very dusty houses and sometimes ill in apparently clean ones – the eye is easily deceived when it comes to dust mites (see p. 115). That is also true of pet allergens, particularly cat allergen, which can be found in buildings that have no resident cats (see p. 119). Some cats are more allergenic than others so don't rule this out on the basis that you are fine with certain cats.

Irritants in the air should be the second suspect. Indoor air is often polluted by a variety of irritating substances (see pp. 221–6), and pollutants from industrial sources (see pp. 212–3) or traffic (see pp. 207–11) are also a possible trigger for asthma attacks. Ozone usually originates with traffic exhaust, but reaches its highest levels where one would least expect it, in rural areas (see pp. 208–9).

Occasionally asthma is worse in certain places because those places hold unpleasant memories or represent difficult personal relationships. There may be traumatic events in the past that you do not even remember consciously but which are still there in your unconscious mind, and able to exert powerful effects over you. For example, quite a few asthmatics find that their asthma gets worse when they go back to their family home. This might be the effect of the family cat, the mould in the bathroom, or the build-up of mites in an unventilated bedroom, but it can sometimes be due to the tensions between parents and children that exist in most families, or even to something deeper and more traumatic (see p. 41). Talking to a counsellor or psychotherapist may help to sort this problem out. Things from the past always cause far more trouble if they are hidden away in the unconscious mind: the key to escaping from the bad feelings they cause is to confront them, not run away from them.

'For me it's worst in winter . . .'

Dan lives in Melbourne, and developed asthma as a child. 'My periods of allergy are linked to various eucalypts being in bloom. For most people in central Victoria – which has one of the highest rates of asthma among children in the world – the worst period is spring when there are very high pollen counts, particularly of rye grass. But for me it's worst in winter when a eucalypt called an ironbark starts to bloom. Because of the Australian ecology the eucalypt trees take it in turns to come into bloom, so there's a succession of trees flowering and the pollen season goes on for a long time. My asthma is always bad at this time, and if I'm doing anything like sweeping the driveway it gets worse. Once I've been set off by this, then I respond to other things more, like traffic fumes or cold air.'

WHY DOES EXERCISE TRIGGER ASTHMA ATTACKS?

Vigorous exercise makes anyone pant and feel out of breath. Muscles make extra demands for oxygen when they work hard, and breathing faster is just a natural response to this. For healthy people, the panting and breathlessness slowly subside once the period of intense exercise is over. But for those with 'exercise-induced asthma' (EIA) it's a different story. When they stop exercising, the breathlessness actually gets worse, and doesn't even *begin* to improve until more than ten minutes after the exercise ended.

Most asthmatics suffer from exercise-induced asthma, and tend to find it difficult to distinguish between this and the normal breathlessness caused by fatigue. Many with EIA are never diagnosed, especially those who have no obvious asthma symptoms *except* when they exercise. Unfortunately, many athletes come into this category, and they may struggle with EIA for years without even realizing that they have a medical problem.

The cause of this common problem is now understood. Breathing faster during exercise causes moisture to evaporate from the airways. This leads to other changes in the delicate airway lining, which ultimately triggers sensory nerves that make the muscles around the airways contract. Narrowing of the airways by these muscles produces an asthma attack.

Research shows that, if moist air is provided, people with EIA can exercise very vigorously without suffering an attack afterwards. In fact, some doctors have made a mask that always supplies warm moist air, whatever the external conditions, and this effectively prevents EIA. They have been disappointed to discover that their patients are too embarrassed to wear it in public.

Asthmatics need exercise

Exercise is good for everyone, and for asthmatics it is particularly important. Without strenuous exercise, the lungs and airways are never called on to stretch to their maximum extent. In time, they lose more and more of their elasticity, through never expanding fully. This can only make the asthma worse.

The less fit you are, the more you pant with the least bit of exertion. You have to take more breaths because your heart and lungs are not working with maximum efficiency. Getting fit – by taking exercise while keeping your asthma under control (see below) – will improve the efficiency of your heart and lungs. Then you pant less, which makes the exercise-induced asthma less troublesome. It does not get rid of the problem entirely, but it does mean that you can run a short distance without getting an asthma attack, whereas before you could not. This means that the ordinary exertions of life – running upstairs or walking the dog – are less likely to trigger an attack.

Being overweight tends to make asthma worse, because your breathing muscles have to work so much harder to expand the lungs. If exercise helps to keep you slim, that too will have beneficial effects on your asthma.

Exercise is particularly important for asthmatic children, physically and psychologically. It keeps the airways flexible, develops the breathing muscles and stimulates the production of growth hormone. Missing out on playground games and sport can make the asthmatic child very isolated socially, and this should be avoided at all costs.

Diagnosing exercise-induced asthma

The diagnosis of this problem is usually quite simple. But if there is any doubt about the diagnosis, the doctor may want you to go for a special exercise test.

Stopping your asthma drugs before the test is especially important, and some drugs have to be stopped for longer than others. Make sure your doctor tells you exactly when to stop each drug. On the day of the study you should avoid drinking coffee or tea.

If you are an athlete, it is important that the testers know this. The exercise routine used for most asthmatics will have to be adjusted to allow for your greater fitness. It is also necessary to take an additional measurement in athletes (*the forced expiratory flow rate through the middle portion of the vital capacity*), because any reduction in this flow rate can reduce your maximum exercise performance. Make sure this test is carried out.

Other medical problems can mimic EIA. Occasionally, top athletes with what looks like EIA actually have vocal chord dysfunction (see p. 311). The stress of competing plays an important part in this condition. The clues that it is not asthma are:

• The symptoms occur during exercise more than afterwards.

- The symptoms vary from one occasion to another despite similar conditions.
- Asthma drugs do not help much.

Biofeedback (see p. 449) has proved useful in treating this problem.

When food and exercise interact
Some people suffer severe EIA, but only when they have eaten certain foods before exercising. For reasons that remain a mystery, the food that most commonly has this effect is celery. A few people are affected in this way by *any* kind of food.

If you have ever had a reaction of this kind, you should be careful to avoid it happening again. A severe reaction called anaphylaxis (see pp. 48–9) can happen in this situation. It can produce total collapse and even be fatal.

Coping with exercise-induced asthma
What to do when you get an attack
The most important thing is to stop exercising immediately. It is dangerous to continue, or to start exercising again before you are back to normal. This is because your lungs are over-inflated (see p. 33) and the level of oxygen in your blood is abnormally low. Trying to carry on exercising in this state is damaging in many different ways. People have died from EIA, so treat it with respect.

Use your short-acting B-2 reliever as soon as you can. Have two or three inhalations, allowing a couple of minutes between each one. If the attack is severe, you can have up to ten puffs. The recovery positions shown on p. 54 may be helpful. Don't go off to the changing-room until you feel better. Should you get worse, you'll need somebody around. If you are not improving and are at all concerned, ask someone to get medical help.

Preventing exercise-induced asthma
Choosing where and when to exercise
Dry air is much worse than moist air, so choose your sporting activity carefully. Swimming is often the least problematic form of exercise because the air breathed is moist, although chlorine can be a problem for some (see p. 295). Ice-skating and skiing are more likely to provoke attacks because very cold air is extremely dry.

Avoiding polluted air may be advisable, especially if you exercise outdoors in an area which sometimes has high levels of ozone, diesel fumes or sulphur dioxide (see pp. 204–15).

When you have a cold or chest infection, EIA is more likely to occur because the airways are already inflamed and irritable. Either wait until you are better, or take extra precautions before exercising.

If you are allergic to pollen, choosing the right time of day to exercise can make all the difference during the pollen season (see p. 171). Drink plenty, so that you are not dehydrated.

Using your peak-flow meter
When your peak-flow is less than 75 per cent of its normal value (that is, the average value when your asthma is well controlled), you should *not* exercise. Take your preventer medication as advised, and make an appointment to see the doctor or asthma nurse.

Using asthma drugs
The main drugs used to treat EIA are B-2 relievers (bronchodilators) and cromoglycate-type drugs.

- You will probably be advised to take one or two puffs of your short-acting B-2 reliever (see pp. 371–2) about 15 minutes before you start to exercise. Having another puff of B-2 reliever at half-time (if you need it) is usually considered safe, but ask your doctor or asthma nurse for advice. If you always need another dose at half-time, this suggests that your asthma is not well controlled and you need more preventer (see pp. 334–41).
- Many doctors now give patients a cromoglycate-type inhaler to use 30 minutes before exercise. This is particularly valuable for children (see p. 338). It is an extremely safe drug, and especially valuable if it reduces the number of puffs of short-acting B-2 reliever needed each day.
- If you only have a *long-acting* B-2 reliever at present (see p. 344), and the doctor is concerned that you should not use any extra B-2 reliever, then cromoglycate-type drugs are useful before exercise. Talk to your doctor about this.
- For those who are still troubled by EIA, and whose asthma is not well controlled at other times, the doctor may wish to prescribe inhaled steroids to calm down the inflammation in the airways. Many asthmatics worry about these inhaled steroids, but they

are very safe at low or moderate doses (see pp. 326–8). The benefits of steroids will not appear instantly. It may take weeks or even months for your EIA to become less severe.

- For some asthmatics, using inhaled steroids will mean that they do not need to take a puff of B-2 reliever before exercise. For others, however, even though the steroids control asthma perfectly well at other times, there are still problems with exercise and a puff of reliever beforehand remains necessary.

Other asthma drugs:

- B-2 relievers *taken as tablets or syrup* have no effect on EIA, even if taken well in advance of exercising.
- Anti-cholinergics, when used alone, only prevent exercise-induced asthma for a tiny minority. But when used in addition to B-2 relievers and/or cromoglycate, they can be helpful.
- Theophylline-type drugs are not particularly useful for EIA.
- The leukotriene antagonists (see p. 340) are helpful for EIA, though not widely prescribed yet. It may be worth asking your doctor about these.
- Terfenadine, a type of anti-histamine, is not considered useful for asthma – except in Japan (see p. 332) – but several studies have shown that terfenadine *does* work for EIA in some people. Unfortunately, you need a large dose, and you have to take it two to four hours before exercise begins. Although this drug can be bought without prescription, you should talk to your doctor before taking it: you may need to undergo medical checks on your heart first. If taking this drug, don't drink grapefruit juice, as the two interact in unpleasant ways.

Warming up

The standard advice for those with EIA is to warm up before beginning vigorous exercise. What is rarely said is that not all types of warm-up work. Exactly how you warm up is really important. The two routines that have been shown to work well are:

- Seven very short sprints of 30 seconds each, with breaks of 2.5 minutes between each sprint. The protection against EIA lasts for at least 20 minutes after the last sprint.
- A leisurely, untaxing 30-minute run. This too gives at least 20 minutes of protection against EIA.

Another study found that warming up for just three minutes did *not* give protection against EIA.

Some people find they can achieve a warm-up effect just by starting out in a very leisurely way and slowly building up to more intensive exercise. Others say they are able to 'run through' their EIA by simply keeping going, but we would advise strongly against trying this unless you are already sure it works for you – ignoring EIA can be dangerous.

Using the 'refractory effect'

About half of those with EIA experience the 'refractory effect': having exercised once, they can exercise again within 30–90 minutes without any problems. Make the most of the refractory effect. You can use it to make sure you are in top form for an important match or race, for example.

Some drugs can block the refractory effect. The drugs concerned are aspirin and other non-steroidal anti-inflammatory drugs (see p. 258). If you take one of these drugs – for a headache, a cold, or the pain of a sporting injury, for example – you will not experience the refractory effect for many hours afterwards. This can seriously affect your performance, so check carefully on all the medicines you take (see pp. 258–9).

Hypnotherapy

One study showed that two brief sessions of hypnotherapy (see p. 450) reduced EIA substantially.

'. . . swimming opens up my airways really well'

Mo Wakeman is 58 and has had asthma most of her life, and brittle asthma for the past 25 years. 'I've always been very active and I want to go on being active now. I swim a lot, because swimming open up my airways really well. I can go in the pool with a peak flow of about 90 and come out at about 250, sometimes 300 if I swim a lot. Swimming is the only thing that I can find now to help me. So I go swimming four times a week, and do about 40 lengths, which really helps.'

WHY IS ASTHMA WORSE AT NIGHT?

A great many people with asthma find that their symptoms are worse at night, and they may wake up gasping for breath in the small hours – a terrifying situation. Other do not wake up in the night, but find their asthma is worst first thing in the morning – in other words, the airways have deteriorated during the night and this is noticed on waking up.

Some asthmatics – those who are not woken up by their asthma – are so used to feeling awful in the morning that they do not realize what the problem is. They have learned to move around very slowly in the morning so that they don't get too breathless, and they just accept this situation as normal. Having a peak-flow meter (see p. 315), and using it morning and evening, can help to reveal how much the airways have narrowed in the night. Treatment can then be adjusted to get the asthma under better control.

A few asthmatics have asthma *only* at night, and have apparently normal airways during the day. This can be a problem for doctors trying to make a diagnosis (see p. 309).

The effects of nocturnal asthma

Controlling nocturnal asthma is vitally important, even for asthmatics who are not woken up at night and have got used to feeling dreadful in the morning. The majority of asthma deaths occur at night, or follow on from asthma attacks that began during the night. So it is important to treat nocturnal asthma and get the inflammation in the airways under control.

If you have nocturnal asthma every night, this is considered by doctors to be severe asthma.

Nocturnal asthma also affects daytime performance. A study published in 1998 showed that children who are frequently woken up by asthma are sleepy in the daytime and do not perform as well in memory tests as non-asthmatic children. These asthmatic children are more likely to be depressed and have psychosomatic symptoms, and some have learning difficulties and behavioural problems. The good news is that when nocturnal asthma is successfully treated, and children wake up less often with asthma attacks, their memory improves and they feel less depressed.

Nocturnal asthma can affect adult asthmatics in the same way, making them tired and under-par by day.

Why does asthma get worse at night?

There are several different reasons why asthma gets worse at night:

- Natural changes in the body, which affect everyone during the night, tend to make the airways narrower in asthmatics. These changes include:
  - a fall in body temperature
  - a fall in the level of the natural anti-inflammatory hormone, cortisol
  - a fall in the level of adrenaline, a hormone which opens up the airways by relaxing the airway muscles
  - increased activity of the parasympathetic nervous system (see p. 418), which tends to narrow the airways
- Allergy to house dust mites, which are abundant in mattresses, duvets and pillows (see pp. 115–6). Unfortunately, many doctors seem to overlook this possibility when treating nocturnal asthma.
- Allergy to feathers, if using feather pillows or eiderdowns. Allergy to cats, if the cat sleeps on the bed, either by night or day.
- In a few cases, a delayed reaction to something encountered during the day, occasionally to a substance inhaled at work (see pp. 268–86).
- Where there is sinusitis (see p. 240), drops of mucus from the sinuses being inhaled during the night and making asthma worse.
- Where there is gastro-oesophageal reflux (see p. 254), tiny drops of acidic liquid from the stomach being inhaled during the night, which irritates the airways and makes them narrower.
- Sleep apnoea: stopping breathing momentarily while asleep (see p. 256).
- Very occasionally, there are psychological explanations for asthma being worse at night (see p. 41).

Treating nocturnal asthma

Drug treatment

The natural changes that occur in the body at night (see above) are each opposed by certain types of asthma drugs:

- The fall in the level of cortisol is opposed by steroid preventers (see pp. 335–8).
- The fall in the level of adrenaline is opposed by B-2 relievers (see pp. 342–5).

- The increased activity of the parasympathetic nervous system is opposed by anticholinergic drugs (see p. 345).

Regular nocturnal asthma suggests that the airways are inflamed, so the doctor will probably suggest increasing your dose of inhaled steroid preventers (see pp. 390–1) or adding them to your treatment if you are not already taking them. These drugs are much safer (when inhaled) than most people imagine (see pp. 326–8) and we would strongly recommend that you use them.

Although inhaled steroids control nocturnal asthma well for many people, there are others whose night symptoms do not improve, even though their daytime asthma is much better as a result of the steroids. For such patients, a *long-acting* B-2 reliever inhaler (see p. 344) such as salmeterol, which is taken regularly rather than 'as needed', can be useful. It is important to get the dose right, as too much can make you jittery and keep you awake.

There are also special tablets containing sustained-release forms of short-acting B-2 reliever. These release small amounts of the drug at regular intervals for several hours. The prolonged effect should last through the night. However, your doctor may be reluctant for you to take B-2 relievers in tablet form (see p. 365).

The part played by the parasympathetic nervous system (see above) in nocturnal asthma suggests that anticholinergic drugs such as Atrovent might be helpful. Unfortunately, these drugs wear off after three to six hours, which reduces their usefulness. If you are woken up by asthma at night, and have trouble getting back to sleep, it may be worth having an anti-cholinergic inhaler to use when you wake up, in addition to your other medicines. For some people with nocturnal asthma this makes a significant difference. Asthmatics who get wide awake if they take a puff of B-2 reliever may prefer anticholinergics at night because they don't have this side-effect. Ask your doctor about prescribing this additional treatment.

A dose of theophylline (see p. 346) before going to bed can also prove useful, especially the slow-release forms such as Theo-Dur.

Avoiding allergens
The most common allergy in nocturnal asthma is house dust mite. First you need to be sure that house dust mite really is the problem allergen for you or your asthmatic child. You can use the checklists on

pp. 115–6, or ask for skin-prick tests (see p. 125). Once the allergy is confirmed, follow the anti-mite programme described on pp. 127–55.

If feather allergy is the problem, simply get rid of everything stuffed with feathers or down. Pet birds should be kept outdoors or, preferably, found a new home.

In the case of cat or dog allergy, banning the pet from the bedroom is essential, and it would be best to find it a new home. You will need to follow this up with some very thorough cleaning of the bedding and the room itself (see pp. 156–60).

Treating other medical conditions

Sinusitis can be difficult to treat, especially if you have had it for some time. The full treatment programme may seem daunting (see pp. 240–5) but it could produce very valuable improvements in your asthma, both by day and by night. Gastro-oesophageal reflux can be treated in various ways (see pp. 254–5) and this can result in a striking reduction in asthma symptoms. Sleep apnoea is also a treatable condition (see p. 256).

'He'd start wheezing and honking within two minutes . . .'

'My husband developed asthma in his forties. After a bit, we noticed that getting into bed, or turning over vigorously at night, would bring on the asthma. He'd start wheezing and honking within two minutes of putting his head on the pillow.' Symptoms like these are often due to dust mite allergy (see p. 115.)

'My asthma has definitely improved . . .'

'I've got a continuous positive pressure machine at home, because I stop breathing when I'm asleep. I found this out when I fell fast asleep at the wheel of the car. I mentioned this to my consultant, and he did tests which showed that I stopped breathing at night. My asthma has definitely improved since I've had the machine.' For more on sleep apnoea, see p. 256.

5

The asthma epidemic – and how to beat it

> ### '. . . we thought we had made a mistake . . .'
>
> When researchers in Germany decided to look at the number of children with asthma, and compared the numbers in a West German city with numbers in two highly polluted cities in East Germany, they expected to find more asthma in the East. They did find more coughing and wheezing in the East, but when it came to asthma, the results were exactly the opposite. Initially the researchers reacted with disbelief. 'We checked all the data entries again because we thought that we had made a mistake,' said the research team leader, Dr Erika von Mutius of the University Children's Hospital in Munich. The children in West Germany had far more allergies than those in the East, and therefore more asthma, despite breathing cleaner air.

WHY IS ASTHMA ON THE INCREASE?

There is no doubt now that asthma truly is on the increase. At one time it seemed possible that doctors had just become more inclined to diagnose asthma, rather than, say, 'wheezy bronchitis' or 'a cough', producing an artificial increase in the asthma statistics. New research shows that, although this diagnostic shift has happened, there is also a genuine and sizeable increase in the number of asthma sufferers. Between 1975 and 1995, asthma rates in children doubled in many parts of the world, and the rates for adults also rose sharply. It is no exaggeration to call this an epidemic.

A Western epidemic

The asthma epidemic is affecting all the rich, Westernized countries of the world. It is also affecting immigrants to Western countries arriving from places where asthma is rare. For example, when people from the Polynesian island of Tokelau move to New Zealand, their chances of getting asthma double. Similar increases have been seen among Filipinos moving to the USA, and Asians from East Africa moving to Britain. The new cases of asthma occur among adult immigrants, as well as their children. For black South Africans moving to Cape Town, rates of asthma in the next generation are *20 times higher* than in the rural villages where the people originated.

Chinese people in Taiwan, who have stayed in the same place but gradually adopted a Westernized lifestyle, now have eight times more cases of childhood asthma than they had in 1974. In Ghana, the wealthier people living in the cities are also experiencing more and more asthma, whereas the poor people *living in the same cities* have far less asthma, and people in the remote villages have *little or none*. Research has revealed the same thing in Zimbabwe. All these communities have also experienced rising levels of other allergic diseases.

Looking at all this research, it is obvious that the asthma epidemic is being caused by some factor or factors in modern Westernized life. Whatever the factors are, they seem to have appeared in the early 1960s and they affect rich and poor alike in Britain and other Western countries, but failed to affect people in East Germany before German unification.

Another puzzling fact about the worldwide distribution of asthma

is that rates seem to be very high in parts of Latin America, particularly Brazil and Peru, and not just among the wealthier classes.

What is causing the epidemic?

Air pollution is usually blamed, but the case against air pollution just
doesn't stand up. Although it can make asthma worse for people who
already have the disease, and it may produce a *small* increase in the
number of people developing asthma, there is no way that air
pollution is the major cause of the asthma epidemic. Some places
with extremely clean air, such as New Zealand, have very high rates of
asthma (see pp. 205–6). The poor urban children in Ghana (see
above) are breathing the same polluted air as the rich urban children,
but suffer much less from asthma.

So what is the cause? There is no simple answer to this question,
but many different factors have been identified. Some of these are
universal in Westernized countries and communities, others are not.
It looks as if the factors in question vary from one country to another,
from one region to another, and even from one asthmatic to another.
So some of the factors listed below may be relevant to you and your
family, and some may not.

Bear in mind that all these factors will probably make no difference
to a person who does not have the inborn tendency to develop
allergies and/or asthma (see p. 25). It is primarily those with the
inherited susceptibility to asthma who will be affected by these
changes in lifestyle.

It is interesting that the large differences between East and West
Germany (see p. 78) only occurred in the generations born after 1961:
before that, West Germans had as little asthma as those in the East.
The same is true when people in Sweden are compared with those in
Estonia. As one researcher points out, 'Living conditions in the
formerly socialist countries of Europe are, in many respects, similar
to those that prevailed in Western Europe 30–40 years ago, including
the type of air pollution, the panorama of childhood infections, types
of immunizations, building standards, and food.'

Looking at the worldwide picture, there is a general link between
asthma and affluence, but within developed countries such as Britain,
asthma rates are the same in all social classes. In other words, the risk
factors are shared by rich and poor alike in the West. This would fit in
with risk factors such as a high-salt diet (for example from crisps and

other salty snacks), sedentary indoor lifestyle, altered patterns of childhood infections due to sanitation and medical care, and poorly ventilated housing leading to allergen build-up. Such factors are shared by rich and poor alike in developed countries, but are still rare in rural Africa and Asia where asthma rates remain very low.

These are some of the likely causes of the asthma epidemic:
A change in diet: A high intake of salt, and relatively few fresh fruits or vegetables, may make people more likely to develop asthma. Diets rich in fat, especially saturated fat, and low in important minerals such as selenium and zinc, could also increase the risk (see pp. 96–104). One of the problems with such a diet is that it tends to promote inflammation. The diet that women eat when pregnant may also affect the baby's chance of developing allergies, but this is not well understood yet (see p. 28).
Less ventilation and more heating: All those tightly fitting windows and money-saving draught excluders have reduced the air-flow through our houses, so that allergens, which are one cause of asthma (see p. 110), can build up to very high levels in the air. With less ventilation there is also more condensation and damp, which encourages mould growth (see p. 117). Warmth and damp are also ideal for house dust mites, one of the most common causes of asthma (see p. 115).
More fitted carpets and upholstered furniture: Given poor ventilation and greater humidity (see above), fitted carpets increase the levels of house dust mite allergens in our homes. Thick curtains (drapes), and sofas and armchairs covered with fabric rather than leather also contribute to the problem. House dust mites live in carpets and soft furnishings in their millions. You cannot see them because they are extremely small, but they are there. Old-fashioned homes, with wooden floors, a few rugs, rattling windowpanes and ferocious draughts, harboured far fewer mites (see p. 147).
Changes in washing temperatures: Clothes, bedding and furniture covers are now washed at much lower temperatures. The introduction of detergents that wash at lower temperatures was good news for house dust mites as they are only killed by temperatures of 55°C (131°F) and above (see p. 131).
Soft toys: Children have more soft toys, and they often sleep with their faces snuggled up against them, inhaling all the allergens from

the millions of house dust mites living happily in the toys (see p. 137).
Pets: More dogs, cats and other furry pets are now kept and they are
more likely to live in the house rather than outside, often sleeping on
their owners' beds. If children are exposed to pets during their first
year of life they are much more likely to become allergic to them, and
this increases the risk of asthma later, when they are two years old or
more (see p. 29). All pets, apart from fish, can provoke allergies and
asthma (and some people become allergic to the ants' eggs used for
fish food).

Moulds and cockroaches: In run-down housing, there are more
moulds and, in warmer climates, cockroaches. Being exposed to
airborne allergens from moulds or cockroaches during the first year
of life raises the risk of asthma developing in children (see p. 26).
Allergy to cockroaches probably explains the very high levels of
asthma in American inner-city areas.

More time spent indoors: Most of us now spend much more time
indoors than out, and children, in particular, spend far less time
playing outside than they did in the past. A child slumped on a sofa
watching a video or playing a computer game is breathing very
shallowly, as well as inhaling large quantities of indoor allergens,
especially dust mites. Children running around outside are not only
breathing better air, they are also exercising their lungs which
increases the capacity and elasticity of the airways and therefore
helps protect against asthma (see p. 68).

Changing patterns of indoor pollution: Breathing high concentrations of nitrogen dioxide gas from gas cookers and gas fires, in
combination with high levels of allergen, increases the risk of asthma
in young children (see pp. 207–8). Old-style indoor pollution, on the
other hand, may have protected against asthma. Studies from
Britain, Germany and Australia all show that using coal or wood
to heat the house may reduce the risk of asthma. This could be due
to increased ventilation reducing house dust mite numbers, but some
think that the smoke itself might, indirectly, reduce the risk of
asthma (see pp. 211–2).

Cigarette smoking: More women now smoke, and many continue
smoking during pregnancy and afterwards. Babies born to smoking
mothers are more likely to develop asthma, and allergies in general
(see p. 89). Other adults smoking in the house after the baby is born
may also increase the risk of asthma.

A change in the pattern of childhood illnesses: Several different lines of evidence link increased rates of allergy and asthma with smaller families and more hygienic conditions. A study in East Germany found that children living in overcrowded conditions were much more likely to have had parasitic infections, and much less likely to have allergies. Overcrowding in Estonia and Poland is also associated with lower levels of allergy and asthma. Parasitic worm infections seem to protect against allergy (see p. 27). Other research shows that children who wash more run a higher risk of asthma (see p. 93) and in this case infection with harmless soil-living bacteria may be responsible (see p. 27). One African study suggests that measles infection protects against the development of dust-mite allergy, but measles vaccination does not. On the other hand, some common viral infections causing chest infections in young children may promote allergic reactions (see p. 93), and these viral infections are probably more common today.

Frequent courses of antibiotics during childhood: Antibiotics, if given to babies under two years of age, increase the risk of asthma (see pp. 92–3).

More sexually transmitted infections: One particular infection of the urinary and genital tract can be transmitted from the mother to the baby during birth, and the child is then three or four times more likely to develop asthma in later life (see p. 88). The bacterium may cause no obvious symptoms in the mother. About 50 per cent of Western women are carrying this bacterium, and most are unaware of it. Levels of infection were probably lower 40 or 50 years ago.

More traffic pollution: Some types of traffic pollution may *very slightly* increase the risk of allergies and/or asthma developing in children (see pp. 207–11). Note that this effect might boost the number of asthma sufferers a little, but, taken alone, it cannot account for the vast scale of the epidemic.

Exposure to pesticides: A study in Ethiopia showed that use of one insecticide almost doubled the risk of allergy while research in Canada has linked asthma with carbamate insecticides (see p. 223).

Exposure to other chemicals: There is a small piece of indirect evidence on this point: a Canadian study showed that children living in newer houses were more likely to develop asthma (see p. 225).

Other theories about the asthma epidemic – true or false?

Are house dust mites alone causing the epidemic?

There are people, including some experts in this field, who seem to be claiming that house dust mites are the major, if not the sole, cause of the current asthma epidemic. Don't you believe it! A study in Los Alamos, New Mexico, a high-altitude region where there are virtually no dust mites, found that rates of asthma were just as high as elsewhere in the USA.

Studies in the former East Germany found that people had high levels of dust mite infestation in their houses, yet relatively low rates of allergy to dust mites, before German unification when the standard of living was low. People in West Germany, with a far more affluent Western lifestyle, had fewer house dust mites, but they were more likely to become allergic to them.

What about vaccinations?

You may have heard that vaccinations, particularly for whooping cough, increase the risk of asthma developing later in childhood. The evidence on this is conflicting (see pp. 94–5), suggesting that vaccinations only make a difference if certain other factors are present or absent.

Could car travel cause asthma?

A doctor in Tasmania has suggested that, for unborn babies, the rise in stress hormones that occurs when their mothers travel by car increases the risk of asthma after the child is born. His evidence is simply that rates of asthma in Australian children have increased roughly in line with the time women spend travelling by car. No one has taken this theory seriously, so it has never been tested. Many other changes in society have occurred at the same time as increasing car travel.

Slightly more impressive evidence comes from Ethiopia, where, in one small country town, adults who owned a car had *four times* the risk of becoming allergic to house dust mites (and dust-mite allergy increased the risk of asthma ten times). But this link could be explained in many other ways. Those with a car were a tiny minority, and were probably more Westernized than their neighbours in a great many other ways as well.

> *'Before 1930, carpets were never left down,*
> *and they were regularly beaten.'*

Professor Tom Platts-Mills is an allergist working at the University of Virginia in the USA. 'Before 1930, carpets were never left down, and they were regularly beaten. Carpets were unusual in housing of low-income families, and they were put in storage from May to October in middle- or upper-class houses. Thus Edith Wharton wrote in 1905 in *The House of Mirth* that Mrs Peniston was "as much aghast as if she had been accused of leaving her carpets down all summer or of disobeying one of the equally cardinal rules of good housekeeping". After 1930, the vacuum cleaner was introduced. Vacuum cleaner sales people, then and now, convinced the public that carpets can be cleaned while on the floor, which is only partly true . . . Allergists have attempted to keep up with the pace of change in the outside world and in housing . . . In the next ten years, the objective of doctors who treat patients with allergic diseases should be active involvement in the design of houses, in their flooring, heating, ventilation and furniture.'

> *'We have been losing the war against smoking in young*
> *women . . .'*

There are many factors involved in causing the current asthma epidemic in Western countries. 'We have actually been losing the war against smoking in young women of child-bearing age,' says Dr Kenneth Chapman, director of the Asthma Centre at the Toronto Hospital. 'We put together infants living in nice, warm, humid, insulated homes with pets and dust mites and a few more mothers who smoke, and we have the stage set for sensitizing young airways.'

'After I'd been there about three weeks I started having asthma . . .'

John is in his 70s, and has had asthma for over 40 years. 'My mother had asthma, and my brother died of it, but I was a pretty vigorous young lad, working on the farm. Then I went off to university in Auckland, but I still had to work in the vacations, on farms, or on the wharf or in a factory. I was a healthy young person, always working hard, biking around, going everywhere really fast.

'When I got my second teaching job I had one year of good board with a fellow staff member, and then I had to move on. It was hard to find really cheap lodgings but eventually I got a cheap place with this rough sort of family. After I'd been there a week I wanted to have a bath. And they thought that was a great joke – a man having a bath! In their bath they stored a big bag of sugar and a big bag of salt, so I had to haul all these things out first. When I wanted a bath *again* the next week, they just thought this was *crazy* – imagine, a chap having *another* bath. That was the kind of place it was.

'I was given a bed which had this huge kapok mattress, a great billowing home-made thing, where you just disappeared into the kapok. After I'd been there about three weeks I started having asthma. I think it must have been the bed that did it. My body had some tendency to asthma, it was in the family, but in my case it took this dusty old kapok mattress to bring it on.

'I was about 30 and I had a terrible time from then on. I used to have these asthma attacks in the early hours of the morning. I'd get up and it would gradually disappear so I'd go to work, but it was difficult to teach having had almost no sleep. I've had asthma ever since.'

As John's case shows, massive exposure to an allergen – in this case probably dust-mite allergen from the mattress – can bring on asthma in a sensitive person. Someone who is already asthmatic can also acquire new allergies in this way, and make their asthma worse. So it is sensible to be choosy about where you sleep, and to avoid any other situations that involve high allergen exposure.

CAN PARENTS PREVENT THEIR CHILDREN
FROM GETTING ASTHMA?

There is much that parents can do to reduce the risk of their children developing asthma, and some of it can be done quite simply and cheaply. Other measures may be a nuisance, and cost a certain amount of money, but compared to the hassle and expense of having an asthmatic child to take care of for the next 10 or 15 years, they are nothing at all.

However, you should bear in mind that all these measures do is *reduce the risk*. They can reduce the risk quite substantially, but even so there is no way to make absolutely sure that a child does not become asthmatic. If you decide to follow the recommendations here, you must remember that you may still have an asthmatic child in spite of everything you have done. But the asthma may well be less severe than it would otherwise have been, so your efforts will not have been totally in vain.

Who should consider carrying out these measures?
- Any parents-to-be who have asthma themselves. If you have asthma or other allergies yourself, the chance of your children becoming asthmatic is higher than for an average parent, because the tendency to develop allergies is inherited (carried in the genes and passed on from parent to child – see pp. 25–6). Should your partner have asthma as well, the risk is higher still.
- Anyone who already has children with asthma or other allergies. This shows that the genes which produce allergies are present in your family.
- Those who have relatives with allergic diseases. The symptoms of allergies and asthma can skip a generation, but the genetic tendency to allergy may still be there, and can be inherited by your children. So even though you and your partner have no allergic symptoms yourselves, it would probably be worthwhile following these measures if one or both of you come from allergy-prone families.

How soon should these measures begin?
They should begin before you even become pregnant, if possible. But if you are already pregnant as you read this, take heart because the

most crucial time to make changes is from the fifth month of pregnancy until the child's first birthday.

If you are reading this late in pregnancy, then there is still much you can do. Even if you have not begun by the time your child is one year old, do not despair: you can still make useful changes to the home environment at any time during childhood.

How to reduce the risk of asthma

These are the measures which, as scientific research has shown, will reduce the risk of asthma developing in a child.

Planning the pregnancy

1. Delay having children until you are in your late twenties or older. Research shows that mothers less than 21 years old are two-and-a-half times more likely to have a child with asthma as mothers over 30. The risk gradually declines with age, so that it is about twice as high for mothers in their early twenties (compared with those over 30), and one-and-a-half times as high for mothers aged 26 to 30. The placenta functions differently according to the mother's age, and this appears to affect the development of the unborn child's immune system.

2. If possible, plan for the birth to take place in the winter or spring (December–May), and avoid the summer months (June–August). In Britain, children born in the summer are a little more likely to develop asthma than those born in winter or spring. This is probably due to the large amounts of grass pollen in the summer air. (Babies born in autumn have a slightly higher chance of developing dust-mite sensitivity, but this will not matter if you are ousting dust mites from your home – see below.)

In Scandinavia, spring is the most risky time for births, because of the pollen from birch trees. There is no research, as far as we know, relating to other countries, but the grass pollen season is probably best avoided everywhere.

3. Ask your doctor to test both you and your partner for a bacterium called *Ureaplasma urealyticum*, which causes non-specific urethritis, an infection of the genital and urinary tract which may or may not produce symptoms. This infection can be passed from women to their babies either in the womb or during childbirth. Recent research shows

that if babies are infected by it, they tend to be wheezy as infants, and they have three times the chance of developing asthma later on in childhood. The infection must be treated in both the mother and father (who can re-infect the mother during sexual intercourse) with an antibiotic called clarithromycin. The antibiotic commonly used for non-specific urethritis, erythromycin, is not effective against this bacterium.

4. If you smoke, stop now. Women who smoke while pregnant substantially increase the risk of asthma developing later in their unborn baby. The products of the cigarette are carried in the mother's blood and reach the placenta and the unborn child. Smoking may increase the risk of allergies generally, not just asthma. Fathers and other household members should also give up smoking, or smoke outdoors.

5. Have your blood pressure checked now. Mothers with higher blood pressure before and during pregnancy are more likely to have babies who develop asthma-like symptoms. Again, this may be explained by an effect on the placenta.

Improving the baby's environment
These measures can be taken before becoming pregnant or during pregnancy: the sooner the better.
1. If you live directly under a high-voltage power line, or within 20 metres (22 yards) of one, consider moving house. Living this close to a power line trebles the risk of asthma, for reasons that are not understood. If you live very close to a main road, especially one with a lot of diesel vehicles (buses, lorries and trucks) it may be advisable to move further away, although in this case the risk is relatively small.

2. Decide on the baby's room now, and take the following steps to reduce the dust-mite allergen in the room:
- Buy a new mattress and quilt for the cot. If possible, cover the mattress with an anti-allergy cover (see p. 133).
- Either remove the carpet or take steps to kill the mites that live in it (see p. 143).
- Remove soft furnishings, thick curtains, clothing, blankets and anything else that can harbour dust (see pp. 143–4).

- Reduce the humidity of the air, both in the nursery and elsewhere in the house (see pp. 139–40 and 166–8).

If you decide to take these measures during pregnancy, someone else (not the expectant mother) should do the dusty work of removing the carpets and curtains.

3. In other parts of the house, such as the sitting-room, where the baby might play or crawl about when it is a few months old, it is a good idea to remove the carpet or give it a regular anti-mite steam treatment (see p. 143) that will kill the mites and inactivate the allergen. Make sure you get the right equipment – the temperature has to be high for it to work.

4. Buy a vacuum cleaner of the kind which retains the dust-mite allergen rather than spraying it out into the air (see pp. 477–9). Otherwise the baby will be breathing large amounts of mite allergen every time you hoover.

5. Find another home for your dog, cat or other pets (except fish). If you cannot bear to part with them for ever, find them a temporary home until the baby is one year old: sensitization to the allergen seems to occur in the first year of life. Clean the house thoroughly after their departure (see pp. 156–60).

6. During the first year of its life, or at least the first six months, try to avoid taking the baby to houses where there are cats.

7. If there is damp and mould in the house (see pp. 168–9), or cockroaches, deal with these problems now.

8. Increase the ventilation in your house, so that any allergens blow away rather than accumulate. (Air conditioning is an expensive option, but it too reduces the risk of asthma.)

9. If you have a gas cooker, consider changing it for an electric one, or fitting an extractor hood to take out the nitrogen dioxide fumes, because these may increase the chance of asthma and allergies developing (see pp. 207–8). You should also replace gas fires, especially older models, as these can produce nitrogen dioxide too.

Taking care of yourself during pregnancy

1. If possible, buy a new mattress for your own bed, and fit it with a mite-proof cover (see p. 133). The risk of allergy to dust mites is thought to be reduced by minimizing the mother's exposure to dust-mite allergen from the 22nd week of pregnancy onwards.

2. Attend ante-natal classes regularly. Mothers with little or no pre-natal care are more likely to have asthmatic children.

After the birth

1. Keep the baby's room dust-free by wiping down all surfaces with a wet cloth regularly, and wet-mopping the floor (if you have got rid of the carpets). Use the anti-mite steam cleaner regularly if you are keeping the carpets.

Breast-feed the baby rather than giving bottle-feeds. Children who are breast-fed are less likely to become allergic to house dust mite and less likely to develop persistent wheezing or asthma. If this is your first baby, you may not realize that there are many obstacles to breast-feeding, which does not come naturally to all women, and which may be discouraged or undermined in subtle and unintentional ways by nursing staff in the maternity hospital. There are many organizations that promote breast-feeding (see p. 463): contact one of these for advice.

In particular it is important to ensure that babies are not given supplementary bottle-feeds by nurses, as this disrupts the pattern of breast-feeding and the delicate balance of supply-and-demand that is being established between mother and baby. Make it absolutely clear in advance that bottle-feeds must *never* be given. You may have to put a notice on the baby's cot yourself.

Cracked nipples get extremely sore and are a major obstacle to breast-feeding. You can avoid these by toughening up the skin of the nipples in the months before the birth – rub them daily with a rough cloth, and later, when they have got used to this treatment, with a nail brush.

2. If you do need to bottle-feed, it may be better to use a type of formula known as a hydrolysate, which is less likely to produce allergic reactions. Talk to your doctor, health visitor or chemist about these hydrolysate formulas. Soya milk is not recommended – it is just as likely to cause allergies as cow's milk.

3. If you are concerned to prevent allergies in general, not just asthma, take special care about the foods you eat while breast-feeding, and about introducing solid foods into the baby's diet. The general guidelines are:

- Continue breast-feeding for as long as possible.
- While breast-feeding, do not eat any eggs, fish, nuts, milk, yoghurt, cheese or other dairy products. (You will need a calcium supplement.)
- Delay introducing solids until the baby is six months old.
- Do not introduce eggs, fish, nuts, milk or other dairy products, wheat, soya or oranges before the baby is one year old. Introduce these new foods gradually, one per week, and notice whether there are any reactions to them. If there are reactions, take this food out of the baby's diet. Keep peanuts out of the diet until three years of age.
- Check with your doctor or health visitor that the baby's diet is adequate.

Some research suggests that these measures do reduce the risk of asthma, but most studies find no effect. If there are any benefits they are likely to be small, compared to the benefits of other measures such as dust-mite reduction. However, being careful about the baby's diet in the first year of life is *very* effective in reducing the risk of eczema and food allergy. Since children prone to asthma are also likely to be prone to other allergies, you may feel that this is worthwhile.

4. When introducing solid foods, try to avoid those that are fatty or salty, so that the baby does not get accustomed to these tastes (see pp. 100–1). Make sure there are plenty of fresh vegetables and fruit in the diet (see pp. 98–100).

5. During the first two years of the baby's life, if the doctor wants to prescribe antibiotics, first ask whether this is absolutely necessary. Is the doctor sure that the baby has a bacterial infection, rather than a viral one? (Antibiotics do not work against viral infections.) If the antibiotics are essential, ask if the baby can be given some type of penicillin, rather than another antibiotic. One recent British study has found that children given antibiotics before the age of two have an

increased risk of asthma later in childhood. (This effect was not, incidentally, anything to do with the infections suffered – it was clearly linked to antibiotic use.) The asthma risk is greater with macrolide antibiotics (erythromycin) or cephalosporins. Penicillins seemed to be safer than other antibiotics: although they also increased the asthma risk, the effect was not as large.

6. Don't worry too much about cleanliness. Recent research in Britain has shown that cleaner children run a higher risk of asthma. For children who have two baths a day and wash their hands more than five times a day, the risk of getting asthma is 25 per cent, compared to a risk of only 14 per cent for children who have one bath every two days and wash their hands less than three times a day.

There are some risks that you simply cannot guard against. For example, there are viral infections which babies catch (called Respiratory Synctial Virus or RSV infections) which may make asthma more likely to develop, although the link has not been established for certain. The symptoms of these infections are like those of a cold, if mild, but there may also be coughing and wheezing, and some children develop bronchitis or pneumonia. This virus is highly infectious and, unfortunately, is often picked up in hospitals.

As the child grows older
1. When the child is old enough to move into a 'big bed', buy a new mattress, duvet and pillows and enclose them in mite-proof covers (check these are safe – see pp. 470–3). (Enclose any upholstered box-springs too.) You could, alternatively, enclose the existing mattress in a mite-proof cover, but you must then inspect the cover regularly for holes, and be sure that the zip and seams are completely sealed.

2. Provide plenty of the foods that protect against asthma and avoid foods that increase the risk (see pp. 96–104).

3. Make sure that the child is outside a lot and gets plenty of exercise, to expand the airways and keep them flexible (see p. 68).

4. Continue to be relaxed about cleanliness (see above).

5. Take care that the child does not become overweight, as this increases the risk of asthma in adults, and probably does so in children too.

6. If your child develops tonsillitis, and there is a possibility of the tonsils being removed, discuss the pros and cons carefully with your doctor. In one Canadian study, children whose tonsils had been taken out were almost three times as likely to develop asthma later. Note that this does not necessarily demonstrate cause and effect: it is possible that whatever increases the risk of asthma also increases the risk of severe tonsillitis. But until doctors are sure about this, it would be sensible to avoid removing a child's tonsils unless absolutely necessary.

7. Avoid moving house too often. Some studies suggest that children who move several times may be more likely to get asthma. This could be due to all the dust-mite allergen that is stirred up when moving house. Or it could be that children who move often also tend to live in newer houses: this seems to increase the risk of asthma (see p. 225).

What about vaccinations?
You may have heard reports that the normal childhood vaccinations can increase the risk of asthma. There was some research which suggested that whooping cough vaccine could do this, but more recent studies in Sweden have shown that, at least for the Swedish children studied, this is not so. Indeed, work in Ethiopia shows that vaccination for whooping cough in that country *reduces* rates of allergy and wheezing by 30–50 per cent. (Other types of vaccination, including polio, measles, diphtheria and tuberculosis, were also linked with lower rates of allergy and wheeze in the Ethiopian study, whereas in Guinea-Bissau, children who suffered measles were much less likely to develop allergies than children who were vaccinated against measles.)

However, a recent study in Oxford found that for British children, whooping cough vaccination did increase, by about 70 per cent, the risk of asthma developing later. The reason for the difference from one country to another may be that the *overall pattern* of childhood infections, vaccinations and medical treatment is what matters, and that the effect of an individual factor will depend on this larger pattern (see pp. 26–8).

Note that the increased asthma risk for whooping cough vaccination found in the Oxford study is only 70 per cent, which is not that large. However, the same study found that giving antibiotics to babies also increased the risk (see pp. 92–3) and when a baby had both whooping cough vaccination *and* antibiotics before the age of two, the risk of asthma more than doubled. Even so, the increased risk of getting asthma has to be set against the possible danger to a baby from catching whooping cough, or going without antibiotics when these are needed. These are issues that you need to discuss in detail with your doctor – whatever his or her advice, please follow it.

Did you know?

A study of children in California found, unexpectedly, that having more than five plants in the house was associated with a much lower rate of asthma – there were about twice as many cases in houses with few or no plants. Despite this finding, you should steer clear of house plants if you have mould allergy (see p. 117) or if you are trying to reduce moisture and dust-mite levels in the house (see p. 115).

'It's so much a part of everyday life now.'

'In the area around Melbourne where we live asthma is incredibly common now. I can't think of *any* of our friends where there isn't at least one member of the family with asthma, and often it's both children.'

'If you go to a primary school sports day, you'll see the teachers going along the line of kids, saying "Have you taken your asthma medication?" It's so much a part of everyday life now.'

CAN A GOOD DIET PROTECT AGAINST ASTHMA?

Twenty years ago, the idea that eating a healthy diet would protect
against asthma – or improve matters for those already suffering from it
– was almost unheard of. Ten years ago such an idea was highly
controversial, and most doctors would have dismissed it as cranky and
way-out. Today, there is evidence from research studies that several
aspects of our diet definitely affect asthma, and others are suspected
of having an effect. But do not be surprised if your doctor or asthma
specialist still does not mention diet to you – it will probably be
another decade before this becomes part of conventional asthma
treatment or prevention.

Why does it take so long for such useful evidence to be put to good
effect? Some doctors still believe that until there is overwhelming
proof for the role of diet, and precise information on the exact
amounts of the different nutrients needed (so that they can prescribe
a particular dose of, say, Vitamin C) asthma patients should be left in
the dark about this development. Obtaining overwhelming proof
would require dozens of first-class research studies all getting pretty
much the same answer – and that is something that will take many
years, possibly decades, to complete.

We think it is wrong to keep asthma patients in the dark. Given the
scale of the current asthma epidemic, anything that can prevent
asthma from developing, or reduce the suffering of those who already
have it, should not be kept a secret.

Besides which, the dietary changes indicated by the research are all
very valuable ones for general health. The changes in diet that are
thought to protect against asthma have many other benefits – other
research suggests that they could also help ward off high blood
pressure, heart disease, stroke, rheumatoid arthritis, osteoporosis
and several forms of cancer. Is it any coincidence that several of
these diseases are also typical 'diseases of civilization' – and that some,
like asthma itself, are at epidemic levels in Western society?

Could the changes in diet that have accompanied affluence and
industrialization be responsible, or partly responsible, for causing such
diseases? Although it is by no means proven yet, this possibility seems
increasingly likely.

The anti-asthma diet

These dietary recommendations are for those with asthma (who probably won't recover by changing their diet, but may find that their symptoms are less troublesome), and for any healthy person who wishes to avoid getting asthma.

Children from families with a tendency to allergy and asthma may benefit enormously from a diet of this kind: it could make the difference between them developing asthma and staying healthy, although other preventive measures, such as allergen avoidance and exercise (see pp. 87–95), are extremely important as well. The earlier children begin this type of diet the better, because their tastes are shaped by the foods they eat early on in life.

Changes to make to your diet (and your children's diet):
1. Eat plenty of fresh fruit.
2. Eat plenty of fresh green vegetables, especially peas, broccoli, spring greens, dark green cabbage, parsley and zucchini.
3. Eat plenty of tomatoes, drink tomato juice, or use lots of tomato sauce, ketchup and paste in cooking.
4. Reduce the amount of salt you eat. This is particularly important for men and boys.
5. Use sunflower oil for cooking, or sunflower margarine, or eat a handful of sunflower seeds every day.
6. Eat less fat and oil overall, especially saturated fats such as cream, butter, lard, fatty meat and full-cream milk.
7. Reduce the amount of meat you eat, especially red meat, and kidney, liver and other forms of offal, but don't cut out meat entirely.
8. Eat cheese, milk, nuts, lentils and shellfish regularly. Choose low-fat milk and cheese.

This diet has nothing to do with food allergy or intolerance

Note that the diet recommended here is one which reduces inflammation in the airways and is therefore useful for *anyone* with asthma. It is a diet with long-term effects not immediate ones.

The question of food allergy and food intolerance – which only affect a minority of asthmatics – is a completely separate issue; it is dealt with on pp. 179–196. Obviously, if you are allergic or intolerant to any food listed above you should ignore the recommendation to eat this food.

Some foods and drinks can bring on an asthma attack

The anti-asthma diet described above is about long-term treatment or prevention of asthma. In addition, it obviously makes sense to avoid foods that aggravate asthma in the short term. There are several reactions to food that can make asthma worse shortly after they are eaten. These reactions are not allergic ones, but they do vary from one person to another.

- Steer clear of any food that gives you heartburn as this can aggravate asthma (see p. 254).
- Foods and drinks containing sulphur-based preservatives should generally be avoided as they give off the irritant sulphur dioxide (see p. 180). Some asthmatics are more sensitive than others.
- Some aspirin-sensitive asthmatics need to avoid mint and peppermint (see p. 234). A low-salicylate diet may also be beneficial in a few cases (see pp. 259–60).
- Some asthmatics are affected by the smell of food cooking. They may need to eat quite bland food that has been prepared by someone else, unless drugs such as cromoglycate (see p. 338) or anti-cholinergics (see p. 235) can block the reaction.
- Alcohol makes the airways contract for some asthmatics, but relaxes the airways for others. Individual alcoholic drinks may have different effects (see pp. 265–6).
- Some asthmatics need to avoid foods containing histamine (see pp. 179–80).

What is the evidence for the anti-asthma diet?
Fruit

A Dutch research study has shown that people who eat more fruit are more likely to do well in a test that measures the health of the lungs and airways, while a British study showed that they are less likely to develop asthma, bronchitis or emphysema.

In addition, there are many studies showing a link between Vitamin C – the major vitamin in fruit – and asthma prevention. This is not surprising because Vitamin C is an antioxidant: a substance which mops up pro-inflammatory substances (called oxidants) before they can produce inflammation in the airways. Oxidants are found in cigarette smoke, traffic exhaust fumes and the polluted air from gas cookers and fires.

Vitamin C also seems to lead to the production of a natural bronchodilator (airway-widening substance), and it may be especially valuable for children whose asthma follows on from colds and chest infections.

However, it is clear from several research studies that Vitamin C is not the only useful item to be found in fruit. The orange pigment beta-carotene, which is another antioxidant, may also help in preventing inflammation. It is found in mangoes, apricots and several other fruits, and is very plentiful in carrots, hence its name. Beta-carotene is thought to be important in preventing other diseases, including some cancers and rheumatoid arthritis. Natural beta-carotene is always preferable to beta-carotene supplements, which may do more harm than good.

The other crucial ingredient found in fruit is fibre which, according to one study, is responsible for healthier airways. How fibre has this effect is unknown at present.

Fresh green vegetables
One Australian study showed that wheezy children ate fewer vegetables. Green vegetables, especially dark green vegetables, are a good source of the mineral magnesium, and among adults in Nottingham, England, those with healthier airways were found to have a higher magnesium intake. Magnesium is believed to protect against asthma by helping the muscles of the airways to relax. You need to eat fairly generous helpings of green vegetables to get enough magnesium; peas, broccoli, courgettes, spring greens and dark green cabbage are the best sources. If you cannot bear green vegetables, or cannot eat them in sufficient quantity, then a magnesium supplement might be a good idea. Chelated magnesium is less likely to upset the bowels than ordinary magnesium supplements.

Dark green vegetables also contain beta-carotene (see above) and, if eaten raw, or only lightly cooked, vegetables provide Vitamin C.

Finally, vegetables also provide fibre, which benefits the airways (see above).

Fibre is best obtained from fruit and vegetables, not from bran-based breakfast cereals, which tend to block the absorption of important minerals.

Tomatoes, tomato sauce, juice, paste, ketchup, etc.

This finding came from one American study where, unusually, individual foodstuffs were examined for their particular effects. Drinking tomato juice and eating tomato sauce were both associated with a lower risk of developing asthma. So was eating pizza, presumably because of the tomato paste used. Tomatoes contain Vitamin C, beta-carotene and fibre, but none of these seemed to account fully for the beneficial effect of a high-tomato diet: so far the magic ingredient remains unidentified.

Salt

Salt probably affects the muscles of the airways directly, making them more likely to contract. A number of different studies have shown that increasing the amount of salt eaten can make asthma worse, while reducing salt can produce an improvement in symptoms. Asthmatic women seem to be less vulnerable than men to the effects of salt.

Additionally, a study from Kenya showed that children eating a high-salt diet were at a 60 per cent greater risk of developing asthma. Keeping children away from crisps and other salty snacks, and not adding too much salt when cooking, may be the way to reduce the levels of asthma in the coming generation.

Sunflower oil, sunflower margarine and sunflower seeds

Sunflower seeds are by far the best natural source of Vitamin E, which is another antioxidant (see p. 98) and therefore helps to prevent inflammation. Vitamin E seems not to be as important as Vitamin C in asthma prevention, but one American study showed that middle-aged women were less likely to develop asthma if they had been eating foods containing plenty of Vitamin E. (Vitamin E taken in supplements did not seem to be beneficial in this study, so you should stick to natural sources.)

Oil and fat, especially saturated fat

The evidence for this comes from a study of adult men in Malmo, Sweden, and another of villagers in Scotland. At present, no one knows why eating too much oil and fat should increase the risk of developing asthma.

Meat

The evidence is not as strong here as it is for some of the other recommendations, but a study of Australian children showed that they were more likely to wheeze if they ate lots of red meat or offal (kidney, liver, etc.). A separate study of American adults found that, of those eating meat less than once a week, fewer suffered from asthma.

We do not suggest that meat should be cut out entirely because several different studies have shown that a shortage of some minerals – zinc, magnesium, manganese and selenium – may be linked with asthma (see below). Of these, zinc is plentiful in meat, especially lean, red meat. Meat is also a good source of manganese and selenium.

All these minerals can be obtained from cereals and vegetables as well, but there are problems with getting them from these sources. Zinc and manganese are more difficult to absorb from plant foods.

In the case of selenium, the amounts present depend very much on levels in the soil. Levels in vegetable foods may be low in countries where selenium is naturally scarce, such as China, Finland, Sweden and New Zealand. Meat and fish are more reliable sources of this mineral. Those most at risk of selenium deficiency are vegetarians (particularly vegans) living in countries whose soil lacks selenium, and relying mainly on local produce.

For those who are already vegetarian or vegan, a mineral supplement might be advisable (see p. 103).

Nuts, cheese, eggs, milk, lentils, fish and shellfish

These are good sources of one or more of the minerals that may be lacking in asthmatics: magnesium, manganese, zinc and selenium. If you are cutting down on meat, you should eat plenty of these foods to make sure you get enough minerals.

Zinc is found in shrimps, clams and oysters, and in smaller amounts in cheese and egg yolks. Nuts, lentils and beans are fairly good sources (but note that soya protein tends to block zinc absorption).

Manganese is found in milk and eggs, in small amounts, but in a form that is easily absorbed. (Although green leafy vegetables, wholegrains and tea apparently contain more manganese, these are not good sources because so little is absorbed.) Lentils are a fairly good source of manganese.

Selenium is found in fish.

Magnesium is fairly plentiful in sardines, peanuts, hazelnuts, walnuts and lentils. Other fish, lean meat, milk, cheese and bananas supply smaller amounts of magnesium.

Would supplements do instead?

The short answer to this question is 'No' – it is always best to get the nutrients you need from food. But there are exceptions:

- **For those who are eating a poor diet**, and who have real difficulty in changing their diet, taking supplements would be preferable to doing nothing.

  The simplest and cheapest action is to take a Vitamin C supplement. See p. 103 for further details.

  The next step up would be to take a multi-vitamin and mineral supplement. If you decide to do this, make sure that the daily dose contains all of the following:

  1. Vitamin C: 500 mg
  2. Vitamin E: at least 7 mg natural Vit E (d-alpha tocopherol), preferably more, but no more than 270 mg (400 iu)
  3. Selenium: 75 μg
  4. Magnesium: 300–500 mg
  5. Manganese: 4 mg
  6. Zinc: 15 mg

  Adjust the amount of zinc according to your particular needs:
    ○ An extra 1 mg a day is needed during pregnancy, and 2 mg a day when breast-feeding.
    ○ Men lose 1 mg of zinc in semen with each ejaculation.
    ○ Steroid tablets increase the losses of zinc in the urine, and a high zinc intake (20 mg a day) is advisable to compensate for this.

- **During a short period of high air pollution**, supplements of Vitamin C and Vitamin E could be used as a protective measure. Several studies have shown that a combination of Vitamin C and Vitamin E protects against ozone, sulphur dioxide and nitrogen dioxide.

  For Vitamin C, a dose of between 500 mg and 1 gm per day

could be taken for three to four days. There is no value in taking the very high dose supplements (1 gm/day) on a long-term basis: they can cause disturbed sleep and provide far more Vitamin C than the body can use.

For Vitamin E, we would recommend at least 75 mg natural Vit E (d-alpha tocopherol), and no more than 270 mg (400 iu).

- **Vegetarians and vegans** should consider taking a multi-mineral supplement, in view of the difficulties in ensuring an adequate intake of zinc and other minerals from vegetable food.

General advice on supplements

Vitamin C: For long-term use, take no more than 500 mg per day. Avoid chewable Vitamin C tablets which play havoc with tooth enamel. If taking a Vitamin C supplement, don't stop suddenly, as the body takes a while to adjust, and you can actually get Vitamin C deficiency (scurvy) if you stop abruptly. Reduce the dose slowly over a period of several days. The longer you have been taking the supplement, the more slowly you should reduce the dose.

Minerals: Several minerals interfere with the absorption of other minerals. For example, an iron supplement will reduce zinc absorption, and high-dose calcium or iron supplements tend to inhibit the absorption of manganese. A complete mineral supplement should be balanced by the manufacturer to overcome these problems. Another way around this problem is to take iron in the morning and zinc at night.

Omega-3 oils: Do not take supplements that include omega-3 oils (also called ω-3 oils, concentrated fish oils or EPA and DHA). Several studies have shown that these are of little or no benefit to asthmatics, and at high doses omega-3 oils can even be harmful, making asthma symptoms worse for some people. Those who are sensitive to aspirin are most likely to be affected. (Other studies show that eating fresh oily fish once or twice a week – which gives a very low dose of omega-3 oils – may benefit asthmatics a little, but high fish intake could be harmful.)

Beta-carotene supplements (often sold as part of 'antioxidant supplements'): We would advise against anyone taking beta-carotene in supplement form. Trials in which cigarette smokers were given a high-dose supplement (50 mg per day) showed that, rather than preventing lung cancer, the beta-carotene appeared to encourage the growth of tumours in some people. Current thinking is that beta-carotene might help to guard against cancer at normal intake (the sort of dose derived from food) but that it has the opposite effect at high doses.

'in those days no one knew how to treat it . . .'

Stephen is 75. 'I have asthma, but it's not bad now. Since the steroid inhalers came in, I'm pretty good really. I do get bronchitis sometimes now, and then I'm a bit wheezy, but it's not like having bad asthma, the way I had it when I was in my 30s and 40s.

'I had a brother who died with it. He was three years younger than me and I think my mother probably was overworking before he was born. They had to find the money to buy their farm that year, and they were working like crazy, night and day. This baby was born, and he was sickly and then he had a severe rash – eczema – as well as having the asthma. My mother thought later that she'd got his formula wrong, that she'd put too much water in, but when I told my doctor this story many years later, he said "No, it would be genetically conditioned". But my mother always felt it was her fault.

'My brother's asthma was always severe, and in those days no one knew how to treat it. They tried all kinds of things – herbal treatments and injections of something or other, but it didn't help.

'In the end he had a bad attack that killed him. His heart had already been affected by the asthma, and he had a heart attack as well. They couldn't get to the doctor in time and he died. He was about 33.'

WHAT DOES THE FUTURE HOLD FOR ASTHMA TREATMENT?

Asthma treatment has improved enormously since the mid-1960s, first with the introduction of B-2 relievers and cromoglycate-type drugs, then with the development of steroid inhalers. But the advances have really done little more than keep pace with the epidemic, and there is a great need for better and more convenient asthma treatments, especially among those with severe and brittle asthma. Within the next ten years, a revolution in asthma treatment seems likely, as new drugs and vaccines come on the market that have been designed with a specific understanding of what goes wrong in asthma.

It is vitally important that such advances do not squeeze out, even further than at present, non-drug treatments and preventive measures. Being truly healthy and in peak condition is something that drugs alone can never give anyone – and something that makes life worth living. It is a matter of eating well, breathing clean air, exercising, resting and avoiding things that cause ill-health. This is true as much for asthmatics as for non-asthmatics, and should be a recognized part of medical care for everyone with asthma.

New drug treatments

In response to the asthma epidemic, huge amounts of research money are being poured into the development of new drug treatments for asthma. The first fruits of that research are now reaching the market, in the form of new drugs that reduce inflammation in the airways by opposing pro-inflammatory messenger substances called leukotrienes (see p. 340).

The development of this type of drug is based on a detailed knowledge of how the immune system works to produce inflammation. Such knowledge gives medical scientists the key to creating specific drugs, tailor-made to block inflammation.

Leukotrienes are only one small part of the complex interaction of cells and messenger substances which produces inflammation. The fact that there are dozens of different agents at work in inflammation means that there are many different possibilities for making new anti-inflammatory drugs.

One of the promising new drugs in this area is called Nuvance, which binds to a pro-inflammatory messenger substance called Interleukin 4. This stops Interleukin 4 from binding to immune cells and triggering further inflammation. Trials carried out so far suggest that Nuvance can replace steroids, and can be taken in tablet form just once a week – a considerable advantage over all existing drugs.

Another approach to stopping inflammation is to tackle the immune cells called eosinophils which flock to the airways of asthmatics. Some researchers believe that they can do this by reducing the action of another group of immune cells, called T-helper cells, which issue the signals that attract and excite the eosinophils. Studies using this approach with severe asthmatics have had some success so far.

Drugs that block the allergic reaction

For anyone with allergies, there is another possible approach to treating asthma – blocking the allergic reaction. Since allergies may be the basic cause of the inflammation in these asthmatics, this is a better solution than damping down inflammation, because it tackles the whole problem at an earlier stage.

Of the asthma drugs currently available, only the cromoglycate-type drugs prevent the allergic reaction itself, and they do not work for everyone.

There are at least two potential new drugs in the pipeline that can switch off the allergic reaction. Both work by blocking the main allergy antibody, called IgE. The first is itself an antibody, made by the biotechnology company Genentech, which binds specifically to IgE and so inactivates it. The second is, at present, a much more speculative idea – a drug which reduces the amount of IgE available, by increasing levels of a substance called CD23 which regulates IgE production.

Drugs that treat specific problems

There is much excitement about the recent discoveries concerning colds and asthma (see p. 237). Knowing why colds and chest infections trigger asthma attacks could open the way to developing drugs which break this link, thus helping millions of asthmatics get through the winter months more easily.

Another specific problem that might be tackled with drugs is the production of hard mucus by asthmatic airways. This unusual type of mucus can narrow airways even more, and sometimes block them completely. Medical researchers are currently asking why this hard mucus is produced, and how it could be reduced or stopped.

Managing drug treatment automatically – 'smart' inhalers

An advantage of many of the potential new drugs is that they could be taken in tablet form. But these drugs will take time to come on the market, and for now most people will have to go on using inhalers. So any advance in the design of inhalers, which improves drug management of asthma, would be welcome. One interesting new product is the SmartMist inhaler, already available in the USA, which measures peak flow and gives instant feedback on inhaler technique, dispensing the dose of drug automatically when the breathing rate is correct. It also records peak flow and drug usage, and can even transmit this information to the doctor's computer records, via a telephone line, so that treatment is reviewed regularly.

A vaccine against asthma?

Understanding more clearly how allergies and asthma develop (see pp. 26–8) has allowed research scientists to dream of an even more radical treatment – a vaccine that would prevent children from developing allergies. The focus of interest now is on early exposure to certain diseases, and the protection this seems to give against developing asthma or allergies later. This protection probably comes about because the balance of the T-helper cells is shifted away from Th2 cells and towards Th1 cells (see p. 27), and researchers believe they can devise a vaccine that does the same thing. Work is already underway at the University of Southampton on a vaccine that achieves this, and Professor Stephen Holgate, who is heading the research team, believes that a vaccine could be available in three to four years' time.

Better methods of desensitization

Research continues into ways to improve the effectiveness and safety of conventional desensitization (see pp. 197–200). This would be very welcome to many asthma sufferers, especially if the treatment could also be made less lengthy. The two newer methods of desensitization (see pp. 200–2) deserve much more research funding and wider acceptance, as both offer the possibility of a far quicker and safer route to desensitization.

Breathing exercises

The popular success of the Buteyko Method (see p. 423), and the results of scientific trials of these and other breathing exercises (see pp. 430–445), suggest that much more could be done with improving the breathing of asthmatics. It would be good if more research funds could be channelled into this area, so that the different forms of exercise could be understood more fully, and compared with each other.

Making asthma treatment more holistic

There are many different factors playing a part in asthma, and many ways it can be tackled, yet conventional treatment focuses almost exclusively on drugs. If you follow just some of the suggestions made in this book, you will almost certainly have less trouble with asthma symptoms, and there is no reason why the same suggestions for self-help should not be given to patients in the doctor's surgery. It is true that many patients prefer to hand over responsibility for treatment to the doctor, and rely entirely on drug treatment, but there are also many others who want to be as healthy as possible while using a minimum of drugs.

One useful way in which asthma management could develop is to broaden the range of treatments available, and to take account of the whole person, not just their airways – in other words, to make asthma treatment more holistic. Perhaps in the future there will be asthma clinics where, at the outset, everyone will get a full assessment of their breathing pattern, a comprehensive set of allergy tests, screening for other diseases (e.g. sinusitis) that can aggravate asthma, advice on allergen avoidance, diet and lifestyle, breathing retraining if needed, physiotherapy to drain mucus from the chest, tuition in exercises to strengthen the breathing muscles, sports training, counselling for emotional and social problems, and the opportunity to attend yoga or relaxation classes. Asthma drugs would, of course, still be needed, but to a lesser extent than now.

6

Allergies

'. . . people don't need to have asthma . . .'

Dr John Maunder is head of the Medical Entomology Centre in Cambridge, where house dust mites and their effects on asthma are studied. 'A policy for asthma which relies on drugs, not one of which has ever cured asthma or prevented asthma, is a national disgrace, especially when it costs half a billion pounds a year. We now know enough about asthma, and the allergens that cause it, to control most cases of it environmentally. Those people don't need to have asthma.'

'. . . we must try to reduce allergen levels in the home.'

Dr Adnan Custovic is a doctor and researcher at the Wythen-shawe Hospital in Manchester. 'Why is asthma increasing? What has changed? There are more pets, certainly, and we have also made our homes into the perfect habitat for house dust mites.
'Are we also more susceptible? I don't think there's any doubt that we are. All kinds of things could be responsible for that including our diet, antibiotics and many other things. However, one thing is for sure, if there were no allergens, nothing would happen: there would be nothing to become allergic to and asthma probably wouldn't develop in most children. That is why I believe we must try to reduce allergen levels in the home.'

ASTHMA AND ALLERGIES – WHAT'S THE CONNECTION?

Many people with asthma also have allergies, and the allergies are usually playing a part in producing the asthma. This is especially true of children: about 90 per cent of asthmatic children are allergic to something, and that is either the main cause of their asthma or an important contributor.

But not all asthma is associated with allergy. In particular, people who first develop asthma when they are adults are much less likely to have an allergy playing a part in their asthma.

To summarize the link between asthma and allergies:

- Some people have both allergies and asthma, with the allergies contributing to the asthmatic reaction.
- Some people have allergies (as shown by symptoms such as hay fever or eczema) but no asthma.
- Some people have asthma but no allergy, especially those who did not have asthma as children.

What is an allergy?

If you have an allergy, your body has taken objection to something completely harmless, such as house dust or peanuts or the pollen produced by grasses, and reacts very badly whenever it comes into contact with it. The thing that provokes your allergy is referred to as your *allergen*.

The immune system (whose proper job is to defend us from bacteria, viruses and parasites) is responsible for this reaction. It attacks the allergen – the dust, peanuts, pollen or whatever – as if it were a dangerous parasitic worm. During the attack, immune cells congregate around the allergen and cause inflammation – swelling, soreness and reddening of the same kind that develops around a deep cut once it begins to heal.

The tendency to develop allergies is inherited – it runs in families. Someone who is allergic to one thing (e.g. house dust mite) is also at risk of developing new allergies (e.g. to moulds or pets) if they are exposed to very high levels of an allergen. So it makes sense for those with allergies not to get into situations where there is a very high allergen load. This may affect choices about jobs (see pp. 280–3), leisure activities, home improvements and pets. One asthmatic, who successfully reduced his exposure to dust mites and became much fitter as a result, decided to renovate his house. A lot of the work needed was in the cellar, which was damp, and he developed mould allergy as a result, making his asthma as bad as it had been originally. It would be sensible to read all the information on pp. 115–26 so that you know what places and activities involve high allergen exposure.

How does allergy produce asthma?
Allergens in the air
Many allergens are found floating around in the air, so they come into the airways when we breathe in. They are all tiny particles, which can only be seen with a microscope (see pp. 158–9). Airborne allergens include things such as house dust mite droppings, moulds, cat allergen, dog allergen and pollen. If you are allergic to one of these and it lands on the surface of your airways, then there is a direct reaction which makes the airway inflamed. There is swelling of the airway lining which reduces the flow of air through the airway. The inflammation also signals the muscles of the airways to contract, producing even more narrowing.

For some people, removing the allergen makes all these effects disappear. This is what happens to asthmatics who get asthma only during the pollen season. But for other asthmatics, the inflammation of the airway lining continues all the time, and the arrival of the allergen just makes matters worse.

Other allergens
Although inhaled allergens such as pollen and dust are the main offenders in asthma, allergens in food and from other sources can also play a part:
- Asthma may be linked to a true food allergy, which is a prompt and often quite severe reaction to food. The more severe type of reaction is known as **anaphylactic shock** or **anaphylaxis** (see pp. 48–9). For some people it is the combination of eating an allergenic food and taking exercise that provokes anaphylaxis, while others have anaphylaxis caused by bee or wasp stings, rather than by food. Anti-venom, given for snake bites, may also provoke anaphylaxis in those who have had anti-venom before. Those with latex allergy are vulnerable to anaphylactic shock during surgery if latex gloves

are used (see p. 282). Anaphylaxis is potentially life-threatening, especially in asthmatics because they often experience a very severe asthma attack during anaphylactic shock. This condition must be treated by a specialist (see p. 301).

- Less dramatically, eating a particular food day after day, often a common food such as wheat or milk, may be contributing to asthma or even be the sole cause. This is not a true allergy but is known as food intolerance. It is rarely obvious that there is any link between the food and the asthma, but there are usually other symptoms that suggest food intolerance (see p. 182). Those with brittle asthma may be more likely to have food intolerance.

'It just seems to be an accumulation of things.'

'My asthma began when I was building an extension on our house. My wife started smoking again about then too and we got a couple of kittens. We'd had a cat before, and I'd never had any problem with that one, but with these kittens, sometimes after I'd been playing with them, I'd notice my eyes were itchy and red. Not every time I play with them though, which I don't understand. They don't seem to give me asthma as such, but I wonder if they do affect it in some way.

'It's a job to find any particular situation that *always* triggers the asthma off. It just seems to be an accumulation of things. When it began I think it was probably a combination of the wood dust and the cigarette smoke, and maybe the cats. Now it never really goes away, but sometimes it's worse than others.'

It is very common for asthmatics to respond to several different triggers and allergens, but only to respond when there is more than one of these factors present. It is as if the airways can cope with just so much, but become overwhelmed by the presence of several different challenges at once.

HOW TO TELL IF ALLERGIES
ARE AT THE ROOT OF YOUR ASTHMA

For some people, identifying their allergens is easy. If wheezing begins every time there is a cat in the room, but never occurs when there are no cats around, then the diagnosis is obvious. But for many asthmatics, it is not so clear-cut as this, and careful detective work is required to work out if allergies are really playing a part, and to identify the particular allergen or allergens that are responsible.

The checklists given here should help in pinpointing the allergens that are affecting you or your asthmatic child.

Before using these lists, it may be a good idea to write down all the places, times of year or activities that seem to trigger asthma attacks, make attacks more frequent, or reduce peak flow. Make the list as complete and comprehensive as possible, then compare it with the checklists and try to find the allergen or allergens that are the best match.

Note that this section deals only with allergens found in the air, not with those in food (see pp. 179–96 for these). Allergens that are only likely to be encountered at work are dealt with on pp. 280–3.

Why not just have allergy tests?

There are several tests for allergy, the simplest being the skin-prick test (see p. 304). If you are referred to an allergist, you will certainly be given these tests. Unfortunately, not everyone is referred to an allergist (see p. 301).

That is one reason why these checklists are valuable for identifying allergens, but it is not the only reason: the tests are not completely infallible. Although they usually give the right answer, *occasionally* they fail. They may suggest that an allergy is present when it isn't (a false-positive result), or they may fail to detect an allergy that really does exist (a false-negative result).

In the case of a false-positive result, the body is mounting the first stage of an allergic response to the allergen (the stage which involves producing an antibody to the allergen) but it is then finding ways to prevent this antibody from initiating a full allergic response.

In the case of a false-negative result, the skin fails to react because, for the person concerned, the antibodies that produce the specific allergic reaction (to dust, or pollen or whatever) are present only in the airways and not in the skin. If this is the case, they may not be in the blood either, so the sort of allergy tests that rely on a blood sample, such as the RAST (see p. 305), may give the same false result.

The only test that is infallible is a provocation test (see p. 305) and few doctors will do this because of the risks involved.

In short, skin-prick tests and blood tests are very useful if you can get them, but they are not entirely infallible, so using the checklists to understand your symptom pattern can give valuable assistance in identifying allergies. If, after using the lists, you still feel that skin-prick tests would be useful, turn to pp. 125–6 for more information.

General guidelines for using the checklists
Keep the following points in mind:

- Not everyone with asthma has allergies. They are less likely if you did not have asthma as a child.
- Even if you have allergies, other factors may sometimes trigger your asthma, such as cold air, exercise, colds and irritants in the air. Take these factors into account – they could explain some of your attacks. There is a comprehensive list of potential triggers on pp. 2–3.
- You can be allergic to more than one allergen.
- There can be more than one explanation for an asthma attack in a particular circumstance. For example, a pillow might affect you because you are allergic to house dust mites which thrive in pillows, or because the pillow is stuffed with feathers and you are allergic to birds. (There can even be psychological explanations for reactions that occur whenever you get into bed – see p. 41.) One common source of confusion is the fact that houses which are warm and humid favour both moulds and house dust mites, so you will need to take a detailed look at other circumstances that trigger attacks.
- Although the reaction to allergens usually comes on pretty quickly, there can also be a 'late reaction' which begins four to twelve hours later and lasts for a day or more. During this time you may be more sensitive than usual to triggers such as cold air or exercise. Sometimes the late reaction is more severe than the immediate one.

The checklists
House dust mites

For the vast majority of people who are allergic to dust, it is not the dust itself which is the problem, but the tiny mites that live in it, eating the moulds and human skin scales that they find there. These mites are too small to be seen with the naked eye. They are not parasites, and they do no harm unless you have allergies to them. The allergic reaction is produced, not by the mites themselves, but by their droppings. These can crumble into tiny fragments which float around in the air.

Very occasionally, people who react to dust are allergic to fibres of sheep wool in the dust, and not to house dust mites. There may also be pollen and mould spores in dust, which can account for some people's allergic reactions in dusty situations, and occasionally people develop allergies to carpet beetles or other household pests whose allergens are found in dust. But house dust mites are by far the most common cause of asthmatic reactions to dust.

Appearances can be deceptive in the case of house dust mites. A house may be thick with dust but, because the windows are open a lot and there is a roaring draught under the front door, it will not have a very high population of house dust mites. The house next door may look all spick and span, but if it is thoroughly draught-proofed, warm and slightly humid, the carpets, curtains and upholstery will be seething with mites. Indeed, vacuuming and dusting every day, if done with an ordinary type of vacuum cleaner and a dry duster, will stir up the allergens and ensure that the air is full of them for much of the time. So an asthmatic with mite allergy would breathe far more easily in the dusty house than the clean one.

Symptoms are most likely to occur:
- In bed, unless the mattress and pillow are brand-new, because mites thrive inside mattresses and pillows. The allergens are forced out when you first get into bed, and when you turn over.
- When sitting in an old armchair or sofa, unless leather- or vinyl-covered. There are millions of mites in the upholstery.
- In houses with carpets that are more than a year or two old (especially fitted carpets) because mites inhabit the gaps between the fibres.

- When doing housework, especially dusting or vacuuming.
- Just after housework has been done, or a carpet has been shampooed, because the allergens are stirred up.
- When lying or playing on the carpet (especially if it has recently been vacuum-cleaned or shampooed).
- When putting on an old sweater that has not been worn for a long time.
- When the central heating comes on at the beginning of winter.
- In autumn (when mite numbers are often very high). In winter if in a well-heated house. During damp weather, if warm.
- In any house with a damp problem, and in houses near to rivers, lakes or the sea, because of the humid air. Seaside hotels are particularly troublesome owing to damp air outside and en-suite showers. Ground floor and basement rooms are also likely to be damp and have more mites.
- In holiday homes that are locked up for the rest of the year, because the mites flourish and the allergen builds up in the unventilated building.
- In rooms that have not been used for months (for example, college students often get worse when they come home for the holidays because their unused bedroom is full of mites).
- In houses with central evaporative cooling systems ('swamp coolers').
- In buildings/bedrooms heated by hot air ducts.

Symptoms are likely to be less:
- In houses without fitted carpets, especially if there are no rugs, or if the rugs are beaten and hung in the sun regularly
- In cold, draughty houses
- In mountain regions. In the European Alps, for example, mites are scarce above 1700 metres (5600 feet)
- In desert regions
- In hospital
- During the summer, as long as it is dry

For detailed information about house dust mites, and how to avoid them, see pp. 127–55.

Moulds

Moulds are fungi that grow on decaying food and dead leaves, and on walls and windows in damp houses. They produce millions of microscopic spores, which float about invisibly in the air, and it is these that provoke allergic reactions.

When looking around for moulds, remember that they vary enormously in colour. Those on stale bread and other foods are green or white. You may see black moulds growing on the walls of badly ventilated bathrooms, around the rubber seals of refrigerators, around window frames (where they just look like dirt) and in the patterned glass of bathroom windows. Shower curtains and cubicles may have black or pinkish-red moulds growing on them. Old vegetables and dead leaves may have grey furry moulds on them, while garden plants and crops can have black moulds or bright orange moulds (called 'rusts') on their leaves. Mushrooms and other fungi often have white moulds growing on them, and cheeses such as Brie, Gorgonzola and Stilton are rich in moulds – it is moulds that make blue cheeses blue. Finally, there are plenty of moulds you cannot even see, such as those growing on the surface of the soil around a house plant.

However, you should also bear in mind that you are unlikely to be sensitive to *all* moulds. Some people are allergic to only one species, some people to two, three or four, but the chances of you being allergic to every mould you encounter are extremely remote. So you may react in some of the situations listed below, but not in others.

Symptoms are most likely to occur:
- Around compost heaps, damp straw or hay, piles of grass clippings or fallen leaves, all of which are full of moulds.
- When raking up fallen leaves or fruit and when removing dead leaves or flowers from plants.
- When watering the garden because mould spores are released when water hits the dry soil.
- When mowing lawns, if the grass clippings were not raked up after the last mowing, because they tend to go mouldy.
- In the vicinity of fields of ripe wheat or other cereal crops, especially at harvest time, because the harvesting machines disperse the spores from moulds growing on the cereal leaves.
- In late summer and autumn, when there are lots of moulds growing outdoors, especially in forests and old orchards.

- Just after the first frost of autumn, as this stimulates spore release by fungi in the soil.
- In winter, when there are more likely to be moulds growing indoors because of condensation.
- In damp houses, or in houses or rooms with humidifiers because moisture encourages mould growth.
- In churches and church halls, since these are often damp.
- In bathrooms, unless well ventilated, owing to the condensation. In cellars, basements, greenhouses and conservatories. In rooms that are left unheated, as these tend to suffer from condensation.
- When in contact with clothes, curtains or furnishings that smell mildewy: even if now dry they will still be full of mould spores.
- In houses that are near lakes, rivers or the sea, because of the moisture in the air.
- In houses with dry rot or wet rot: some mould-sensitive people react to the spores of these timber-rotting fungi.
- In houses where old timber floors or walls are being removed, as this stirs up old spores.
- In houses where central heating has just been installed, as this warms up the moulds in the house and encourages them to release their spores.
- In houses with lots of house plants.
- At Christmas, if you have a real Christmas tree, as microscopic moulds can grow on the needles. When the tree is brought indoors, the unaccustomed warmth stimulates these moulds to shed their spores.
- When handling old vegetables or fruit.

Symptoms are likely to be less:
- In deserts and other climates that are fairly dry and warm all year round.
- In spring and early summer.

Other fungi
Some asthmatics may be allergic to the spores from fungi other than moulds. A study in New Zealand found that 16 per cent of asthmatics in Auckland were sensitive to a large bracket fungus that grows on

dead trees, called *Ganoderma*. This fungus can produce over 5 kg (11 lbs) of spores a week in mid-June, and asthmatics are advised to avoid them. The allergic potential of other large fungi has, for the most part, not been studied.

Cats, dogs, horses, mice and other animals

These animals are grouped together here for convenience only. Generally speaking, people are allergic to one particular species. So if you are allergic to cats, you are probably *not* going to be allergic to dogs or horses or other animals.

People are often misled by the fact that they did not develop symptoms when they first obtained a pet or first began working with animals. In fact, symptoms may not appear until many months after close contact with the animal begins. Sometimes it takes as much as a year.

Most people who are sensitive to cats are sensitive to all kinds of cat, and the same goes for dogs, but a few people are sensitive to one breed of cat or dog, and not to other breeds. You might also find that some cats trigger off your asthma, but not others: this is because individual cats vary, and some produce far less allergen than others (see p. 161).

Another confusing factor with cats is that their allergens are extremely persistent, lingering on in houses where no cat has lived for years. These allergens are also very small and lightweight, so they stay airborne indefinitely, prolonging allergic reactions among sufferers. (By contrast, pollen and dust-mite allergens settle quite quickly in still air – see p. 162). Cat allergens are also carried about on people's clothing, and in this way they turn up in cat-less houses, schools and public buildings. Note, however, that you would have to be extremely sensitive to react to the tiny amounts found in such situations.

Sensitivity to rats, mice and other rodents may be brought on in several different ways: by having them as pets, by working with them, or because they are present as pests in rundown housing.

Symptoms are most likely to occur:
- When the animal is present.
- *After* being with the animal: for some people, a brief exposure to the animal can cause quite mild symptoms at the time, but a much more severe reaction later on. This delayed reaction can last for days, or even a whole week.

- In a room or house where the animal spends a lot of time, even though it is not present. Poor ventilation will add to the problem.
- When close to other people who have been touching the animal, or when in contact with their clothing. Only a minority of people who are highly sensitive to their allergen will react in this way. Cats and horses are more likely to provoke such extreme sensitivity than other animals.
- In the case of rats, mice, hamsters and other small animals, when in contact with the urine or bedding, because airborne particles from the urine are usually the allergen.
- For someone who is very sensitive to horses, when sitting on a sofa stuffed with horse-hair, or lying on a horse-hair mattress. (Only very old furniture and mattresses are likely to contain horse-hair).

Symptoms are likely to be less
- In well-ventilated houses, even though the allergenic animal is present, because a good draught flushes out the allergens that are floating in the air. This will only work for people who are *not* extremely sensitive to their allergen.

Pollen

Pollen is the very fine powder produced by flowers for fertilization. Brightly coloured garden flowers are rarely the problem, as their pollen is mostly heavy and sticky and is spread to other flowers by insects, not by the wind. The pollen that causes allergic reactions is usually from grasses, trees or other plants with inconspicuous green flowers. They are 'wind-pollinated' which means that they shed millions of lightweight pollen grains into the air in the hope that some will find its way to other flowers of the right kind.

If you have hayfever, and you also have asthma, there is a good chance that pollen is contributing to the asthma symptoms. But even for those asthmatics who do *not* have hayfever, it is possible that there is an allergy to pollen playing a part in their asthma.

No one is allergic to all the potentially allergenic pollens. Some people are allergic to pollen from one species of plant only, others are allergic to a set of related plants such as several different grasses, while the really unfortunate ones are allergic to a whole variety of plants including some trees, some grasses and various other species such as docks, plantains and ragweed.

Each plant species has its own pollen season, usually lasting a few weeks. The more species you are allergic to, the more weeks of the year you will encounter allergenic pollen in the air and suffer symptoms.

In many parts of the world, pollen allergy is diagnosed on the basis of having symptoms in spring and/or summer only. This works quite well, as long as you are not allergic to something else as well, which keeps the symptoms going all through the winter. In this case your symptoms will simply get worse in the pollen season, and will gradually return to normal some time after the season ends.

The other problematic situation concerns those living in winterless climates, where the offending pollen is in the air for most of the year. In Queensland in north-eastern Australia for example, there is grass pollen in the air almost all the time. In other areas with year-round warmth, such as the rest of Australia or the southern states of the USA, particularly California and Florida, the seasons for allergenic pollens are long and overlapping, and often quite variable. All this makes diagnosis difficult without skin-prick tests (see p. 126).

Symptoms are most likely to occur:

- At a particular season of the year, usually spring or summer in temperate regions. (Some people have hayfever as soon as pollen is in the air, but only develop asthma gradually as the season progresses.)
- When driving on motorways, as the air turbulence created by the traffic tends to churn up all the settled pollen.
- On hot dry days, when plants prefer to release their pollen.
- Out of doors.
- In the early hours of the night, especially if the bedroom windows are open (see p. 172).
- When the pollen count is high – assuming that the count refers to your particular allergenic pollen (if not stated, counts are usually for grass pollen in Britain, but for ragweed in the USA). However, in certain weather conditions, the actual amount of allergen in the air can be much higher than the pollen count suggests, because soluble allergen leaks out of the pollen grains, including grains that have accumulated on the

ground and other surfaces. This leakage of allergens often happens during thunderstorms or when rain follows a long dry spell (see pp. 228–30). Other factors, such as ozone, can heighten allergic reactions to pollen.

Symptoms are likely to be less:
- On damp cloudy days, as plants are less likely to release pollen.
- After rain, which washes pollen out of the air (but there are exceptions – see above).
- In winter, although there are exceptions: around the Mediterranean, for example, cypress trees pollinate in winter.
- In an air-conditioned building or car, as the filters of the air conditioner take out pollen. You should get more symptom relief from air conditioning than anything else.
- Indoors with the windows closed, but allow time for the pollen to settle (about four to five minutes for intact pollen grains).
- At the coast, when a strong sea breeze is blowing, as this brings in pollen-free air.

Identifying the species of plant concerned
For some countries, this can be done on the basis of when the symptoms occur. In the northeastern USA, the earliest pollens are those of trees, such as birch and hazel, which can begin in February or March, and usually peak in April. The grass pollen season is from late May to July, with the peak in early June. Docks, nettles, plantains and mugwort (collectively called 'weeds' by the medical profession) start pollinating in July and continue through September. Symptoms that begin in midsummer and continue into the *late* autumn are more likely to be due to moulds.

To confuse matters, one species of mould, *Cladosporium herbarum*, begins spore production in June in Britain, and can roughly coincide with the grass pollen season. Allergy to this mould can easily be mistaken for grass-pollen allergy. Symptoms that are out of step with the day-to-day variations in the pollen count are the main clue, but you will need skin-prick tests for both *Cladosporium* and grasses to confirm the diagnosis.

For more detailed information about allergenic pollens and their pollination seasons for all parts of the world, see the comprehensive pollen calendars in *Hayfever*, by Jonathan Brostoff and Linda Gamlin, published by Bloomsbury.

These pollen calendars may help you in identifying your problem pollen, and they can be extremely useful in planning holidays once you have identified the culprit.

There are additional clues for those allergic to grass pollen. Symptoms are likely to be worse when close to long grass, unmown lawns where the grass has flowered, or hayfields. Mowing the lawn can also provoke symptoms, because tiny droplets of grass sap are dispersed by the mower and can be as allergenic as the pollen.

A special note about oil-seed rape

Asthmatics are often made worse by being near fields of oil-seed rape, the yellow-flowered crop that is now widely grown in Britain and other European countries. People tend to assume that they are allergic to the pollen of this plant, but in most cases their airways (and their noses) are simply being irritated by airborne chemicals (volatiles) that the oil-seed rape produces (see p. 175). These irritants affect many people, not just those with allergies.

Cockroaches

In some inner-city areas in the southern USA, cockroach droppings and skin particles are the most common cause of allergies and asthma. They are also a cause of asthma in Japan, Taiwan and parts of France. Allergy to cockroaches is generally found in warmer climates, since they do not fare well in cold winters. However, cockroaches do occur in Britain (for example, in some blocks of flats in London), with numbers increasing in the summer months and declining greatly in the winter: this might lead to seasonal symptoms which could be mistaken for hayfever.

Symptoms are most likely to occur:
- indoors
- in housing that is badly maintained, especially in inner-city areas
- during summer, if you live in a cooler climate

Symptoms are likely to be less:
- in the country, away from inhabited areas
- in mountain regions

Other insects

Occasionally people develop allergies to other insect pests found in the house, such as carpet beetles or house flies. Insects encountered at work, including silk worms and insects reared for biological pest control, can also cause allergies.

Insects kept as pets, such as stick insects, might lead to allergic reactions especially if kept in poorly ventilated bedrooms. Outdoor insects are unlikely to provoke allergies, but problems with midges have been reported from Japan.

Less common allergens

There are a great many other things to which you might be allergic, but which do not affect as many asthmatics as the common allergens. Among these rarer allergens are:

- antibiotics
- enzymes from washing powder
- henna (tends to affect hairdressers)
- mink urine
- allergens encountered at work (see pp. 280–3). Some of these, such as flour or sawdust, may also be encountered at home, and may then provoke reactions
- fibres of wool, cotton or other textiles

Dust from soybeans or other beans

An allergy of this kind usually begins through exposure at work (see p. 281) but can be acquired in other ways, as in Barcelona in the 1980s, when a great many new cases of asthma appeared. The fact that there were periodic outbreaks of severe attacks among these asthmatics alerted doctors to some widespread environmental cause, and the outbreaks were eventually linked with the delivery of soybean products to the Barcelona docks. Clouds of soybean dust were being released over the city as the processed soybeans were poured into huge storage silos. Those who developed asthma as a result tended to be older people who either smoked, or had smoked in the past.

Latex

Sensitivity is usually acquired at work, although children who have had a lot of surgical operations (for example, those with spina bifida) can also develop latex allergy. Once sensitized, there may be a reaction to rubber articles at home such as balloons, elastic bands, condoms and rubber gloves. Fortunately latex sensitivity is still rare at present, except among hospital workers (see p. 282). If you have latex sensitivity, it may be advisable to wear a Medic-Alert bracelet (see p. 459).

Getting skin-prick tests

Despite their limitations (see pp. 304–5), skin-prick tests can some-times be very helpful in pinpointing allergens. If you need skin-prick tests you should be offered them on the NHS, but this often does not happen (see pp. 301–2). If you cannot get the tests on the NHS, or if the waiting list is excessively long, you could have them done privately.

A full set of skin-prick tests is time-consuming and therefore costly. By using the lists in this section, you can find out a lot about your allergies and narrow down the suspects considerably, so that the number of skin-prick tests you need is greatly reduced. (You can also investigate your allergies by making various changes – see pp. 127–78 – and observing the results.)

If you do want skin-prick tests, ask your GP to refer you to a consultant allergist for private treatment. Should you have trouble finding out where tests can be obtained locally, ring the British Allergy Foundation (see p. 452).

Another option is to find an alternative therapist in your area who does skin-prick tests. Some homeopaths do them, as do many alter-native therapists with a special interest in allergies, but bear in mind that some of the other diagnostic methods and treatments they use could be of doubtful benefit: these therapists tend to offer a mixed bag of proven and unproven methods.

If you are taking anti-histamines, be sure to stop taking them for at least two days before the tests, and much longer for *astemizole* (brand-names include: Hismanal, Pollon-eze). These will interfere with skin-prick tests by inhibiting the reactions to the allergen.

Skin-prick tests for dust

If you think you are allergic to dust, ask for separate tests to be done for house dust itself and for house dust mites. If you react to the former but not to the latter, then clearly you are allergic to something else in the dust, not the mites. Possible candidates are sheep's wool, mould spores, pollen, cockroaches, carpet beetles and other house-hold insects. Individual tests should be made for each of these.

Unfortunately, it is not yet possible to test separately for the different allergens produced by house dust mites, Der p1 and Der p2.

Skin-prick tests for pollens

If you are getting skin-prick tests for pollens, ask for specific pollens to be tested if possible. Quite often, tests are done with 'mixed tree pollens', or 'mixed weed pollens', or 'mixed weed and shrub pollens'. Each of these mixtures contains several different species that pollinate at the same time of year. If you get a positive result, all it tells you is that you are reacting to pollens that appear at a certain season. Although this can be helpful in distinguishing late-summer pollens from mould spores, the information it supplies is very limited in its usefulness. If you are going to the trouble of having skin-prick tests, you may as well find out exactly which tree or 'weed' you are allergic to. Such information may be very helpful in avoiding the pollen, especially when travelling abroad (see p. 178) or choosing trees or other plants for the garden (some of the 'weeds' are closely related to garden plants). The individual extracts for the different allergenic plants are available, so just ask that they be obtained.

You should also have a skin-prick test for *Cladosporium* mould (see p. 122).

Skin-prick tests for moulds

The skin-prick tests are unlikely to include all possible mould allergens. Over 20 different moulds produce allergic reactions in Britain alone, and there are many more worldwide. Most people with mould allergy react to more than one mould, but a few react to one type of mould only, and if that type is not included in the testing, there will be no reaction. This will not happen often, but it is a possibility.

' . . . they know they'll have a great influx of asthma sufferers . . .'

Sarah is a nurse in Melbourne. 'The hospitals here gear up now, if they know there's been a high pollen load, a dry day, and a thunderstorm is on the way, because they know they'll have a great influx of asthma sufferers once the storm breaks.' The interaction of pollen and thunderstorms is explained on p. 229.

AVOIDING HOUSE DUST MITES

If you or your child have an allergy to house dust mite, reducing the levels of mite allergen in your home can make asthma more manageable, improve the quality of life and reduce the need for drugs.

Research shows that the levels can be reduced substantially using a few simple measures. But it is important to take the *right* measures – there is a lot of bad advice on the topic of house dust mites, which could waste your time and money without producing any improvement. Indeed, if you followed some of the advice given you could easily make matters worse!

Who should be avoiding dust mites?

Before reading any further, are you sure you should be concerned about dust mites? The idea that *everyone* who has asthma should avoid house dust mites – an impression often given by advertisements for expensive anti-mite products – is mistaken.

You only need to avoid dust-mite allergen if:
1. You or your child are allergic to dust mites. The checklist on pp. 115–6 will help you decide if there really is an allergy to house dust mites. Skin-prick tests (see p. 304) can be helpful in distinguishing dust-mite allergy from allergy to something else found in house dust (see below).
2. You are expecting a baby and your family has a tendency to asthma or allergy (see pp. 87–95).

Know your enemy

A minority of those allergic to dust are not allergic to house dust mites, but to some other component of dust. This can be checked using skin-prick tests (see p. 125). In such cases, it is necessary to get rid of dust itself or whatever component of dust that is the problem.

For the majority of people, it is house dust mites that are the problem – or rather the mites' droppings, which are the source of the allergen. It is vital to remember that *mites are the enemy – not dust itself*. Your house can be the cleanest one on the street and still be seething with dust-mite allergen. Fanatical vacuuming and dusting will be of no use whatever if your home provides comfortable hideaways for dust mites where the vacuum cleaner cannot reach them –

and most modern houses do. Since the mites cling on to the carpet fibres very firmly when the vacuum cleaner passes overhead, about 65 per cent of them remain afterwards, in addition to all those lurking inside mattresses and upholstered furniture. Indeed, vacuuming regularly with an ordinary vacuum cleaner *will make matters worse* (see p. 478).

Skin scales, which we shed all the time, are the mites' staple diet. They get right inside mattresses, pillows, bedding, armchairs, sofas, cushions and soft toys – and they settle deep down in the pile of carpets. These hiding places provide luxury conditions for the mites: huge supplies of skin scales to eat, and a warm, humid environment.

There are four important aspects to any mite reduction programme:
- Eliminating the mites' hiding places, or at least preventing the allergens from leaking out of them and into the air.
- Making your house less congenial to mites, by making the air drier.
- Getting rid of existing mite allergens, or inactivating them so that they can no longer cause allergic reactions.
- Changing your cleaning tactics, so that you both discourage mites and avoid dispersing their allergens into the air. This is mostly a case of 'working smarter', not working harder.

Making the air drier may seem like a bad idea if you are one of those who finds moist air beneficial during a severe asthma attack. Steam inhalations (see p. 349) can be used to provide moist air directly to the airways during an attack, without increasing the day-to-day humidity of the bedroom. Generally speaking, if you reduce your exposure to allergens, your airways will be less inflamed, so dry air will be a lot less problematic.

The clean-sweep vs. the piecemeal approach
If you know for sure that you or your child have mite allergy, if the asthma symptoms are really bad, and if you are committed to doing something about it, you may want to go for the 'clean-sweep' approach. This means doing everything you can to control house dust mites all in one go. Be aware that it is going to involve quite a lot of money, time and energy. But the rewards could be huge.

Alternatively, there is the piecemeal approach, where you make a few changes and see what effect that has, then make some more changes, and so on. This can be cheaper in the long run, but there are some disadvantages as you will see if you read through all the steps listed below. We suggest that you start with all the steps in Phase One and Phase Two.

We imagine that most people will choose the piecemeal approach, so we have presented the advice in a step-by-step form. If you want to go for the clean-sweep approach, you should do everything listed here at once. Either way, read right through to p. 155 before you start.

Not making matters worse

A lot of dust will be churned up during some of these procedures, especially if you take up carpets or haul old mattresses out of the house. Even bundling up a duvet to take it to the dry-cleaners or taking blankets off beds to wash them will produce invisible clouds of dust-mite allergen. Needless to say, this will make any dust-allergic person worse. Not only should they not do the work, they should not be in the house until the work is complete, the cleaning-up afterwards is all done, and the dust has settled. If there are no family or friends who can do the work, consider paying someone else to do it, or look around for a local 'helping-hands' group who will do it for you free of charge – ask at a nearby church or community centre.

If you are asthmatic, and you have absolutely no choice but to do the work yourself, or to be present, then you should get a good-quality mask and wear it throughout. Make sure that the mask is capable of filtering out the tiny particles that carry the allergen (see p. 481). An ordinary dust mask is not good enough. Ensure that you can breathe well through the mask when physically active.

Did you know?

A human being sheds one gram of skin particles a day. This is enough to feed 10,000 house dust mites for six months.

Spot the mistake!

'*As far as dust mites are concerned, wool carpet is a hostile environment, providing none of the conditions they require to thrive.*'

'*Dust mites in the air cause allergic reactions in an estimated 15–20 per cent of the population . . .*'

'*The mattress protector completely surrounds your existing mattress. This means that any dust mites inside the mattress will eventually die when you put the cover on, because they can neither feed nor escape.*'

All these statements come from advertising or promotional material – and from very reputable sources, including a respected department store, a national trade organization and a university department developing a commercial product. They are all intended to persuade you to spend your money in particular ways – on wool carpets, on an air filtration system, or on a particular kind of mattress cover. Each of these statements is wrong or seriously misleading, as you will realize if you read this section in full. Dust mites will live very happily in wool carpets, they hardly ever become airborne, so very few will be eliminated by an air filter, and if sealed inside an old mattress they will survive for many years on the skin scales already there.

Combating dust mites is now big business, and false claims are common. Some stem from ignorance and wishful thinking on the part of the advertiser, while others are deliberately misleading. It's a question of 'Let the buyer beware', so make sure you know the facts about dust mites before you buy.

Basic facts about mites and their allergens

Dust mites feed on skin scales, but only if they have been broken down first by moulds. Not all moulds suit dust mites – some make them ill. High humidity (70–90 per cent) favours the mould that suits dust mites best (*Aspergillus repens*). This is one reason why humid air benefits mites.

The mites themselves do not drink, but absorb water from the air. When the relative humidity falls below 50 per cent, the mites gradually dry out and are killed.

Dead skin is the main food for the common house dust mite *Dermatophagoides pteronyssinus*, but they also like dried semen (leading some researchers to suggest that using condoms, or laundering sheets 'the morning after', could help to reduce the number of dust mites in beds). Dust mites known as *Dermatophagoides farinae*, which infest stored food, are also found in houses, where they eat biscuit crumbs and other specks of food in carpets. There are several other species of mite found in houses, and the exact mix of species varies from one part of the world to another.

The dust-mite allergens come from its droppings or faecal pellets – the allergens are found in the proteins that coat the droppings. There are two main allergens in this protein coating, called Der p1 and Der p2. Der p1, which is the troublesome allergen for many asthmatics, is inactivated by heat, but the temperature needed is close to or above boiling point, so steam is necessary. Der p2, which may be the major allergen for some people, is not affected by heat.

Dust mites are very widespread, and are carried about in clothing. Even if you could eliminate all the mites from your house, new ones would continually be brought in from outside. This is why you need ongoing measures to prevent recolonization. A new mattress will be colonized by dust mites within four months.

Adult dust mites live about two to four months. The females lay one to two eggs a day, and these take a month to reach adulthood. Very high temperatures will kill eggs as well as adult mites, but chemical sprays will not.

Mites are killed by temperatures of 55°C (130°F) and above. In practical terms (with washing machines where temperatures are given in degrees Centigrade) this means washing clothes at 60°C (140°F). Washing at lower temperatures will not kill mites (unless a pesticide or some essential oil is added to the wash) but it will wash away the mite allergens. Even washing in cold water (with detergent) will remove some allergens, but warm water is more effective. Washing will also remove human skin scales, depriving the mites of food.

Dry-cleaning fluid kills mites, and removes at least some (20–70 per cent) of the allergen.

If you want to know more about mites, an excellent book, *House Dust Mites* by Des Whitrow, is published by Right Way Books.

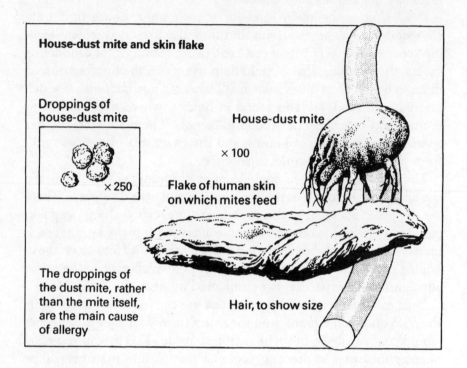

House-dust mite and skin flake

Droppings of house-dust mite

× 250

House-dust mite

× 100

Flake of human skin on which mites feed

The droppings of the dust mite, rather than the mite itself, are the main cause of allergy

Hair, to show size

Phase One: beds and clothing

The best place to start is with the bed, because you spend more time there than anywhere else – every time you turn over in bed, your weight pushes a great blast of air out from the mattress, and with that air comes a large allergen dose.

Some people find that simply reducing the mite levels in the mattress, pillows and bedding will give them excellent relief from asthma, and they stop there. The good effects are felt in the daytime too, not just at night. Because the airways are not being challenged by a huge dose of allergen while in bed, they become less inflamed and sensitized generally.

By also making the simple changes to the bedroom listed in Phase Two – designed to reduce the humidity in your bedroom and keep mite allergen out of the air – you will get the maximum benefit from these improvements to your bed.

Option A: Replacing the mattress and bedding

If you can afford it, this is one of the best ways to tackle the mite problem in your bed. It will get rid of all the existing mites, and prevent recolonization of the bed.

A1. Buy a new mattress and new pillows. It doesn't matter what kind of pillow you buy. It's a myth that pillows with synthetic filling are better than feather pillows – indeed, recent research shows that polyester pillows grow more mites than feather ones, but since you are covering them it won't matter. (If expense is no object, a waterbed is worth considering as it has no upholstery to harbour mites.)

A2. Buy anti-mite coverings for both mattress and pillows. These keep both skin scales and mites out of the mattress and any existing mite allergens in. In the case of a new mattress or pillow, they should prevent it becoming recolonized by dust mites. For details about these coverings see pp. 470–4: don't buy without getting clued up about the products first, as there are a lot of false claims being made. These anti-mite covers will need wiping down weekly to prevent a build-up of dust mites on the outer surface, unless you are following step A11.

A3. Alternatively, you could buy a new mattress and pillow with ready-fitted anti-mite covers (see p. 474). Where the asthmatic is a small child, these may be safer, posing no threat of suffocation unlike loose covers – but check this point with the manufacturer.

A4. Either buy a new duvet (comforter) or wash your existing one, or get it dry-cleaned. Washing must be done at a temperature of 60°C (140°F) or more (too high a temperature for most duvets, but check the label) or at a lower temperature using a mite-killing wash (see p. 475)

A5. Buy an anti-mite cover for the duvet (see p. 472.)

A6. Alternatively, buy a duvet and pillow that can be washed at 60°C (140°F), and wash them regularly, once a month. You must have a tumble-dryer, or have access to one, if choosing this option, because the bedding must be dried out completely after washing. If you leave any moisture in the bedding, this will quickly lead to a flourishing mite population.

A7. What is underneath the mattress? If you have an upholstered bed base with enclosed box-springs, these will also contain a few mites. A simple wooden or metal bed frame is preferable. If replacing the bed is out of the question, then you should enclose the upholstered base in a mite-proof cover. You may need to construct your own cover from plastic sheeting and heavy-duty tape (see p. 471). Make sure you seal the cover around the legs of the bed – there should be no openings.

A8. Wash all sheets and blankets at 60°C (140°F) or more, or have blankets dry-cleaned, or buy new ones. You could buy blankets that can be washed at high temperatures (see p. 475). From now on, wash sheets once a week and blankets once every two weeks. You may be able to wash the blankets less often if you follow step A11 every day.

A9. Get rid of any patchwork quilts, eiderdowns and fleecy under-blankets. Alternatively, you can dry-clean them, but this will have to be repeated regularly, at least once a month, unless you follow step A11 every day.

A10. Electric blankets can be cleared of mites by washing them at 60°C (140°F). If yours cannot be washed, consider buying a new washable one. Alternatively, leave the electric blanket on at full setting for twelve hours, covered by bedding so that the temperature builds up. (Take care if you have bought mite-proof bedding covers – see below). This will kill the mites but not remove the existing allergen, so you may want to spray with tannic acid or polysaccharide (see p. 476) to inactivate the allergen. Heat the blanket thoroughly and air it after spraying.

A11. If you don't already have an electric blanket, consider buying one, as they can be used to keep the bed free from moisture. This is valuable in preventing mites from setting up home in the *outer* surface of your new mite-proof covers, so that you do not need to wash the covers, sheets, under-blankets, etc. so frequently. Put your electric blanket on at a high setting in the morning, after you get up, while the bed is being aired. Before you go out, make the bed, but leave the electric blanket on. It should stay on for at least twelve hours while covered with a duvet or blankets: this dries the bed thoroughly and makes in inhospitable to mites. *Note that some mite-proof covers may be damaged by this proce-dure.* Check with the manufacturer if it is safe to heat up the covers in this way. If you have not yet purchased any covers, the special mite-proof Egyptian cotton covers (see p. 473) would be a good choice as they can definitely tolerate this level of heat without damage. You should also check that the wiring on the blanket is safe and there is no fire risk from leaving the blanket on all day. Do not use this treatment with vinyl-covered mattresses.

Option B: Killing all existing mites and preventing recolonization
This option relies on a new process which may not be available in all parts of the world.

B1. Arrange for a contractor (see p. 479) to heat-treat the bed, mattress and all bedding: this treatment is designed to kill all mites, even those in the mattress, and neutralize the allergen.

To prevent recolonization, you can *either* have this treatment repeated every three months, *or* carry out the following measures:

B2. Buy anti-mite coverings for the mattress, pillows and duvet. See step A2 (p. 133).

B3. From now on, wash sheets once a week and blankets once every two weeks. See step A8 (p. 134).

B4. Get rid of any patchwork quilts, eiderdowns and fleecy under-blankets or dry-clean them regularly. See step A9 (p. 134).

B5. Use the electric-blanket treatment every day. See step A11 (p. 134).

Option C: Keeping the existing allergen away from your airways
This approach will work reasonably well and is much cheaper.

C1. Buy new pillows with built-in anti-mite covers (see p. 133), or new pillows and separate covers (see p. 133)

C2. Buy an anti-mite cover for the mattress. *You must get someone who is not asthmatic to put this on*, as there will be a lot of allergen expelled from the mattress in the process. For those on a tight budget, a mattress cover can be made from plastic sheeting and tape (see p. 471). If the bed base is upholstered, you must seal this in plastic sheeting too.

C3. Buy an anti-mite cover for the duvet, and get someone else to put it on.

C4. Wash all sheets and blankets at 60°C (140°F) or more, or at a lower temperature using a mite-killing wash (see p. 475), or have blankets dry-cleaned. You will need to repeat this every week for sheets and every two weeks for blankets, unless you are using the electric-blanket procedure (step C7).

C5. Get rid of any patchwork quilts, eiderdowns and fleecy under-blankets. Alternatively, you can dry-clean them, but this will have to be repeated regularly, at least once a month, unless you follow step C7 every day.

C6. Treat electric blankets, as described in step A10 (p. 134).

C7. Use the electric blanket procedure as in step A11 (p. 134) daily to prevent reinfestation of sheets, blankets, etc. If you have made your own mattress cover from PVC sheeting, you should *not* use this heating treatment. If you have made it from another plastic, such as polythene, it may not be able to withstand the heat, or it *may* survive with a thick blanket or two between the plastic sheet and the electric blanket. Experiment very cautiously. Air the bed and the room well after you turn the electric blanket off and before going to bed, in case the plastic releases fumes when heated.

The drawback of the cheaper option is that hordes of mites and their allergens are still inside the mattress, and if the slightest tear occurs in the anti-mite covering, the allergens will start to come out. (Even with a new mattress and pillows, you do need to be careful not to tear the coverings, but the immediate consequences of doing so are not as bad. In the long term, however, you will get build-up of mites inside a new mattress with a torn cover.)

For the maximum improvement, we would strongly suggest that you back up these measures with the changes to the bedroom listed on pp. 139–141.

> ### *Did you know?*
>
> As much as 10 per cent of the weight of an old pillow may be made up by human skin scales, live mites, dead mites, moulds and mite droppings.

Special points about children's beds and toys

- If there is more than one child in the room, all the mattresses and bedding should be dealt with in the same way.
- No asthmatic child should sleep in the lower half of a bunk bed, even if all the mattresses and bedding have been changed, because mites and their allergens will shower down from the upper bunk.
- Discourage children from having pillow fights or trampolining on the beds, even if anti-mite covers have been fitted.
- Soft toys can be full of house dust mites. There are three different ways to combat this:
  - Toys that can be washed at 60°C (140°F) or more should all be washed once a week, drying them very thoroughly and speedily – preferably in a tumble-dryer – afterwards.
  - Alternatively, soft toys should spend at least six hours in the freezer once a week, to kill the mites. The first time you do the freezer treatment, wash the toys at the highest possible temperature immediately afterwards to remove any existing allergen. Once you get going with the weekly freezing regime, you only need to wash the toys occasionally. Again, they must be thoroughly dried.
  - Toys that are not washable can be heated in a tumble-dryer weekly to kill the mites. This will not remove or destroy allergen, so the treatment must begin when the toys are new, before any build-up of allergen can occur.
- Avoid buying fabric story books or soft building blocks. Dolls' clothes and dressing-up clothes should be washed at 60°C (140°F) regularly, or at a lower temperature with a mite-killing wash (see p. 475). Keep other toys free of dust by storing them in a cupboard and wiping them with a damp cloth periodically.

- 'Comfort blankets' can also be full of dust mites. The washing/ freezing treatments described for soft toys can be used. If your child is completely inseparable from the blanket, you could try cutting it in half when he or she is asleep, so that you can clean one half, while the other remains in use. Then swap the two halves over.

Mites live in clothing too . . .

Clothes are often full of mites, especially thick items that are not washed often, such as sweaters, and clothing that has to be dry-cleaned, such as coats and woollen trousers. One study showed that there was 18 times as much mite allergen in such garments as in clothes that were washed regularly.

1. Dry-clean all your sweaters and woollen trousers, or wash them at 60°C (140°F), or at a lower temperature using a mite-killing wash (see p. 475). From now on, keep them in a warm dry airing cupboard so that they are always *very* dry.
2. Have all coats and jackets dry-cleaned and make sure they hang somewhere really dry from now on. A small 'space heater' of the kind sold for greenhouses, placed underneath your coat rack, will keep the air round the coats dry.
3. In future, when it rains, make sure that wet coats, sweaters and hats are put in a place where they can dry out quickly and completely to reduce the numbers of mites living in them.

. . . and even in your hair

Dandruff consists of skin flakes, and may help to feed mites in pillows and clothing. Mites can also live in the hair itself, and on the scalp. Using an anti-dandruff shampoo may help some asthmatics.

Protect yourself from dusty jobs and places

From now on, be careful about exposing your airways to dust. If you are asthmatic, you should never be the one to empty the vacuum-cleaner bag. If you live alone and have to do this job, wear a good mask (see p. 481).

If you need to get things from an attic or a spare room, wear a mask, or ask someone else to do it for you. When it comes to decorating, think in advance about which activities will stir up dust. If you are stripping wallpaper, for example, wash it down first to remove dust.

Moving house stirs up huge amounts of dust, as does spring-cleaning, turning out cupboards or moving furniture. The asthmatic should not take part, nor be around, unless wearing a good mask.

'. . . they're nothing but jelly babies on legs . . .'

As head of the Medical Entomology Centre in Cambridge, Dr John Maunder has become a world expert on house dust mites. 'When you see scanning electron microscope pictures of house dust mites it makes them look as if they're covered in great thick armour, like prehistoric monsters – but that's an illusion. If you look at them under the light microscope, the light shines right through them. They're translucent – they're nothing but jelly babies on legs. They're not armoured and invincible. Just dry the air out around them and they're finished. All it takes is ventilation. So we've got to put the ventilation back into houses.'

Phase Two: Essential changes to the bedroom

Whichever option you are following for Phase One, at the same time make the following improvements to your bedroom:

1. If there are damp walls in the bedroom, due to structural problems such as cracks, a leaking roof or rising damp, get these fixed. See p. 166 for further details.
2. Make sure moisture from the bathroom and kitchen do not get into the bedroom: close the kitchen door and open the window when you are cooking, for example. Curb moisture production in the house by putting lids on boiling saucepans, venting your tumble-dryer outside, etc. (see pp. 166–8).
3. If your bedroom has an en-suite shower, fit a powerful extractor fan, or open a window wide during and after showers, or just stop using this shower. En-suite basins may also generate a lot of moist air, which can be combated in the same way.
4. Air your bedroom very thoroughly whenever it's dry and sunny outside.

5. Remove any sources of moisture in the bedroom such as pot plants and fish tanks. If you have a humidifier in your bedroom, get rid of it.

6. Don't dry clothes in the room and don't shampoo the carpet, as this leaves a lot of moisture behind. (Ignore advertisements for 'anti-mite shampoos' – research shows these to be ineffective.) The same goes for the widely advertised 'professional steam-cleaning' treatments. These mostly use very hot water, not steam, and the carpet stays wet for some time. These commercial treatments are not the same as the specialized anti-mite steam treatment system described on p. 143.

7. Avoid using calor gas heaters, as these produce a lot of moisture, and fan-heaters because they churn up mite allergens from the carpet. Convector heaters are not quite so bad, but they can also make more allergen airborne.

8. Seal off any hot-air ducts from centralized heating systems, as these blow mite allergens around the room. Several different studies have linked this type of heating with more cases of asthma.

9. Unblock any air bricks or other fresh-air vents, to improve ventilation.

10. When dusting, use a damp cloth and rinse it out regularly, or use a special duster with an electrostatic charge that holds the dust (see p. 479). If damp-dusting, you can add a few drops of eucalyptus oil which deters mites. Never flick the dust into the air with a dry duster or feather duster.

11. Make sure your vacuum cleaner is not filling the bedroom air with allergens.
    • If possible, invest in a vacuum cleaner that keeps in all the allergens, or vents them outside, rather than spraying them out into the bedroom air. Make sure that the vacuum cleaner you buy really does its job well – a lot of machines now claim to be 'allergy' vacuum cleaners but they are not all equally good (see pp. 477–8).
    • If you cannot afford a good cleaner, fit a filter to the exhaust of your existing vacuum cleaner. Cover the bed with a clean sheet and open the windows whenever you vacuum, leaving them open for half an hour afterwards.

After closing the windows, allow the dust to settle for another half-hour, then carefully remove the dust-cover from the bed before the asthmatic comes back into the room. This system is less than perfect, so if the asthmatic has to do the vacuuming, a good mask (see p. 481) should be worn throughout the procedure.

12. Once you have sorted out a new vacuuming system, spring-clean the bedroom. Get rid of any thick dust under beds, along skirting boards or picture rails, on top of wardrobes or behind furniture. If there are things stored under the bed find another home for these, so that vacuuming is easier in future. While this spring-cleaning is in progress, completely cover the bed with a dust-sheet and remove it carefully afterwards.

'I have never felt better . . .'

Tricia used to feel that asthma and other allergic problems were ruining her life, until she decided to deal with the dust-mite problem. 'I no longer have endless sleepless nights due to asthma attacks, rhinitis and sinusitis. Having found out that I was allergic to dust mite, I bought a powerful dehumidifier, anti-mite covers for the bedding and a marvellous vacuum cleaner. The change that they have made to the quality of my life has been enormous. It is so wonderful to finally find things that actually do what they claim to. I have never felt better.'

Dealing with bathroom carpets

While you are making these changes to the bedroom, you may want to think about the bathroom too. If it has a fitted carpet, this will be heaving with dust mites, thanks to the humid air and rich supply of skin scales. Get rid of the bathroom carpet and replace it with tiles, vinyl flooring or linoleum. At the same time, you could install an extractor fan to take out bathroom moisture – this will benefit the whole house.

Things that won't work

A lot of the published advice about dust mites is well-meaning but wrong. None of the following measures (all taken from highly reputable sources) will help, and some will make asthma worse:

'*Pillows should be aired by hanging them outdoors.*' (Unless you live in the Sahara, this won't help much. The mites will survive by migrating towards the centre of the pillow.)

'*Mattresses should be aired by regularly turning them.*' (This won't affect the mites one tiny bit, but it will blast huge amounts of mite allergen out of the mattress and into your airways.)

'*Vacuum-clean mattress and pillow twice-monthly.*' (This will make little or no difference to the amount of allergen you inhale while in bed.)

'*Wash sheets, pillow cases and duvet covers once a week. It is especially important to wash these weekly if the mattress, pillow or duvet is not covered.*' (If they're not covered with anti-mite covers, washing the bed linen will make little or no difference.)

'*Run central heating a few degrees lower (especially in bedrooms).*' (Mites don't mind cooler temperatures that much – in fact they thrive in chilly spare rooms. Having the bedroom cooler than the rest of the house can lead to condensation and damp, making the mite problem worse.)

'*All you need to do to ensure your home stays well ventilated is to open a window or use a fan to aid air flow.*' (A fan won't ventilate or dehumidify the house if the windows are closed, but it will churn up allergens from the carpet and furnishings, so that you inhale more.)

'*Vacuum bedrooms and living room daily.*' (Vacuum cleaning trebles the amount of mite allergen in the air, unless you are using a special vacuum cleaner designed to keep the allergen in. Daily vacuuming with an ordinary vacuum cleaner can make allergic symptoms substantially worse.)

Have the changes done any good?

Once you have completed all the changes listed for Phases One and Two, you should wait for several weeks – or even a few months – before deciding how effective the measures have been. For many people, the asthmatic airways will take time to respond fully, because the inflammation (see p. 22) only settles down slowly. In one study, although there were some improvements within four months, it took *eight months* for the full benefits of an anti-mite campaign to be seen.

Keep a record of your peak flow drug usage and symptoms, starting before you introduce the measures and continuing afterwards.

Phase Three: Creating a virtually mite-free bedroom

If Phases One and Two have done some good, but not enough for your liking, or if they have had no effect but you know for certain that dust mites are the allergen, go on to Phase Three.

Option 1 – For those who don't mind housework

1. Eliminate mites in the carpet, in one of two ways:
   - *Either* remove the bedroom carpet and replace it with a polished wood floor, cork tiles, vinyl flooring or linoleum.
   - *Or* invest in a special anti-mite steam cleaner (see p. 479) that kills mites in the carpet and 'cooks' the main dust-mite allergen Der p1, making it harmless. You might imagine that such a treatment would leave a lot of moisture in the house, but in fact the steam is at such a high pressure and temperature that it is far less moist than the steam from a kettle. The carpets dry within half an hour. Choose a dry day for the steam treatment and air the room well for an hour afterwards.

     Neither option is cheap. Bear in mind that if you decide to go for the first option, you will need to mop the floor very regularly (see below) as the dust will quickly build up, and is easily made airborne from an uncarpeted floor. One of the advantages of carpet is that it does 'hold' dust at floor level and stop it being swirled around by every current of air.

2. Wash the curtains at 60°C (140°F), or at a lower temperature using a mite-killing wash (see p. 475), or dry-clean

them, or – and this is the best option – remove the curtains and replace them with blinds of a kind that can be easily dusted, preferably wet-dusted. Velvet curtains are the worst for holding dust – even if you don't like blinds, at least replace velvet with curtains made of a thinner fabric. Curtains should be washed regularly, every two to three months. If you have bought an anti-mite steam cleaner for the carpet, this can also be used on the curtains every two to three weeks. (It is safe with most materials, but not chintz or antique velvet.)

3. Remove all dirty clothes from the room, clean out drawers and shelves, and dry them thoroughly. From now on, store nothing but freshly laundered clothes in the room. All coats, hats and sweaters should be kept elsewhere.

4. If you have any upholstered items in the room, such as padded headboards, cushions, armchairs or stools with padded seats, remove these.

5. Remove any padded coat-hangers, draught excluders, fabric lampshades and anything covered in velvet or plush material. Look around the room carefully for any other likely mite hideaways.

During this stage, you may be stirring up a lot of dust mites and their allergens, especially if you take down curtains or remove the bedroom carpets. Unfortunately, these allergens and mites will settle on the beds with their clean new anti-mite covers. To avoid this happening, either remove the beds and bedding to another room first, or cover the beds and bedding really well with a large sheet of flexible polythene (e.g. a shower curtain) tucked in all round – an ordinary cotton sheet will not be enough in this instance, because mites may land on it and crawl through on to the bed below. Allow the dust to settle for several hours afterwards before uncovering the beds. (One advantage of the clean-sweep approach is that you take the carpets up first and avoid these complications.) Needless to say, asthmatics should not do this work themselves (see p. 129).

Once you have made these changes, you should adopt the following cleaning routine:

• Damp-dust (or use an electrostatic duster – see p. 479)

regularly, at least three times a week, to reduce the build-up of skin scales that are the mites' food supply. You may want to remove as many ornaments, pictures and other dust-gathering items as possible, to make thorough dusting easier.

- If you have eliminated carpets, you must mop the floor regularly, preferably every day, but at least two or three times a week, including under all the beds. Either use a wet mop (drying the floor very thoroughly afterwards) or an oiled mop.
- If you have kept the carpet, repeat the steam-cleaning treatment once a month. You should also vacuum-clean once or twice a week, preferably using a vacuum cleaner of the kind that retains allergenic particles (see pp. 477–8) or vents outside (see p. 478).
- If you have got rid of fitted carpets and want to have rugs, make sure they can be washed regularly, preferably at 60°C (140°F) (lower temperatures will require a mite-killing wash – see p. 475). Hanging rugs outside in the sun and beating them is another option as mites hate sunshine and dryness, but the asthmatic should not have to do the beating, unless wearing a good mask (see p. 481). Three hours' strong direct sunlight is needed to kill mites. Freezing conditions in winter will also do the trick. Sheepskin and other animal-skin rugs are likely to be crawling with dust mites, so get rid of them.

Option 2 – For those who hate housework
You can escape all this repetitive cleaning and still have a mite-free bedroom by using a dehumidifier. You need a really powerful one, especially designed for killing mites. This makes the air too dry to breathe (its relative humidity or RH goes down to 25 per cent), so you can't have it on when you are in the room. The idea is that you leave it on in the bedroom during the day, allowing it to get the air really dry. Mites cannot tolerate desert conditions, and after a few months the population of dust mites will dwindle away to nothing, except perhaps in the deepest recesses of mattresses and armchairs. With a dehumidifier, you can have enough dust on the dresser to write your name in, but no dust mites!

A dehumidifier will be quite expensive (see p. 477) and you need to remember to put it on and close the bedroom door every day. You also need to have fairly tight seals around your windows and doors, otherwise moist air will come in from outside and spoil things. But if you can meet all these conditions, the dehumidifier will be very effective. Some dehumidifiers also act as air filters (see p. 152) which is useful if you have pollen or mould allergy as well.

In the evening, be sure to turn the dehumidifier off and leave the bedroom door open for an hour or so before going to bed. If you try to sleep in over-dry air, this in itself could trigger off an asthma attack by drying out the airways.

There is, of course, an alternative to the dehumidifier, which does much the same job and is *absolutely free* – leaving the window open as much as possible (except when it is misty or raining). In other words, re-create the sort of bedroom our great-grandparents endured – cold and draughty. House dust mites hate it.

Should you have a fireplace in your bedroom, you could have an open fire, which will warm things up and increase the ventilation (see p. 148).

If you choose the dehumidifier option, remember that all the allergen which was already there in the bed, carpet, curtains, clothes and soft toys will still be present. You need to work out ways to eliminate or inactivate this allergen or keep it away from your airways. You should also eliminate sources of moisture that will counteract the good work of the dehumidifier. So you need to:

1. Deal with the bed as described in Phase One (any option). You can omit the electric blanket treatment as the dehumidifier will make this unnecessary. And you could get away with keeping a patchwork quilt, as long as you dry-clean it to remove the allergen first – with something fairly thin, the dehumidifier should be able to kill all the mites inside.

2. Make the basic changes to the bedroom described in Phase Two, steps 1–8. Ignore step 9. You will need to follow step 10 at first, but once the dehumidifier routine is established, and there are few dust mites living in the dust, you can relax on this. With regard to step 11: in the early stages, when all the existing allergen is still in the carpet, a special vacuum cleaner will be very useful. However, the expense may not be justified in the long term, unless you can see a role for it in other parts of the house. You may prefer to vacuum with the windows open and the bed covered (see pp. 140–1), or

use a spray that inactivates allergen (see p. 476), or a combination of these two.

3. Wash all clothes, curtains and soft toys to remove the allergen. Wait until the dehumidifier routine has been established for a week or so before doing this. Clean out drawers and shelves on which clothes have been stored. It would also be sensible to give soft toys the freezer treatment before washing them, to kill the mites inside them right from the start. The good news is that once you have got your daily dehumidifier routine going, you do not need to rewash everything regularly because mites will be a thing of the past, so no new stocks of allergen will be produced.

4. If there are armchairs in the bedroom, it would still be advisable to remove these, unless they have been heat-treated along with the bed (Phase One, Option B). The dehumidifier may, eventually, manage to kill off the resident mites deep in the upholstery, but the accumulated allergen will remain. Whenever anyone sits on the chairs, more allergen will be forced out from within.

'Dust-mite infestation is something new . . .'

Dr John Maunder is head of the Medical Entomology Centre in Cambridge, where the life-cycle of house dust mites, and their effects on asthma, are studied. 'The Victorians were crazy about microscopes. They looked at everything under the microscope. But there is only *one* description of a house dust mite from that era. It was Christmas Day 1894, and a chap called Trouessart had just been given a new microscope for Christmas. He was so excited he wanted to look at something straight away, and he decided he'd like to look at the structure of a feather. So he went and got a feather from his pillow, and there was a house dust mite – a species completely unknown to science. No one else saw one until 1922 when there is a description from a microscopist in Belgium. It is absolutely inconceivable that the mite was anything like as common as it is today. We have to accept that dust-mite infestation is something new, that it's because of what we've done to our houses.'

Did you know?

A study carried out in Denmark showed that just fitting allergen-proof covers to mattresses and pillows of asthmatic children with dust-mite allergy produced excellent results. After 12 months the children were, on average, using half as much inhaled steroid, having much less asthma at night, and producing better peak-flow readings.

Phase Four: Simple changes in the sitting-room

The measures listed here are ones that you can carry out without making major changes to the decor or furnishings of your sitting-room. Needless to say, if you are keeping sofas and armchairs that you have had for years, there will still be a significant level of dust mite allergen in the room.

Essential first steps

Follow the steps described for the bedroom in Phase Two (pp. 139–41).

Additional measures

1. *Either:* have an open fire in the sitting room. This improves ventilation considerably: as warm air and smoke go up the chimney, the fire pulls in clean air from outdoors.

   Or: use a powerful dehumidifier designed to kill mites (see pp. 145–6). This makes the air too dry to breathe, so leave the dehumidifier on in the sitting room all night, with doors and windows closed. The room must be effectively sealed for the dehumidifier to get the air really desert-dry, so this is not an option if you have open fireplaces. (Nor is it a good idea if you have antique veneered furniture as this will be damaged by the dry air.)

   If you are buying a dehumidifier for the bedroom you can use it in the sitting room as well. You probably won't want to move it every day, as it is quite heavy, but you can run it every day for a month in the bedroom, then every night for a month in the sitting room, then on to the hall/stairs for a month, then back to the bedroom again. Keep this cycle up indefinitely, and mite levels will remain low throughout the house.

Wash the sitting room curtains once the dehumidifier routine is well established.

The dehumidifier will eventually kill all the mites in the room except, perhaps, those hidden deep in the armchairs and sofa. The open fire will have a similar though lesser effect. But neither will have any impact on the existing allergen, and whenever anyone sits down on the sofa – whoosh! – out the allergens come in a great wheeze-inducing blast. So it makes sense to combine this with measure 3 below.

2. Use a special mite-killing steam cleaner (see p. 143) to destroy the mites in the carpet and curtains, and make their allergen harmless. If you have small children this is a very useful measure, because children spend a lot of time on the carpet, inhaling allergens at close range.

   You can also use the steam cleaner on the outer surfaces of sofas and armchairs, but it will not reach the mites or allergens within the upholstery.

   The carpet will quickly get reinfested from your armchairs, so you will need to repeat the steam treatment once a month.

3. Reduce the amount of allergen inhaled from your sofa and armchairs by ordering made-to-measure anti-mite covers for the removable cushions (see p. 484) and using tannic acid or polysaccharide spray to inactivate the allergens on the fixed upholstery (p. 476). (If you are using a special steam cleaner on the upholstery, there is no need for sprays as well, but the covers will still be valuable.)

   These sprays simply neutralize the allergen, and do not affect the mites at all. They are relatively innocuous and a lot less worrying than the pesticide sprays. Sprays will only affect the allergens near the surface, not those inside upholstery. If using tannic acid, check first that it will not stain your fabrics. Polysaccharide spray is non-staining (see p. 476).

   Take any loose covers off and spray the upholstery beneath. Wash the loose covers and any cushion covers at 60°C (140°F), or use a mite-killing wash (see p. 475).

Even when you have taken these measures, you should avoid sleeping or lying on sofas as this exposes you to a high dose of allergen.

Why not just use sprays?

There are sprays that inactivate allergen, sprays that kill mites, and combined sprays that do both (see pp. 475–6). Any spray that kills mites contains pesticide, and if you have young children, using these is not a good idea. Children are bound to pick up the spray on their skin while playing or crawling on the carpet. Because the chemicals persist, and spraying has to be repeated regularly, steady exposure to the substances in the spray is inevitable.

Although these sprays are theoretically safe, the effect of constant intake over several years by young children has never been tested. No pesticide is completely risk-free, and the idea of constant exposure, year in year out, is alarming, whether for adults or children. This is why we have not recommended spraying with pesticides in the bedroom. Most of us spend far less time in the sitting room, so sprays may have a place in controlling mites here, but the other approaches described are far preferable.

Quite apart from these drawbacks, several studies have found that the pesticides do not always work well. Some of the mites in a carpet survive, often quite a high proportion. No spray can kill the mites that are inside a mattress, pillow or sofa.

Mite-killing chemicals may sometimes have a place as a cheap, short-term measure. If you do decide to use them, leave the spray or powder on for 12–18 hours, and brush it in repeatedly. The instructions on the packet may recommend leaving it on for only 4 hours, but research shows that this does not have much impact on the mites. Vacuum very thoroughly afterwards to remove the dead mites. Unless you have a really good vacuum cleaner (see p. 477), use a spray that inactivates allergens (see p. 476) before vacuuming. Repeat the treatments regularly. Recent studies suggest that treatments must be repeated every 2–3 months to be of any value.

Phase Five: The all-out anti-mite programme

In addition to Phases One to Four, take the following measures:

  1. Eliminate mites in the upholstered furniture.

- *Either* get rid of all your existing upholstered furniture and cushions. Replace with leather-covered or vinyl-covered furniture (impenetrable to mites) or furniture made of wood or bamboo with loose cushions and no upholstered arms or other fixed upholstery (e.g. futon-style sofas, or the type of furniture designed for conservatories). Fit these cushions/futon mattresses with tailor-made mite-proof covers (see p. 484) when new. Then put external covers on top, making sure that these can be washed at 60°C (140°F). All the new furniture should have proper legs, so that you can vacuum-clean underneath.
- *Or* have all upholstered furniture and scatter-cushions heat-treated by a contractor, as described for beds on p. 479. To prevent reinfestation, either have this treatment repeated every three months, or buy a powerful dehumidifier (see p. 476) and use this in the sitting-room at nights.

2. Replace any velvet or other plush materials (e.g. in curtains) with thinner materials having a smooth surface. (If you have a powerful dehumidifier, this is not necessary – just wash the curtains to get rid of the existing allergen.)

3. Eliminate mites in the carpet. (Again, this is not necessary if you are using an anti-mite dehumidifier but you will need to de-activate the existing allergen with a special steam cleaner, or with sprays (see p. 476).)
- *Either* get rid of fitted carpets throughout the house, and replace with smooth flooring (wood, cork, vinyl or lino).
- *Or* invest in a special mite-killing steam cleaner (see p. 479) and treat the sitting room carpets with it once a month, hall and stair carpets once every 3 months.

If you go for the first option:
- Cover furniture etc. with plastic sheeting while the carpets are being removed, to keep dust and mites from settling on them. The asthmatic should be having a holiday somewhere else while this is happening.
- Remember that you will have to wet-mop everywhere very regularly (see p. 145) as there is nothing now to 'hold' dust at floor level (see p. 143).

If you go for the second option:

- You need to vacuum-clean regularly, once a week with a special vacuum cleaner that retains allergens. (Although the steam cleaner has inactivated existing allergens, mites will recolonize the carpet gradually and produce new allergen, unless you are using a powerful dehumidifier.)

Do air filters or ionizers have a useful role to play?

An air filter which simply does that – filters the air – will remove much of the dust-mite allergen from the air you breathe. However, dust-mite allergens come in quite large heavy particles, which don't become airborne all that easily. So the amount actually *in the air* is normally insignificant, and the air filter will not achieve much.

There are many things an air filter will not do. Unless it also incorporates a dehumidifier, it will not kill dust mites. Nor can it stop you from inhaling the mite allergen that comes from the interior of pillows, mattresses, duvets and armchairs – your nose is too close to the source for the filter to make a difference.

So an air filter will not reduce your intake of dust-mite allergen very much. Indeed, if the filter has a powerful fan and is placed at floor level, the fan may churn up mite allergen from the carpet, cancelling out any good effects that it has.

Air filters can be valuable for other allergens, including those of dogs and cats (see pp. 156–65). Filters may also be good for mould spores or pollen, because these allergens come in from outside every time a door or window is opened, and it is useful to be able to clean the indoor air of them, once doors and windows are shut. So if you are affected by any of these allergens as well as house dust, it may be worth investing in an air filter.

Ionizers often make asthma worse, so they are not recommended.

What about air conditioning . . . ?

Conventional air-conditioning units take moisture out of the air, and can play a useful part in reducing the level of dust mite infestation in the home. However, other measures (such as dealing with the bed and bedding) will still be necessary to reduce asthma symptoms.

Unless you live in a very hot and humid climate, air conditioning may be a rather expensive and inefficient way of tackling dust mites. A far cheaper and more effective way of reducing humidity in the house is to increase the everyday ventilation (by allowing a few draughts into the house) and to open windows whenever the weather is dry. However, if you are allergic to pollen as well, air conditioning could be advantageous, as it removes pollen from the air.

One type of air-conditioning unit, called a 'central evaporative cooler' or 'swamp cooler', actually *increases* the humidity in the house and encourages dust-mite infestation.

. . . or mechanical ventilation heat recovery units?

These are the latest high-tech product for fighting mites. The idea is to take the air out of your house and exchange it for cleaner outside air, using a clever piece of engineering to extract the heat from the outgoing air and warm up the incoming air. These units work well in Scandinavia, where winters are cold and dry, but in Britain, the incoming air tends to be too moist. As a result, the unit cannot produce the kind of dry indoor conditions needed to reduce the mite population.

'Thank heavens I did . . .'

Julie has had nocturnal asthma for many years. She recently bought special anti-mite covers for her duvet and pillows. 'I was somewhat hesitant about buying these things because of the not insignificant cost, but I decided to take a chance. Thank heavens I did. I woke up this morning after the first long deep unbroken sleep I've had in years. I really couldn't believe it. I usually wake up gasping for Ventolin by 4 a.m. Sometimes I make it until 7 a.m., but the first thing I do is reach for Ventolin. Today I didn't need my inhaler until after 5 in the evening – an absolute miracle.'

The costs of mite control

Controlling mites can be an expensive business if you buy all the latest products. But it can also be done fairly cheaply if you are resourceful. If you follow Phases One and Two (pp. 132–41) choosing Option C of Phase One and the cheapest versions of each step, the total cost need not be very high. The cheapest measures can also be highly effective, especially if you are prepared to tolerate slightly Spartan living conditions with lots of fresh air and draughts. Children who are brought up this way tend not to mind at all – they are so used to it they think nothing of it, and they are generally very healthy.

In Britain, there may be financial assistance available for some asthmatics who cannot afford anti-mite measures. Contact the National Asthma Campaign (see p. 452) and ask for their Financial Assistance Factsheet, which lists organizations that might be able to help with grants.

For those living in rented accommodation (including, in Britain, council housing), any damp problems that result from structural defects should be put right by the landlord. A test case has shown that the landlord can be considered legally liable if damp causes asthma or makes it worse (p. 170). Compensation may be high, so it makes sense for landlords to take preventive action. Your local department of health should be able to advise you about your legal rights.

Away from home – where mites are found

Quite a few people with asthma and dust-mite allergy had their first major attack of asthma as a result of sleeping on a very old mattress, or under an ancient eiderdown, while away from home. The dose of allergen that you receive while sleeping in the spare room of a friend or relative can be frighteningly high. So if you have dust-mite allergy, be very choosy about where you sleep. Spending the night on an old sofa is also hazardous.

In theory, mites can live in any upholstered material. They can occur in padded chairs in offices, and are sometimes numerous in car seats if the car is kept in a fairly warm garage. Seats on trains and coaches tend not to have too many mites, because the temperature falls so low at nights.

Hotel beds are also a potential source, especially those with en-suite showers which make the room very humid. Some hotels in the USA and Scandinavia now offer low-allergen rooms – let's hope hotels in other countries follow their lead.

Mites in food

There are several different kinds of mite, related to the house dust mite, which live in stored food. Some of these are also common in houses, where they live on crumbs of food that fall to the floor.

Someone who is allergic to house dust mites may also be allergic to these food mites. On the other hand, eating mite allergens in stored food may make people *less* likely to develop an allergy-inhaled mite allergen. Allergens that are consumed by mouth are generally ignored by the immune system, something known as 'oral tolerance'. One immunologist has suggested that improved methods of food storage, resulting in fewer mites in food, have contributed to the current upsurge in allergy to inhaled dust-mite allergens.

Allergies to mites in hay, grain and flour sometimes occur in farmers and other workers who handle mite-infested material. Eczema is the most common symptom, and this is sometimes referred to as 'grain itch'. Asthmatic symptoms are also a possibility.

Cheese is home to other species of mite, and these can cause allergic problems for cheese producers and handlers, usually a form of eczema.

'The windows didn't open properly . . .'

'The first house we lived in after we were married was a miner's cottage, built in the 1890s, a little timber house. That was in the highlands in southern Victoria. The place was just a mass of holes. It was about 500 metres up, in a heavily forested area, with long, cold, damp winters.

'The second house was in Bendigo, in flatter, drier country, with summers much longer and hotter. That was a brick veneer house, only about 17 years old, all pretty tightly sealed. The windows didn't open properly, so there was no through ventilation. In that second house we had much more trouble with asthma, especially from the blankets, pillows and doomas [eiderdowns]. It seemed a much cleaner house than the first one, but we were far less healthy there.'

This pattern of symptoms is related to dust mite allergy: a lot of moisture is produced within our houses and ventilation is vital in combatting mites (see pp. 139–40). Recent research on Melbourne houses has also shown higher levels of dust mites linked to weatherboard walls, wooden floors built on stumps (allowing ground moisture to soak up into the floor), central heating, damp bedrooms and ageing fitted wool carpets.

AVOIDING POLLEN, CATS, MOULDS AND OTHER ALLERGENS

All these allergens can be avoided to some extent – you may not be able to eliminate them completely but you can certainly reduce your exposure. Don't expect immediate benefits from avoiding your allergens. You probably won't notice any benefits for a few weeks, and even then the improvement will be small. It takes several months for the full effects to be felt.

Cats

If you have a cat, and you or your child are allergic to cats, your doctor will probably have advised you to find the cat another home. It is good advice, which we can only repeat. Cats produce highly potent allergens and most cats produce them in staggering abundance. Generally speaking, people with asthma find that although they miss their pet a great deal, especially at first, the huge improvement in their health makes it worthwhile in the long run. If you feel better, and can get out and enjoy life more, the comfort and company that a cat provides may not be missed as much as you expect.

If it is a child that is allergic to the cat, then the importance of freeing your house from cat allergen cannot be emphasized enough: it could make the difference between the child having asthma for life or 'growing out of it' in a few years' time. And if you are hoping to prevent asthma developing in a new baby, not having a cat at home will greatly improve your chances (see p. 90).

Finding a home for an adult cat is often difficult, as most people want kittens, but try advertising locally, in a shop or Post Office, and explaining in your advertisement exactly why the cat needs a new home. Ask around among elderly neighbours – they may value having a mature cat that is already house-trained and doesn't race up the curtains. You could also ask family and friends or your local vet, who may be keen to help if they understand how serious the problem is.

Once the cat has gone

Like the smile of the Cheshire cat in *Alice in Wonderland*, something important will linger on long after your cat has departed. Allergens.

They will be in the cushions, armchairs and sofas, deep in the carpets and stuck to the curtains and walls. They will actually be *inside* upholstery, and mattresses if the cat once slept on the bed, forming a reservoir of allergens that will waft out every time you sit or lie down. Unless your allergy to cats is relatively mild, a serious clean-up operation is called for.

It is important to realize that you can't *see* this allergen. Many people assume that it is cat fur which acts as an allergen, or flakes of skin. In fact the allergen is a protein found in the sweat and saliva of the cat. Although there is some allergen stuck to skin particles and fur, the real problem is caused by microscopic specks of dried allergen floating around in the air. They are extremely small, which means that they don't settle for six hours or more, however still the air (see p. 162). And when they do settle – on curtains, lampshades, shelves and furniture – they are easily disturbed and made airborne again by the least little breeze. Just walking quietly around the room will be enough to churn up the ultra-light cat allergen particles.

The first part of the clean-up involves airing the house very thoroughly, opening all the doors and windows wide and getting a good breeze through. This will get rid of the huge amount of allergen that is just hanging in the air. Having done that, you may want to wait a couple of weeks, and see how much your asthma improves, before embarking on a spring-clean. Obviously, if you are substantially better and needing very few drugs, then you do not need to clean up much. If you still have troublesome symptoms, these are the measures you need to take:

- Wash everything that can possibly be washed: curtains, loose covers, cushions and their covers, duvet covers, pillow cases, bedspreads, etc. Washing at high temperatures has no advantage over washing at cool ones (or even in cold water) for cat allergen, as it is not affected by heat. The objective is to wash the allergen away, so use plenty of detergent and maximize the amount of rinsing the clothes get by not loading the machine as fully as usual. You could run the rinse cycle twice to be really safe.
- Wash duvets, blankets, eiderdowns, etc. As far as we know, no one has carried out experiments to show if dry-cleaning removes cat allergen; it is probably best to assume that it does not do so.

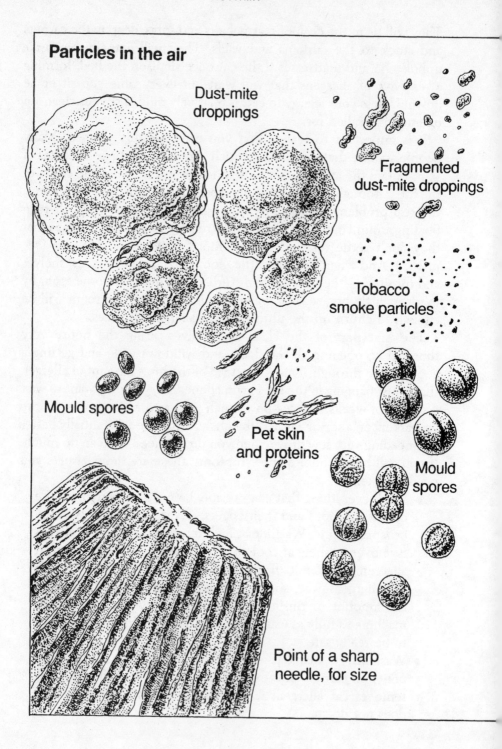

Particles in the air

Dust-mite droppings

Fragmented dust-mite droppings

Tobacco smoke particles

Mould spores

Pet skin and proteins

Mould spores

Point of a sharp needle, for size

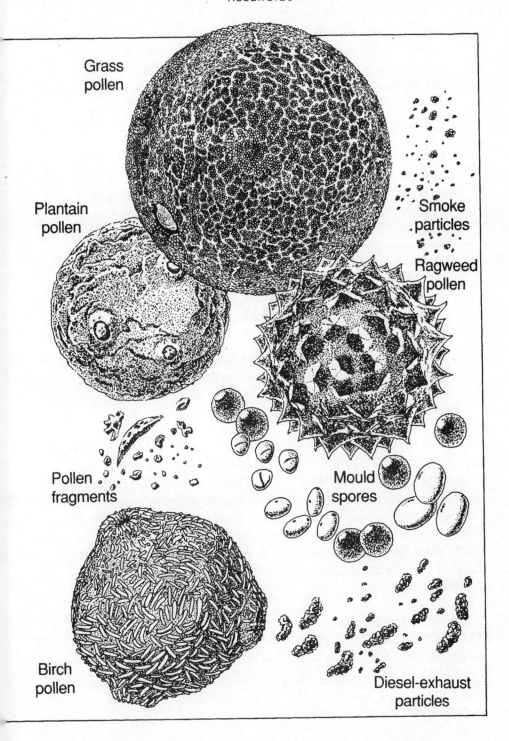

Grass pollen

Plantain pollen

Smoke particles

Ragweed pollen

Pollen fragments

Mould spores

Birch pollen

Diesel-exhaust particles

- If you suspect that there is a substantial reservoir of allergen in your mattress, pillows and duvet, because the cat used to sleep in your bedroom, consider buying new ones. If your pillows and duvet are washable you could wash them instead. Covers designed for dust-mite avoidance (see pp. 470–4) will also help by keeping most of the cat allergen from escaping into the air.

- There are often vast reservoirs of allergen inside the seat cushions of sofas and armchairs, where the cat once snoozed away the day. You could tackle these with a spray that neutralizes allergens, such as tannic acid or a polysaccharide spray (see p. 476). Although the sprays are marketed mainly for dust-mite allergen, they should work on other allergens, including those from cats. However, a lot of cat allergen will overwhelm the tannic acid, and you will need to vacuum-clean very thoroughly first to remove as much allergen as possible, then spray repeatedly to deal with what is left. Assuming the cat has gone, the sprays will only be needed for a few weeks or months, so there will be no long-term build-up of the spray. (Anti-mite steam cleaners, which neutralize dust-mite allergen – see p. 143 – will *not* work for cat allergen as it is not sensitive to heat.)

Most of these tasks (for example, taking down curtains to wash them) will involve disturbing the accumulated cat allergen, so levels in the air will increase vastly for a time. Exposing yourself to this onslaught, if you are asthmatic and cat-allergic, is asking for serious trouble. Someone else should do the work, and you should be out for the duration and for at least six hours afterwards. If you need to come home, even briefly, make sure you are wearing a really good mask (see p. 480) – it needs to filter out the tiniest of airborne particles (see p. 466).

Is it possible to keep the cat?
This is not a good option, and you should only consider it if the allergy to cats is not that severe and your asthma is fairly mild. In these circumstances, if you really cannot bear to part with the cat, you could experiment with some less drastic measures, and see how much improvement there is:

- Increase the ventilation in your house as this will make a huge difference in reducing the amount of allergen in the air. Air the house regularly, and keep a window slightly open whenever the cat and/or the allergic person is indoors. Alternatively, use an HEPA filter to clean the air. These are not much use for dust-mite or cockroach allergens, which are relatively large, heavy particles (see p. 152) but they work in this case because cat allergens are very small lightweight particles which easily become airborne, so there is quite a lot of allergen in the air most of the time. Needless to say, an air filter cannot do anything to protect you from a cat sitting on your lap.

- Prevent the cat from sleeping on the bed of the asthmatic person by keeping it out of the bedroom entirely. If it has been in the habit of sleeping there, wash all the bedding and pillows, and buy a new mattress and duvet.

- Build the cat a little shed or out-house where it can sleep some of the time, to reduce the amount of allergen building up in the house. Make it as warm and comfortable as possible, and feed the cat there sometimes, so that it feels at home. Alternatively, you can confine the cat to the utility room or lobby, giving it a comfortable bed, and perhaps sprinkling a little catnip there to make it seem more attractive.

- Tom-cats produce more allergen than female cats, and the amount declines when they are neutered, so if you have an unneutered tom, have him neutered and see if things improve.

- Individual cats vary enormously in the amount of allergen they produce: if you have more than one cat, you could try housing each one outside in turn to see which is the least allergenic.

- Avoid using fans or fan heaters which churn up allergens from carpets and furnishings into the air. This can defeat your efforts by constantly recharging the air with settled allergen that has been accumulated over the years.

- Get a high-suction vacuum cleaner of the kind that retains allergen particles (see pp. 477–9) so that you can vacuum the furnishings thoroughly – and without spraying the allergen around the room.

- If the cat is still coming indoors, remove fitted carpets and all soft furnishings, replacing the latter with leather- or vinyl-covered armchairs which will not accumulate cat allergen.

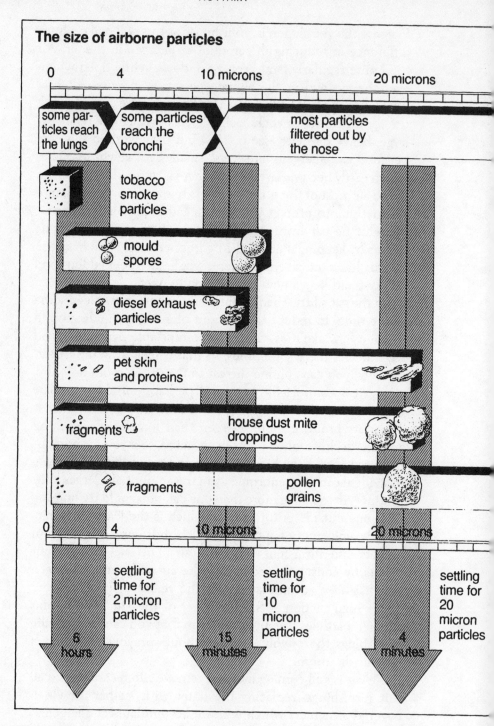

The size of airborne particles

0   4   10 microns   20 microns

some particles reach the lungs

some particles reach the bronchi

most particles filtered out by the nose

tobacco smoke particles

mould spores

diesel exhaust particles

pet skin and proteins

fragments   house dust mite droppings

fragments   pollen grains

0   4   10 microns   20 microns

settling time for 2 micron particles

6 hours

settling time for 10 micron particles

15 minutes

settling time for 20 micron particles

4 minutes

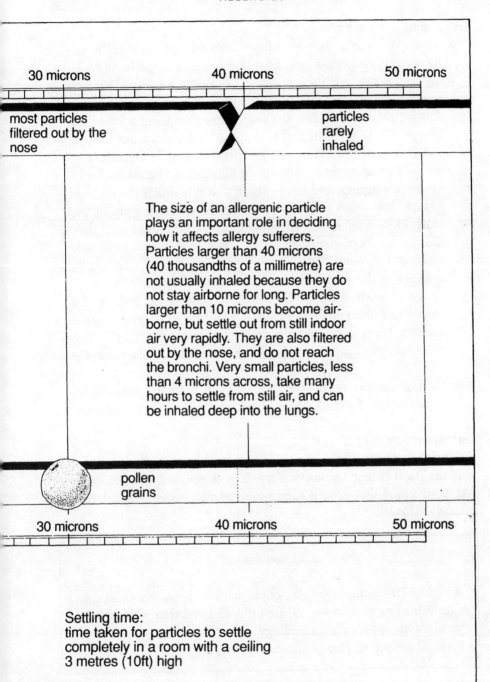

30 microns   40 microns   50 microns

most particles   particles
filtered out by the   rarely
nose   inhaled

The size of an allergenic particle
plays an important role in deciding
how it affects allergy sufferers.
Particles larger than 40 microns
(40 thousandths of a millimetre) are
not usually inhaled because they do
not stay airborne for long. Particles
larger than 10 microns become airborne, but settle out from still indoor
air very rapidly. They are also filtered
out by the nose, and do not reach
the bronchi. Very small particles, less
than 4 microns across, take many
hours to settle from still air, and can
be inhaled deep into the lungs.

pollen
grains

30 microns   40 microns   50 microns

Settling time:
time taken for particles to settle
completely in a room with a ceiling
3 metres (10ft) high

Things that don't work:

- Giving the cat a shower. Many authors, ourselves included, have previously suggested that you wash your cat by drenching it in water and then rubbing it dry with a towel. This was based on research which showed that, after a cat had taken a shower in this way, the washing water contained a lot of cat allergen. It seemed logical to assume that this meant less cat allergen in the air. More recently, researchers in Detroit have actually measured the amount of allergen in the air around a cat after washing, and have shown that it is much the same as before: cats seem to produce an inexhaustible supply of the stuff. However, as the authors of this report point out, they did not try immersing the cat in water, nor did they use any kind of detergent. Other researchers have found that totally immersing the cat in water does make a difference.
- Spraying with Allerpet-C, which is claimed to reduce the amount of allergen released. Full scientific trials by the same Detroit team have shown that this does not work. The manufacturer's claims are based on very weak research methods.
- Dosing the cat with acepromazine, an animal tranquillizer. Again, scientific trials have shown that this does not work.

Untested treatments:

Dosing the cat with Vitamin E. There is one isolated report of this working, so it might be worth a try. The dose used was 100 iu/day. Ask your vet if this dose is safe for your cat (Vitamin E is toxic in excessive doses).

Did you know?

Roughly 20–30 per cent of people with asthma are allergic to cats. Amazingly, a survey in the USA showed that more than a third of people with cat allergy still keep their cat, despite medical advice to find it another home.

Cat allergens away from home

Cat allergen travels around on the clothes of cat-lovers and gets absolutely everywhere. It is found in public buildings, including schools, cinemas and banks, and even in hospital waiting-rooms. A recent study at Wythenshawe Hospital in Manchester found that the padded seats in the waiting area of the chest clinic contained very few dust mites, but significant amounts of dog and cat allergen.

Dogs

Like cat allergens, those of dogs are small and lightweight, so, if you keep your dog, the air will be full of them most of the time. This means that HEPA filters can be very useful, although you also need to take other measures, such as excluding the dog from bedrooms and keeping it outside for more of the time. Washing dogs thoroughly in a bath, using dog shampoo, reduces the amount of allergen in the coat and, hopefully, in the air. Dogs produce less allergen than cats, but you still need to clean up thoroughly.

Mould spores

Spores are produced by moulds and other fungi. They are too small to be seen without a microscope, and they float about in the air. A spore is to a mould what a seed is to a plant – it can grow into a new mould.

Whereas dust-mite allergen is produced exclusively indoors, and pollen exclusively outdoors, mould spores can be produced both indoors and out. Assuming you are allergic to both indoor and outdoor moulds, you will need to adopt a two-pronged strategy: avoid mould-rich places outside, and reduce mould growth inside your home.

Even with careful avoidance measures, you may still be exposed to a lot of mould spores. In some cases, particularly allergy to a type of mould called *Alternaria*, it may be wise to increase your dose of preventer inhaler (e.g. steroid or cromoglycate) during the spore-producing season. One study has shown that severe near-fatal asthma attacks commonly occur during the *Alternaria* season among those allergic to this mould.

Avoiding moulds out of doors

The first six items on p. 117 describe outdoor situations where mould spores are found in abundance. Try to avoid these situations, and any other activities that involve contact with mouldy plant material.

Reducing mould growth indoors

The main task is to reduce dampness and moist air in the house, as this encourages mould growth on walls, around windows, on tiles and shower curtains, in clothes and carpets.

To reduce moisture in the house:

- Sort out any structural problems, such as rising damp or cracks in the walls. Older buildings may lack basic features, such as a damp-proof course, a waterproof membrane in the floor, or waterproof 'sarking felt' under the roof. All these items can be added – even a damp-proof course can be added quite cheaply, by injecting waterproofing liquid into a line of holes drilled in the existing walls just above ground level. Damp patches around windows can sometimes be remedied by spraying a layer of silicon on to the wall externally. Ask a builder, surveyor or architect for an estimate for the work.
- Check behind furniture and in cupboards for any damp patches. If there are persistent damp problems in cupboards, buy silica gel crystals from a hardware shop to dry out the air, or use a low-power space-heater designed for this purpose.
- Get rid of any humidifiers. It is a myth that the air in centrally heated houses is too dry and that this irritates the nose: carefully controlled tests have shown that this is not the case, as long as the air is clean. If you feel your nose and mouth are uncomfortably dry at home, try tackling indoor pollution (see p. 221) or simply turning the thermostat down a little. Far from being too dry, the air in most homes is much too moist. (During a severe asthma attack, some people find that moist air is beneficial to the airways. Steam inhalations (see p. 349) can be used to provide localized moist air in these circumstances.)
- Heat all parts of the house equally well: rooms that are colder than the rest of the house will be vulnerable to condensation. Loft insulation will help to keep ceilings warm.
- Keep lids on saucepans, and turn off kettles as soon as they boil, to reduce steam in the kitchen.
- If your kitchen has an extractor fan, use it whenever you cook. If not, consider having one fitted. Alternatively, open a window while you cook, and leave it open for a while afterwards.

- Dry clothes outside, in a tumble-dryer vented to the outside, or in a well-ventilated utility room. (Most laundrettes have large tumble-dryers which you can use even if you have washed your clothes at home.)
- If you can afford it, fit a powerful extractor fan in the bathroom. If not, open the windows wide after baths or showers, to allow the moisture to escape. During rainstorms, leave the bathroom door open instead: this will disperse the moist air to the rest of the house, which at least reduces mould growth in the bathroom. (But close the bedroom door to keep the steam out of there.) An extra heater in the bathroom, which can be left on after baths and showers, will help disperse the moisture. Wipe down tiles and grouting with an old towel after showers.
- Don't leave towels and bathmats in the bathroom to dry.
- When it is raining, have baths rather than showers as they produce less steam.
- Take down any vinyl wallpaper, and replace it with emulsion paint or ordinary wallpaper. These allow moisture to be absorbed into the wall and eventually to escape to the outside, whereas vinyl paper keeps it on the surface of the paper encouraging mould growth there. This is particularly important in the kitchen and bathroom. Walls should not be painted with gloss or eggshell paints either, as these are impervious to water. Tiled areas should be kept to a minimum.
- Cold windows and window frames encourage condensation. Replace any metal window-frames with wood or PVC frames, and fit double-glazing, which gives a much warmer glass surface.
- Mop up any condensation that does occur around windows, or on windowsills, every day. Dry the cloths outside or in a utility room.
- Above all, ventilate the house. Whenever the air is dry outside – hot or cold – give the house an airing. Open several windows so that a good draught blows through.
- In new houses, or after major renovation work, ventilation is even more important. Up to 1360 litres (300 gallons) of water is used in construction, mainly for plastering. This takes at least nine to twelve months to evaporate under normal con-

ditions. A dehumidifier (see p. 476) may be worthwhile during this period, especially if there is a lot of rain. Beware of speeding up the process too much (e.g. by over-heating the house) as this can cause plaster and concrete to crack, or timber to warp.

Even with all this hard work, you will still have some moisture in your house, so there may be persistent mould growth which you need to combat. And there are the millions of spores left by the moulds of yesteryear which must be eliminated. Needless to say, someone other than the asthmatic should do this work, because exposure to spores will be high.

Combating the growth of moulds:
- Throw out any fabric or furniture that smells mildewy: it is packed with old mould spores.
- Clean the rubber seals around fridges and freezers, going into all the crevices to get out the black mould that lives there. This needs to be done regularly.
- Clean up any mould growing around windows, or in the bathroom or kitchen. White spirit kills it very effectively, without the use of water, and it takes a long time to grow back again. Or you can wash the walls down with dilute bleach. There are also anti-mould sprays that can be used for this purpose. Never brush mould growth off with a dry cloth, as this simply disperses the spores. From now on, keep an eye out for new mould growth, and remove it promptly.
- Replace shower curtains regularly, or clean them thoroughly with anti-mould spray.
- Reduce the number of house plants, and eliminate any that need constant moisture. Learn to love cactuses if you can. Take good care of the remaining house plants: trim off dead leaves and flowers promptly, and scoop out the top layer of soil occasionally (it will be full of moulds), replacing it with fresh soil, sand or grit. Bowls of pot-pourri should also go, as these can be full of mould spores.
- Eat bread, potatoes, vegetables and fruit promptly, and do not leave ripe fruit about for long.

Despite the fact that you have cut down on moisture and condensation and combated mould growth, there could *still* be a lot of mould
spores around, especially in an old house, one that has been very
damp in the past, or one that is near a lake or river. If symptoms persist
in spite of all the measures listed above, and if you are sure you are
allergic to moulds (see p. 117), you will need to take a few more steps.
The hard work you have put in so far has not been wasted – it will all
help in the long run. There would be little point in buying an air filter,
for example, if you had not already reduced mould growth substantially: the filter would be fighting a losing battle.

Keeping mould spores out of the airways:
- There may be a lot of mould spores in house dust. If you are
  asthmatic, you should not dust, vacuum-clean, sweep floors or
  make beds. In fact, you should be out when this occurs, and
  the house should be thoroughly aired before your return.
  Wearing a mask that excludes mould spores (see p. 480) will
  help if this sort of housework is unavoidable. A vacuum
  cleaner designed to retain allergens or vent them outside
  (see p. 477) may also be valuable.
- Consider buying a high-quality air filter to take mould spores
  out of the air in your bedroom or sitting-room, or both. It
  needs to be adequate for the size of the room.
- Where there is a persistent damp problem that you cannot
  tackle, a powerful dehumidifier (see p. 476) used during the
  day in bedrooms, and at night in the sitting-room, will kill off
  most moulds and make it difficult for them to regrow. Shut
  the doors and windows in the room where the dehumidifier is
  operating. Air conditioning will also reduce the humidity of
  the air, but not as much.
- Keep away from damp basements, conservatories and greenhouses. Never sleep in a room which has mould growing on
  the walls or window-panes.
- Avoid using fans or fan heaters, as these churn up mould
  spores from the carpet and other surfaces.

Some pollen telephone lines give mould-spore counts as well (see
p. 459), and you can use these to avoid going out on the days with
very high spore counts.

Did you know?

There are more mould spores in the air than anything else. The record count in Britain is over 160,000 spores per cubic metre of air, whereas the record pollen count is 2800 grains per cubic metre. Fortunately, mould spores are not particularly allergenic, or even more people would be sneezing and wheezing.

If you live in public housing, and there is a problem which is aggravating asthma in some way, such as mice or cockroaches, or dampness due to structural faults which is encouraging mould growth or house dust mite, you can demand to be rehoused. In a test case in the British courts, a boy with asthma successfully sued the local authority because damp housing conditions had aggravated his condition. Your doctor should be able to supply a letter of support to the housing department.

Did you know?

An average human being gives off about 1 litre (2 pints) of water in sweat every night, and more during the day. A family of four is estimated to produce 10–20 litres (18–36 pints) of water vapour every 24 hours. All this water vapour has to be flushed out of the house with good ventilation, or it will encourage the growth of moulds and house dust mites.

Pollen
This is the most difficult allergen to avoid, but there are several measures you can take to reduce your exposure.

Find out which pollen affects you
It helps to know which pollen (or pollens) you are allergic to. You may be able to work it out on seasons alone (see p. 122) or you may need skin-prick tests (see p. 126).

Then learn to recognize the plants concerned: consult a plant field guide.

Know what time of day the offending pollen is likely to be in the air
By understanding the patterns of pollen release and movement, you
will have some idea when your offending pollen is most likely to be in
the air. You can then time your activities accordingly. Aim to be
indoors with the windows closed when pollen counts peak, or (even
better) in an air-conditioned car or building, or an indoor swimming-
pool. If you cannot manage being indoors, at least try to stay away
from obvious sources – such as areas of unmown grass in the morning,
if you are grass-sensitive.

Understanding pollen release and movement allows you to continue with some healthy outdoor activities throughout the pollen
season. If you are grass-sensitive, for example, you can take advantage
of the early sunrise during June, and get up at 6 a.m. for a run, so that
you are safely home by 7.30. Or you can go out in the early evening,
after grasses have finished releasing pollen, and before the evening
'pollen shower' (see below).

Pollen release occurs at different times of day for different plants:
Grasses: In the case of grasses, they release their pollen from about
7.30 a.m. onwards on a warm dry summer morning, but if the ground
is damp, because it rained the previous evening or because there is a
dew, the release will be delayed until the moisture has evaporated.
Unfortunately, a few species of grass wait until the afternoon, so there
will be some pollen entering the air all day.
Ragweed: This potent North American allergy-producer gets going
much earlier than grasses, releasing its pollen between sunrise and 9
a.m., although certain weather conditions can delay release until as
late as 2 p.m.
Birch: This one is an afternoon pollen: release peaks between noon
and 6 p.m.

Unfortunately, there is no information at present for other types of
plants.

Whatever pollen is your allergen, these general points will apply:
- All plants favour warm sunny days for releasing pollen, and
  they all avoid rainy or cool weather.
- During cloudy days there is a build-up of pollen in the flowers,
  so expect a bumper pollen count on the next day of good
  summer weather.

- Pollen goes up – and then it comes down. As the air warms up during the day, it begins to rise, carrying the pollen with it. On a still day, the rising pollen accumulates high up in the atmosphere, where it also mixes and spreads about. When the air begins to cool down after sunset, the pollen is no longer buoyed up by rising currents of air, and it slowly descends again, a thick blanket of mixed pollens that falls indiscriminately on everything. The invisible 'pollen shower' falls quite quickly in the countryside, and most of it reaches ground level between 8 and 10 p.m. In the city, hot pavements and buildings keep the upward air currents going and pollen stays aloft for longer. Most of the pollen lands on the city at about midnight, and some may still be coming down at 2 a.m. This is why you may wake in the middle of the night with an attack of hayfever or asthma, especially if you sleep with the windows open.
- Strong winds during the day will stop the pollen accumulating in the upper atmosphere, as will rainfall, so the late-evening 'pollen shower' will not occur.

Use pollen counts and forecasts to help avoid pollen

The pollen counts, given on radio and television, and on special pollen help-lines (see p. 459 for the telephone numbers) are based on actual counts of pollen made at specific sites earlier in the day, or on the previous day.

Pollen forecasts for the next day are produced by computer models, and they are really no more than informed guesswork, based on the time of year, the present pollen count, the temperature and rainfall over the last few days, the weather forecast for the next day, and an understanding of the behaviour of pollen (some of the principles involved are described in the previous section). At best, pollen forecasts are only as reliable as the weather forecast, and there will be local variations in both weather and pollen that the forecast does not cover.

Pollen outlooks for the next three days are prepared in the same way, and are as reliable – or unreliable – as three-day weather outlooks.

Despite their limitations, pollen forecasts and outlooks can be very useful. If you have a choice about going out or staying at home, use them to help you decide. Some pollen-forecast services are definitely better than others, so shop around, especially if you are allergic to something other than grass. (Too many services still ignore other pollens.) Early-morning TV programmes may give an up-to-the-minute pollen forecast for the coming day.

Pollen forecasts can also be useful in deciding when to increase your asthma preventer drugs (steroid or cromoglycate inhalers) or to start taking anti-histamines for hayfever. The forecasters can now predict the start of the grass-pollen season quite accurately, and pollen telephone lines usually start up in May so that people can find out when the season will begin. The start of the tree pollen season is far more difficult to predict, unfortunately.

Understanding pollen counts:
- The counts are given in number of pollen grains per cubic metre of air. These are intact pollen grains, not fragments (see below).
- If the type of pollen is not specified, the count or forecast probably relates to grass.
- The figures are usually averages for a 24-hour period, which includes both pollen peaks and periods of low pollen. The actual count at peak times will therefore be much higher. Sometimes pollen counts for peak periods are given, but this will usually be stated.
- Some plants provoke symptoms at quite low counts, others only at high counts. In Britain, for example, the highest annual count for grass will be about 150 grains per cubic metre, whereas tree pollens can reach 1000 grains per cubic metre. Despite this, many more people are allergic to grass pollen than to tree pollen.

Reduce the amount of pollen inhaled when outdoors
Reducing the amount of pollen you inhale when you *are* outdoors can have benefits that continue long after you are safely indoors again. By avoiding big doses of pollen, you will not aggravate your airways, so they will be less sensitive to smaller amounts of pollen, other allergens, and irritants in the air.
- If you can afford it, buy an air-conditioned car. Keeping the car windows closed on an ordinary car also helps, but of course the

car will get extremely hot. Fitting a filter to the air intake of an ordinary car (see p. 482) is cheap, and will reduce pollen even further, but not lessen the heat unfortunately.

- Wear a mask that will keep out pollen grains and fragments (see p. 480) during peak pollen times. Even a scarf or hand-kerchief, tied tightly over the mouth and nose, will give some protection.
- If you feel too self-conscious wearing a mask, try smearing a little Vaseline (petroleum jelly) just inside each nostril and breathing through your nose only (this is a very good idea for asthmatics anyway – see p. 418). Much of the pollen coming into your nose will stick to the Vaseline and never reach your airways. This is as effective for hayfever as it is for asthma.

Reduce the pollen count indoors

There is one piece of good news about pollen grains: they are much larger than other allergenic particles, which means that they settle more quickly from the air. In an average room with 3-metre-(10-foot-) high ceilings, all the pollen will settle within four minutes, providing the air is completely still (add four minutes for every additional 3 metres of ceiling height). So all you have to do is close the doors and windows, sit down and wait. After four minutes or so you should be breathing air that is virtually pollen-free. However, because part of the allergic reaction occurs four to twenty-four hours after encountering the allergen (the 'late-phase reaction') you may still have asthmatic symptoms (or hay-fever) for some time, due to pollen that you inhaled earlier in the day or the previous day. Even if you do still have symptoms, you can at least feel that you are helping towards a less wheezy day tomorrow by giving your airways a break from pollen now. Reducing the pollen load for a few hours every day should produce benefits in the long run, with the airways becoming less severely inflamed.

Unfortunately, a few plants produce tiny fragments, much smaller than pollen grains, that carry the same allergens. The plants known to do this are rye grass, ragweed, Japanese red cedar and Australian white cypress-pine. There may be others as well. If these fragments are in the air, the settling time will be much longer – up to six hours. The tiny fragments will behave more like cat allergen (see p. 157) and you will need better air filters, masks and vacuum cleaners to deal with them than you would need for whole pollen grains.

A few plants even produce airborne chemicals, called 'volatiles', that provoke symptoms in those allergic to the plant's pollen. Birch trees do this: the volatiles come from the buds weeks before the pollen is released, and they affect many people who are *not* allergic to birch pollen, as well as those who are. Volatiles cannot be removed from the air by masks or air filters unless these contain an activated carbon filter (see pp. 481–2).

These measures can reduce the amount of pollen you inhale at home:
- Keep the windows closed, especially in the early hours of the night when the 'pollen shower' occurs, those times of day when your allergenic pollen is being released (see p. 171), and any times when you usually have symptoms.
- When you arrive home, change into a set of clothes that you only wear indoors. These will not be carrying the heavy pollen load of your outdoor clothes.
- Rinse your hair, especially if it is thick or long. Hair also carries a large amount of pollen, which you will continue to inhale, especially in bed.
- Avoid any vigorous movement (such as children running around) in the rooms where the asthmatic sits or sleeps, as this will create air currents that stir up pollen from the floor and furnishings.
- Where such air currents cannot be avoided, consider using an air filter, or installing air conditioning. If buying an air filter, make sure that it is adequate for the size of the room, and ask if you can have the filter on a trial basis for a week or two. Air-conditioning units with special anti-allergen filters are available at extra cost, but are probably not necessary: even without such a filter, air conditioning units remove about 95 per cent of the pollen from the air.
- As an alternative to air filters and air conditioners, wet-dusting and vacuuming every day (using a vacuum cleaner with a special filter – see p. 477) will reduce the amount of pollen that is available to be churned up.
- If there are lots of draughts at home, block up the gaps to keep pollen out and the air indoors as tranquil as possible. Be sure to unblock the gaps again at the end of the pollen season, to prevent damp and condensation which encourage moulds and dust mites.

- Keep pets out of the house during the pollen season, as they bring in pollen on their fur. If you can't keep them outdoors, at least exclude them from the bedroom, and avoid stroking them or getting too close. Alternatively, someone other than the asthmatic could brush them thoroughly before they come in.
- Dry all clothes and bed-linen indoors during the pollen season, to prevent them collecting pollen. If you have any sensitivity to dust mite or moulds, a tumble-dryer would be useful for this, as you should avoid moist air in the house.
- During the day, cover your armchair and bed with an old sheet, and fold this up very gently once you arrive home. There will be a thick layer of pollen accumulating on the chair and bed all day, which you would disturb as soon as you sat down or laid down. With the sheet, you can remove most of it safely. Wash the sheet to get rid of the pollen, and dry it indoors so that it stays pollen-free. If you don't have a tumble-dryer, you will need two or three sheets so that you can use a clean one each day. If you are studying, you could do the same for your desk and books when you are not working.

Choose where you live and work to reduce your pollen exposure

Obviously, this is not possible for everyone, but if you do have some freedom of manoeuvre, the advantages of getting away from pollen could be enormous.

- If you are grass-sensitive, living beside a hay meadow, 'set-aside' land, or any other area with long unmown grass is obviously a bad idea. Cereal crops such as wheat and oats, although they are grasses, release little pollen and rarely cause problems. Rye does release pollen, and may affect some grass-sensitive individuals.
- Generally speaking, the city does not have any particular advantages over the countryside, as pollen is blown into town from elsewhere, as well as being generated from city parks, gardens and wasteland.
- High up in a tall apartment building may be one of the worst places, because of pollen rising on warm air currents (see below): pollen counts can be much higher ten storeys up than they are at ground level.

- Living beside the sea would help enormously, as onshore breezes blow the pollen away.
- Try to avoid big cities that have a problem with 'inversions' (air trapped at ground level by a layer of warmer air above). The most notorious ones are Los Angeles and Mexico City. Pollen accumulates in the air under these conditions, as do pollutants.
- Mountain valleys, if deep and enclosed by peaks, can also be affected by inversions, and this can trap pollen produced in the valley. On mountain peaks and ridges, by contrast, the wind tends to blow pollen away.

If you are moving to a new area, you would be wise to research the average pollen levels and pollen seasons in that area. (See Useful Addresses.)

Is it worth planting a 'low-allergen garden'?

There has been a lot of publicity about low-allergen gardens – gardens in which any type of plant that has ever caused an allergic reaction is excluded, along with all scented plants (because the scent can be an irritant – see p. 232). These gardens do have merits for schools, clinics and hospitals, and the idea of planting one around the Olympic village for the 2000 Olympic Games in Australia is excellent.

But for the average private garden, planting a low-allergen garden is like taking a sledgehammer to crack a nut. There will be hundreds of plant species that can, potentially, cause allergic reactions, but do not affect anyone in your family. There is little point in excluding these, and they include some of the most desirable garden plants.

All that is really necessary is to avoid planting (or remove if already planted) any plants causing symptoms. Even if you are allergic to grass pollen, you do not need to get rid of your lawn. Keep the grass short so that it does not flower and avoid mowing it yourself, as droplets of grass juice are sprayed out by the mower and can act as allergens.

Escaping during the pollen season

If you are not too tied down by family or work commitments, you may like to consider getting away at the height of the pollen season. Generally speaking, when the pollen season is in full swing near your home, the same plants will have finished pollinating further south, and not yet started further north. So those in the south of England, for example, could go north to Scotland or Yorkshire, or head south to the Mediterranean.

Alternatively, head for a windy sea coast, or some high mountain peaks. For more specific and detailed information on pollen seasons in holiday spots worldwide, see *Hayfever* by Jonathan Brostoff and Linda Gamlin, published by Bloomsbury.

Did you know?

Italian children with severe asthma are sent to a special school in the Italian Alps, where there is no trace of house dust mites, pollen or animal allergens. After nine months, they have far less trouble with asthma, and blood tests show that they are much less allergic to common allergens. They stay well for a while after returning home, but three months later they are as allergic and asthmatic as before.

Cockroaches

To get rid of cockroaches, it is necessary to:
- eliminate all food scraps and crumbs, and any pools or drips of water which the roaches can drink
- seal all the cracks and holes which roaches come in through
- use bait stations to kill roaches, replacing them every two to three months

It is almost impossible to eliminate roaches from one apartment in a block, because they will come back in from neighbouring apartments. HEPA air filters are of little value with cockroach allergen.

IS IT TRUE THAT FOOD ALLERGIES CAN AFFECT ASTHMA?

Food can certainly affect some asthmatics, but this is not necessarily food *allergy*. It may be a direct reaction to food additives such as sulphites or it could be food intolerance.

Food allergy and asthma

If you have a true food allergy, this produces a very prompt and unmistakable reaction to the offending food, so you will probably have made your own diagnosis long ago.

The best treatment is to avoid the food completely. You may need to carry an adrenaline (epinephrine) syringe in case you eat the food by mistake (see p. 348) and you should be familiar with the signs of anaphylactic shock (see p. 48). Where children suffer from food allergies, and others in the family eat the offending food (e.g. peanut butter), it is important to keep kitchen surfaces clear of the food. Read labels on packet food very carefully, and be extremely cautious about food in restaurants and cafés. Learning more about food allergy (see p. 63) could be a lifesaver.

A few people with asthma and food allergy are so sensitive that even tiny airborne particles from the food can bring on an asthma attack. Someone who is allergic to potatoes, for example, may be affected just by peeling potatoes, while someone who is allergic to peanuts may begin to wheeze if a packet of peanuts or a jar of peanut butter is opened nearby. Fortunately, there is little risk of a life-threatening reaction to airborne particles. (There are also cases of asthmatics reacting to the smell of food cooking – see p. 98 – but this is a general reaction to smells, and a completely separate issue.)

People who are allergic to latex (rubber) may, very occasionally, react badly to food that has been prepared in factories where the workers wear latex gloves.

Alcohol and caffeine

Alcohol and caffeine can both affect asthma, causing the airways either to narrow or to open up (see p. 265).

Histamine in foods

The body produces a substance called histamine as part of true allergic reactions. Unfortunately, some foods and drinks also contain histamine, and some asthmatics are particularly sensitive to it, and will react with an asthma attack. Very ripe cheeses, Continental sausages (the kind that are matured for a long time) and cheap wines are the main sources. Tinned tuna and mackerel sometimes contain histamine if the fish have been stored badly before canning, but they then tend to have a sharp, peppery or metallic taste. Fresh tuna can also contain histamine: if it has been kept too long it tends to look darker in colour. Taking an anti-histamine will block the reaction to histamine in foods.

Food additives
Some food additives can make asthma worse. The main ones are those that release the gas sulphur dioxide.

Sulphur dioxide from foods
Sulphur (or sulfur) dioxide is a gas that can irritate the airways of asthmatics and provoke an asthma attack. Some preservatives give off this gas in small amounts, and it is inhaled during eating. There is no need to avoid these preservatives unless you are sure they trigger attacks.

Most dried fruits are treated with sulphur dioxide and give off the gas when chewed. Dried apricots have very high levels of sulphur preservatives. *This treatment does not have to be declared on the label.* Dried fruit that has not been treated will usually be labelled 'unsulphured'. The following preservatives give off sulphur dioxide:

- sodium sulphite
- sodium hydrogen sulphite
- sodium metabisulphite
- potassium metabisulphite
- calcium sulphite

These preservatives are widely used in wine, beer and cider, and do not have to be declared on the label. Home-made wine is no exception: Campden tablets, sold to wine-makers, contain potassium metabisulphite.

Fresh sausages may also contain these additives. Cod can be treated with sodium hydrogen sulphite to bleach and preserve it. Although sulphites are not allowed on meat, unscrupulous butchers occasionally add them to old meat to give it a 'fresh' red colour. In all these cases, however, the greater part of the sulphur dioxide will be driven off by the high temperatures used in cooking.

A fourth 'hidden source' of sulphur dioxide is restaurant, take-away and cafeteria food. French fries used in the catering trade have usually been dipped in a metabisulphite solution. Prepared salads, avocado dip, shrimps, prawns and lobster are also treated with these preservatives.

Fruit salad, glacé cherries, fruit juices, fruit pie fillings, dried vegetables and soup, fruit squash, pickled onions, jam, fruit jellies and custard are other possible sources of sulphur dioxide in the catering trade. It is not worthwhile avoiding these foods unless you know they trigger your asthma attacks.

Packaged foods often contain sulphites and metabisulphites, but these are easier to avoid as they are declared on the label. Look for the names given above, or for the appropriate 'E numbers'. These are E220–E227.

Taking a supplement of Vitamins C and E may reduce your sensitivity to sulphur dioxide.

A few asthmatics may be sensitive to other food additives, but this is usually a much slower reaction.

Food intolerance and asthma

Food intolerance is a delayed reaction to food which takes many hours to develop. The foods at fault are usually those that are eaten every day (and often those that are liked most and eaten at every meal). Food intolerance tends to cause a range of different symptoms affecting various parts of the body. Asthma may sometimes be caused, or made worse, by food intolerance.

The link between the food and the symptoms is far less obvious in food intolerance than it is in food allergy. This is because the reaction to food is delayed, and because the foods are eaten very regularly, so that the symptoms from one meal tend to 'run together' with those from the next. Consequently, special detective work is called for in diagnosing the problem. This detective work takes the form of an 'elimination diet', where you cut out all the foods you normally eat, and then test them one by one. This is the only truly reliable and accurate test for food intolerance – advertised tests, such as those involving hair samples, are a waste of money.

Should you try an elimination diet? Is it worth it? If you have mild or moderate asthma, and few other health problems, the chances of food playing a part in your asthma are fairly small and it is probably not worth the trouble of investigating this possibility. Those who are most likely to respond to an elimination diet are:

- Asthmatics who also have various other unexplained symptoms, such as headaches, migraine, diarrhoea or constipation, nausea and indigestion, joint pain, excessive tiredness, a general feeling of vague ill-health, mouth ulcers, stomach or duodenal ulcers, rhinitis (a constant runny or blocked nose), glue ear, aching muscles or oedema (water retention). These are all common signs of food intolerance, although they can all be caused in other ways as well. Occasionally there are other effects from food intolerance, such as depression or anxiety, Crohn's disease and rheumatoid arthritis. Some children with hyperactivity have food intolerance.

- Asthmatics who have noticed that a particular food makes their asthma worse. Where there is intolerance to one food, there could well be intolerance to another.

- Those with exercise-induced asthma (see p. 70) who sometimes respond severely to exercise and sometimes have little or no reaction. Sensitivity to a food or foods may be playing a part in the response to exercise.

- Severe asthmatics and brittle asthmatics: recent research has shown that as many as 60 per cent of brittle asthmatics have food intolerance. However, there is a risk of a potentially dangerous asthma attack when foods are tested – if you react to a tested food you may react to it very severely. So it is vital that you arrange for close medical supervision of your elimination diet. Ideally, you should test foods in hospital, staying in for 24 hours after each food test. If this is not possible, stay on the exclusion phase (see below) for a month before testing any foods (to reduce your sensitivity), then test foods very cautiously, starting with a single mouthful, eating two to three mouthfuls the next day, and working up to a normal portion over a period of five days. Stop if there is any reaction or decrease in peak flow. Don't hesitate to call an ambulance if your asthma symptoms get worse.

The elimination diet

The purpose of the elimination diet is to ask your body questions about the foods it has to cope with, and give it a chance to tell you which ones make it ill. In order to hear the answers, you need a period of 'silence' – that is, a period with no symptoms at all. This is why you exclude all foods that are likely to be causing problems at the outset. Eliminating different foods one by one rarely works because most people are sensitive to more than one food: they must *all* be eliminated at once for the symptoms to disappear – to create the 'silence' which you need. (The main exception to this rule concerns very small children, who are eating a limited number of foods anyway, and are unlikely to be sensitive to a great many of them. See pp. 193 for details of investigating food sensitivity in babies and toddlers.)

All elimination diets fall into two parts. First you avoid any food that might be causing trouble and see if the symptoms clear up – the **exclusion phase**. If the symptoms do disappear, then foods are reintroduced, one at a time, to discover which ones produce symptoms – the **reintroduction phase**.

The elimination diet sounds simple enough, although in practice there can be pitfalls and the results are not always clear-cut. This section of the book has been planned to help you avoid as many of those pitfalls as possible. You should read the whole section before you begin.

Do not be put off by the constant references to things going wrong. Only a minority of people will encounter problems such as these, but when they do arise, extra advice is needed.

There is no point whatever in doing an elimination diet half-heartedly – it simply won't work. You cannot have a day off it in the middle, unlike a weight-reducing or 'health' diet – it is a **diagnostic diet**, not a treatment in itself. If you stop for a day – or even for one meal – you will not get a clear result.

It is also a mistake to rush into it because things are more likely to go wrong. Doing the diet again is often very difficult. The process itself can change you – in particular, you *may* acquire new sensitivities to the foods eaten during the exclusion phase, simply because they are eaten more regularly and in greater amounts than before. If you are already sensitive to a wide range of foods, acquiring new sensitivities may prevent you from having a 'second go' at the elimination diet – you need a basic set of foods to which you have no reaction, in order for the diet to work. *The important thing is to get the elimination diet right first time.*

Preparing for the elimination diet
Seeing your doctor
The first, and most essential step, is to see your doctor. Explain that you want to try an elimination diet, and ask for advice. He or she may well have reservations about elimination diets, and you will be better prepared if you have read all of this section and understand what is involved. If the doctor feels that you should not alter your diet for medical reasons, you *must* take this advice.

Keeping a record
As soon as you can, start keeping a daily record of your symptoms. This will prove very useful later, giving you a detailed picture of how you felt before you began the diet – a base-line to which any later state of health can be compared. Record your peak flow (see p. 315) morning and evening.

At the same time, you could also make a record of what you eat. When you come to plan your diet you need to be aware of what foods you eat very regularly. Keeping a food-diary for a week or two can be quite an eye-opener.

Before you start
Some people with multiple symptoms of the kind associated with food intolerance are actually hyperventilating (see p. 419). It makes sense to investigate this possibility before you try an elimination diet.

The contraceptive Pill can play a complex role in food intolerance (as well as increasing the risk of asthma generally – see p. 263). If possible, come off the pill before starting the elimination diet and use some other form of contraception. Stay off the pill for a year at least, and reintroduce it at a time when your health, and your diet, are stable, so that the effects will be obvious.

If you are allergic to pets, house dust, pollen or other airborne allergens, do whatever you can to reduce your exposure to these (see pp. 127–78) before trying an elimination diet.

Planning the diet
Timing is all-important here, as birthdays, Christmas, weddings,

family get togethers and holidays cause immense problems. Ideally, you should plan things so that the diet falls in a quiet period, or postpone celebrations until afterwards. The diet will run for about three weeks if you *don't* respond to the exclusion phase. If you do respond, then it will continue for two to three months. *Any departure from the diet will confuse the result.*

If you are asked out to lunch or dinner, it is not that difficult to take your own food, and you get over the embarrassment fairly quickly. For picnics and days out, cook the foods that you are allowed and take them in plastic boxes.

Don't start the diet without planning what you are going to eat for the first few days, and buying the things you need. It is worth cooking up some meals in advance, so that you can have something ready within a few minutes. A freezer is invaluable – you can cook your special meals in bulk and freeze them in individual portions. A supply of allowed 'snacks' in a cupboard is also helpful – see p. 187 for ideas.

Packaged and tinned foods should be avoided during this diet. You will find that most prepared foods contain excluded items anyway: it may not say 'milk' or 'eggs' on the ingredients label, but it could be there under another name – see pp. 194–5 for the synonyms used. And it is not unknown for labels to omit an ingredient. So it is much better, at this stage, to stick to simple home-prepared foods because you know exactly what has gone into them. Tinned foods should be avoided at first because the lining of the cans, a golden-coloured phenol resin, contaminates the food slightly. Some food-intolerant people are sensitive to this.

The Exclusion Phase
Decide which foods you are going to eat during the exclusion phase. The aim is to come up with a list of at least 12 foods that are obtainable, affordable, and which you have never eaten in any quantity or with any regularity, before. They should include a variety of different items – some fruit, some vegetables, some meat or fish, and some starchy foods. From the following foods, choose those which you very rarely eat (less than once a week):

Vegetables
  Celery, fennel and celeriac
  Avocado pears

Swede (can be eaten raw, grated, in salads, as well as cooked)
Watercress
Spinach
Alfalfa sprouts
Okra (also called bhindi, or ladies' fingers)
Asparagus

Meat and fish
Turkey
Duck
Goose
Rabbit
Pheasant or other game
Lamb
Fish (but not smoked fish or shellfish)

Fruit
Gooseberries
Blackcurrants
Redcurrants
Bananas
Pears
Kiwi fruit
Mangoes
Pomegranates
Lychees
Passion fruit
Guavas

Starchy foods
Millet
Buckwheat
Turnips
Parsnips
Yams
Sweet potatoes
Dasheen
Cassava
Tapioca

Sago
Chestnuts
Chickpeas (also a good source of protein)
Pumpkin

Oils
Olive oil
Sunflower oil
Safflower oil
Rapeseed oil
Coconut oil and creamed coconut

Snacks
Pumpkin seeds
Macadamia nuts
Pistachio nuts
Cashew nuts
Brazil nuts
Pine nuts

Obviously, you should exclude any foods that you suspect of causing symptoms.

This is meant to be a very simple, basic diet, in which you consume nothing but your allowed foods. No herbs, no spices, no flavourings, nothing tinned and no packaged foods of any sort. It is not going to be a gastronomic delight, but the diet does not last long and it may make you much healthier.

Eat only your allowed foods, *remembering to vary your diet, not to eat any one food every day, and not to eat too much of any one food*. Drink only bottled mineral water. You can drink herb teas, but avoid any that you have consumed regularly before. You should also vary them and not drink more than two or three cups a day – you can become sensitive to anything you eat or drink, and herb teas are no exception. Check the label, and avoid those containing orange, lemon or apple extracts.

Continue the exclusion phase for at least ten days. If you are not substantially better by then, it is highly unlikely that you have food intolerance. Keep a record of everything you eat, all your symptoms, and your peak flow.

You should also weigh yourself regularly during this diet, especially if you are not overweight at the outset. Anyone who is underweight should not embark on the diet without medical advice. If you find you are losing weight rapidly, then you should discuss the matter with your doctor. Elemental diets (see p. 192) can sometimes be useful in these circumstances, as a nutritional supplement.

Possible outcomes:
Feeling much worse
This often happens during the first few days of the exclusion phase, and it is generally considered a good sign. These 'withdrawal symptoms' are seen in many food-sensitive patients and seem to be caused by suddenly cutting out the offending food. They should pass by the end of the first week.

Feeling a little worse
This may be a mild version of the withdrawal symptoms, but if it persists after seven days, then it is something else. One possibility is that you were undernourished to start with and the diet has made things worse. If this seems likely, take a nutritional supplement.

Feeling worse, then much better
Once you have felt consistently better for two or three days, you should start the reintroduction phase – see below. Don't delay doing this. Write down exactly how you feel at this point – it may be useful and encouraging to refer back to this later if you suffer a lot of reactions during food testing.

Feeling much better quite quickly
This can happen, especially in young people – they seem to miss out on the withdrawal symptoms. Go on to the reintroduction phase.

Feeling much better, but with one or two lingering symptoms
It looks as if you have cut out your main offending foods, but are still eating something that is a problem (assuming that you have ruled out all other problems, such as airborne allergens, hyperventilation and environmental chemicals). Think again about your previous eating habits – is there anything you used to eat quite frequently and are still eating? Cut all these out.

If your symptoms clear, go on to the reintroduction phase immediately. If they don't, the best option is to go on to a full 'rare-food diet', only eating foods that you have never eaten before.

If the remaining symptoms are mild, and fairly constant from day to day, you could go on to the reintroduction phase – you may get some sort of useful result from testing. If you can discover which foods are the main source of trouble, and establish a diet on which you are reasonably well, then you are in a good position to investigate further. It could be that the remaining symptoms are due to some other problem – such as airborne allergens.

Feeling worse, then much better, then worse again
If you go through the withdrawal symptoms, feel greatly improved for a while, but then begin to go downhill again, this is a rather bad sign. It does not happen to many people, but if it does happen to you, you need to think very carefully about the situation.

The most likely explanation is that you are developing a new sensitivity to something allowed on the exclusion phase – probably something you are eating a lot of. Look at your food record for the exclusion phase, and try to work out what this might be – foods you ate *before* the diet, rather than entirely novel ones, are obvious suspects. Cut out any such foods and see what happens. Meanwhile make great efforts not to eat too much of any one food.

If you get better again, and stay better for two or three days, you can begin the reintroduction phase. Continue to vary your diet as much as possible during this period.

If you are still not well, or if you have unclear results during the reintroduction phase, then one possible solution is an elemental diet (see p. 192), but you should consult your doctor about this.

Feeling about the same
It seems unlikely that food sensitivity is your problem.

Reintroduction Phase
Wait until you have been free of symptoms for two or three days, but don't wait any longer than this. Begin by testing foods that are probably not the cause of any trouble – things you do not eat very often. Choose items that you like – if the foods pass the test, you can incorporate them into your menus, which will allow you to eat less of

the exclusion-phase foods. Throughout the reintroduction phase it is vital that you keep your diet varied and *do not eat too much of any one food*. In particular, *do not eat any one food every day*. Continue to record everything you eat, and your symptoms – if something goes wrong, this record will prove invaluable. You should not test foods if your chest feels tight or your peak flow is already low.

Only test one food at a time. Eat a normal-sized portion of the food in question (unless you have severe or brittle asthma – see p. 182). Notice any changes that occur at the time, or later in the evening, or the following day. If your peak flow is much lower than usual the next morning, that may indicate a reaction to the food. During the first five weeks of testing, test each food for one day only. If you think you may have reacted slightly, but are unsure, test the same food again the next day. If you get a reaction to any food, stop eating it immediately. Allow the symptoms to subside and your peak flow to return to normal before testing any more foods.

After five weeks, your sensitivity may be declining, so you need to test each food more thoroughly, by eating it for three days in succession. If you get no reaction by the fourth day, then the food can be considered safe, but avoid it again for four days (to offset any possible effect of eating it for three days in succession) before beginning to eat it once more.

The reintroduction phase should take about seven or eight weeks. If it takes any longer than this, there is a risk of lost sensitivity: the food-intolerant person becomes less reactive after avoiding the culprit food for a time. If you are still testing foods eight weeks after starting the exclusion phase, then you need to test the foods more rigorously still. This means eating each reintroduced food every day for a week before declaring it safe.

If there are some foods that you have still not tested after 12 weeks, reintroduce all those foods for three to four weeks and see if any symptoms return. If they do, cut all those foods out again, wait until you feel better, then reintroduce them one at a time. Use three-day testing for preference, or one-day testing if you have a lot to get through.

No reaction on testing
A few people recover on the exclusion phase of the diet, but then show no reactions when foods are tested.

There are two likely explanations for this outcome. One is that the diet has had a placebo effect (see p. 36). The other is that the sensitivity has been greatly reduced by simply avoiding the food for a month or two. Further dietary restrictions do not seem to be needed, but it is advisable to keep the diet varied to avoid a recurrence of the problem.

Special points about food testing

Milk and cheese should be tested separately. Test milk first, using fresh milk, not evaporated or dried. If you react to milk you will probably react to cheese and butter as well, although some milk-sensitive people can eat butter. Even if you can drink milk, you may react to cheese, because it contains various chemicals produced by bacteria and moulds during the cheese-making process. Some people can tolerate evaporated milk, but not fresh milk. If you react to fresh milk, you could test 'evap' later, but leave at least a week before you do so.

Citrus fruits should be tested with orange first, then lemon. If you can eat both of these safely you need not test the others.

Test yeast before mushrooms. You can either use yeast extract (e.g. Marmite) or yeast vitamin tablets.

Test wheat before other cereals. Do not test it as bread, because this contains various other ingredients as well. Certain breakfast cereals are pure wheat, notably Puffed Wheat and Shredded Wheat, and these are good for testing – they can be moistened with fruit juice if you are not able to have milk. Some people are intolerant of the part of the wheatgrain that is lost during the production of white flour, so they only react to wholemeal flour and bread. Others are sensitive to white flour only, probably because of the additives in white flour, or the chemical processes, such as bleaching, that are used in its production.

If you react to wheat, allow at least a week to pass before testing any more cereals – test something else in the meantime.

Rye can be tested as rye crispbread, but make sure it is pure rye, because some contain wheat bran. (Also bear in mind that some people who react to yeast also react to malt, which is a common ingredient in crispbreads and cereals.) Oats can be tested as porridge, and maize as sweetcorn or cornflour. Barley can be tested by eating pearl barley – boil about two or three tablespoons of it in plain water or home-made stock. It may seem rather pointless testing a food such as barley if you never eat it normally, but you could have become sensitive to it if you drink beer regularly, or if you are sensitive to wheat. Rye, barley and oats are all quite closely related to wheat and cross-reactions are not uncommon.

Living on a restricted diet
If you do discover that you have food intolerance, and continue on a restricted diet, you must take great care to get enough vitamins, minerals and other nutrients in your diet. A recent study found that people with brittle asthma tended to eat a diet deficient in Vitamins A and E, because many of them had food intolerance problems. It may be wise to take a good multi-vitamin and mineral supplement.

Elemental diets
These are scientifically devised diets which provide all the nutrients you need in a liquid form, free of any food molecules that are likely to cause allergy or intolerance. It is very rare, though not completely unknown, for anyone to be sensitive to an elemental diet. If you do react, it may be to the flavouring used, so ask for an unflavoured version.

For people who are sensitive to many different foods, elemental diets can be useful during an elimination diet, either as the sole form of nutrition, or as a supplement to a very limited range of foods. Anyone who develops new food sensitivities while on the diet may find it helpful to substitute an elemental diet. It is, however, an expensive option, and the taste is not especially pleasant.

Some elemental diets can be bought from chemists' shops without prescription, but you should talk to your doctor before embarking on this kind of diet. If you can arrange to test foods under medical supervision, that would be a good idea, as test reactions can be severe following an elemental diet.

Asthma drugs during the elimination diet
To ensure that the results of food testing are clear, you should try to keep your asthma drugs at about the same dosage throughout the elimination diet. Talk to your doctor about this before you start. It is better to be on a dose of preventer drugs that keeps your asthma really well controlled than to be on a lower dose and risk having a very

severe attack when foods are tested. Even with your asthma well controlled, you should still be able to detect the effect of problem foods when these are tested, especially if you use your peak-flow meter to help track your symptoms.

If you do get a severe reaction to a food, use your reliever inhaler as much as necessary. You may also need to increase your preventer dose for a few days until the reaction subsides, but you should then go back to the original dose.

Are elimination diets safe for children?

This is very vexed question. There is always the worry that children will be malnourished if they are put on restricted diets, especially if they are not having any milk products. Such deficiencies are rare, and usually occur when parents decide that their children are sensitive to certain foods, don't talk to their doctor about it, and put the children on a restricted diet for many months or years, without giving them vitamin and mineral supplements to compensate. A few cases such as this have occurred, making doctors very anxious about any child trying an elimination diet. This is unfortunate, as some asthmatic children do have food intolerance, and can be much healthier and happier if they avoid the problem food.

If an elimination diet is done carefully, with your doctor's supervision, and supplements are given where necessary, there is no real risk to your child. *You must have your doctor's agreement before starting such a diet.*

The asthmatic children most likely to benefit from an elimination diet are those with other symptoms suggestive of food intolerance (see p. 182). Before trying a diet, be sure to reduce exposure to airborne allergens such as house dust mite, if these play any part in the child's asthma.

Children are generally sensitive to fewer foods than adults, so a less rigorous form of the diet is needed. To begin with, try simply cutting out milk, wheat, eggs, fish, oranges and other citrus fruits, yeast, peanuts, soya products, food additives and any food that the child eats every day or has a craving for. For very young children, just try a milk-free diet as a first step.

Foods containing yeast

Main sources of yeast
- bread, including pitta bread and pizza, but excluding soda bread, matzos and chapattis
- buns and cakes made with yeast, e.g., doughnuts
- yeast extract (Marmite, Vegemite, etc.)
- Oxo cubes and most other stock cubes
- Bovril
- anything labelled 'hydrolyzed vegetable protein'
- beer, wine and cider
- vinegar and pickles
- sauerkraut
- vitamin tablets containing B vitamins, unless labelled 'yeast-free'

Secondary sources of yeast
- dried fruit
- over-ripe fruit
- any unpeeled fruit
- commercial fruit juices
- anything labelled 'malt'
- yoghurt, buttermilk and sour cream
- synthetic cream
- soy sauce
- tofu
- any leftover food, unless eaten within 24 hours, or 48 hours if stored in a refrigerator
- whisky, vodka, gin, brandy and other spirits

Other sources of fungi that may affect some people
- mushrooms, puffballs, truffles, and other edible fungi
- Quorn, mycoprotein (meat substitutes derived from fungi)
- cheese, especially Brie and Camembert

Synonyms used on food labels

Arachis oil	*Peanut*
Baking powder	*May contain maize (corn)*

Casein, caseinate	*Milk*
Cereal binder	*Usually wheat*
Cereal filler	*Usually wheat*
Cereal protein	*Usually wheat*
Cereal starch	*Usually wheat or maize* (corn)
Cornmeal	*Maize (corn)*
Cornstarch	*Maize (corn)*
Corn syrup	*Maize (corn)*
Dextrose	*A type of sugar, derived from maize*
Edible starch	*Usually wheat or maize (corn)*
Flour	*Usually wheat flour*
Food starch	*Usually wheat or maize (corn)*
Fructose	*A type of sugar*
Glucose syrup	*A type of sugar, usually derived from maize (corn)*
Groundnut oil	*Peanut*
Hydrolyzed protein	*Usually yeast*
Hydrolyzed vegetable protein	*Usually yeast*
Lactalbumin	*Milk*
Lactose	*Milk sugar*
Leavening	*Yeast*
Lecithin	*Usually egg or soya but, very rarely, peanut*
Maltose	*A type of sugar*
Miso	*Soya*
Modified starch	*Usually wheat or maize (corn)*
Ovalbumin	*Egg*
Starch	*Usually wheat or maize (corn)*
Sucrose	*Sugar*
Textured vegetable protein	*Soya*
Tofu	*Soya*
Vegetable gum	*Can be soya or maize (corn)*
Vegetable oil	*Usually a mixture of oils, often including corn (maize) oil*
Vegetable protein	*Usually soya*
Vegetable starch	*Can be soya or maize (corn)*
Whey	*Milk*

In some foods labelled 'no added sugar', apple juice could be considered as a synonym for sugar, because highly concentrated apple juice has been used to sweeten the product.

Labels on shampoos and cosmetics
Under a new European directive, compulsory from 1 January 1999, all soaps, shampoos, creams and cosmetics must carry a full list of ingredients. To overcome language barriers, the names are in Latin. (Only those people who have a severe life-threatening immediate allergy need to avoid such products.)

Arachis hypogaea	*Peanut oil*
Corylus americana	*Hazelnut*
Corylus avellana	*Hazelnut*
Corylus rostrata	*Hazelnut*
Bertholletia excelsa	*Brazil nut*
Gadi iecur.	*Cod liver oil*
Juglans nigra	*Walnut*
Juglans regia	*Walnut*
Lac.	*Milk*
Ovum	*Egg*
Piscum iecur.	*Mixed fish oil*
Prunus amara	*Bitter almond*
Prunus dulcis	*Sweet almond*
Sesamum indicum	*Sesame*

'As soon as I'd finished my drink I was wheezing.'

Barny is 15 and has hayfever and mild asthma. 'I can't drink orange soda. I get really wheezy on it, especially cheap orange soda. The last time I had it was at my friend Nick's house, about four years ago. That was when we first noticed that it had this effect. As soon as I'd finished my drink I was wheezing. I got really bad, so I haven't had orange soda since then.'

Orange soda is usually coloured with tartrazine, a substance that provokes attacks for some asthmatics. Although Barny reacts to this very quickly, other people may have a much slower reaction to foods and drinks, not feeling any effects for several hours, sometimes not until the next day (see p. 181).

TACKLING THE CAUSE OF ALLERGIES:
DESENSITIZATION TREATMENTS

If allergies are the result of the immune system 'making a mistake' (see p. 110), can the immune system be re-educated, so that it reacts normally to harmless allergens such as pollen or mould spores? For almost a century, doctors have been working on methods to switch off allergic reactions. These are known collectively as 'desensitization treatments' or 'immunotherapy'. There are three main methods currently in use, and many more in development. Unfortunately, this whole field is beset with controversies, particularly in Britain, where desensitization is not available to most of the people who could benefit.

Desensitization treatments are far more expensive, at least in the short term, than asthma drugs, and are certainly more time-consuming. There is no guarantee of success, and even if the treatment works, some asthma drugs may still be needed, and a certain amount of allergen avoidance necessary, so that the desensitization treatment has less to battle against. In spite of these drawbacks, many asthmatics benefit a greal deal from desensitization.

The most orthodox form of desensitization is known as **hyposensitization** or IIT (Incremental Immunotherapy).

The two other form of desensitization therapy are still not accepted, at least in Britain, by conventional medicine. One is known as **neutralization therapy**, the other as **enzyme-potentiated desensitization**. Both are effective for many patients, and, unlike hyposensitization, neither has ever killed anyone.

Hyposensitization

This treatment uses injections of allergen extract just underneath the skin. A series of injections are given, with each one employing a more concentrated allergen extract than the one before. For the first injection, an extremely dilute solution is used, containing only the most minute quantity of allergen. The dose is then increased gradually, which, in theory, allows the body to learn to tolerate the allergen.

In the original version of the treatment, the patient was given between ten and twenty injections, usually at the rate of two a week. Similar treatment schedules are still used by some doctors today, although most draw the line at fifteen injections, and would not go up to twenty unless there were special difficulties. Alternatively, there are now some much shorter courses, where the allergen extract is combined with another substance which speeds up the process. These shorter courses use only three or four injections, given at weekly intervals, and while they can be helpful for some, fewer patients benefit. Unpleasant side-effects, such as asthmatic attacks or anaphylactic shock (see p. 48) may also be more likely. Another approach is to use a large number of injections but to give them at daily or even hourly intervals, known as **rush desensitization**. This too tends to bring on unpleasant reactions more readily. On the whole, the slow and laborious method, using ten, fifteen or even more injections, seems the most satisfactory.

If an injection produces an allergic reaction (other than itching and redness at the injection site), it is clear that the treatment has progressed too quickly, so the allergist administers the same dose for the next injection, or even goes back to a lower one. Infections make people more reactive to the injections, so if a cold or flu strikes during the course, the concentration will be lowered, or kept the same, until it has passed. Set-backs such as these lengthen the whole process.

It is vital that appointments are kept throughout the course of injections because missing a couple of weeks can wipe out all the benefits so far accrued. The success rate seems to depend very much upon the technique used, and the care with which it is carried out. Don't be afraid to ask the doctor or allergist about their usual success rate before you decide on taking the treatment. Once the course is complete, you will probably be given annual booster doses for three to five years, to maintain the good effects.

Despite its advantages, hyposensitization is now very difficult to obtain in Britain due to a ruling by the Committee on Safety of Medicines in 1986. This states that hyposensitization must not be used for severe asthma, and should only be given where there is resuscitation equipment available (which rules out most local surgeries). Patients must be kept there for an hour after the injection, in case of side-effects.

The reason for this ruling was a spate of deaths due to hyposensitization. Between 1957 and 1986, 26 people died during their course of injections, with 11 of the deaths between 1980 and 1986, and five in the 18 months just before the report. Many of the deaths occurred as a result of anaphylactic shock (see p. 48) or a severe asthma attack. Some were due to errors in the way the hyposensitization was carried out, or a failure to give the right treatment when someone reacted badly, rather than to intrinsic problems of the hyposensitization method.

Hyposensitization is still freely available in all other countries, and many doctors now feel that the British restrictions are too strict. When carried out with proper care, the treatment rarely has adverse effects.

If you are having hyposensitization treatment, you can help to ensure your own safety. Never have any injection if you have asthma symptoms at the time, or if your peak flow is less than 70 per cent of your best reading. Ideally your peak flow should be checked before the injection, and again before you leave the surgery. If you are taking beta-blockers (see p. 262) or have a heart condition, discuss the safety issues with your doctor. Thirty minutes is the absolute minimum waiting time after each shot for someone with asthma – if your doctor asks for less, you should probably look for someone who takes a more cautious approach. It is best to stay for 60–90 minutes. If you are receiving desensitization anywhere other than a hospital, ask if the doctor has resuscitation equipment or how he or she deals with emergencies.

Bad reactions can begin some hours after the injection, so stay within reach of a phone for about 24 hours. If you do experience any effects, be sure to tell the doctor when you go for the next injection, so the dose can be adjusted. Also inform the doctor if you have an infection of any kind, as this can alter your reaction.

Research is currently taking place on new and safer extracts for use in conventional hyposensitization.

Limitations of hyposensitization

Needless to say, if you are being hyposensitized with extract of dust mite allergen, when you are actually sensitive to mould spores, the treatment is not going to work. Accurate diagnosis is therefore essential. Before the treatment begins, you will be given a skin-prick test to confirm the diagnosis, but remember that the test can produce a false-positive result (see p. 304). You can save yourself, and the doctor, a lot of time by not embarking on a series of injections with the wrong allergen. Read pp. 113–26, and consider whether the skin-prick test result agrees with the other facts, such as when and where you experience symptoms.

The other major limitation of the technique is that there are only a certain number of extracts available commercially, and if you happen to be allergic to yak sweat or passionflower pollen, you will be out of luck. Assuming your allergen has been identified, and can easily be collected, some allergists may be prepared to make the extracts themselves.

Enzyme-Potentiated Desensitization

This technique is practised fairly widely, and in Britain it may be possible to obtain treatment under the National Health Service, depending on where you live. Ask your doctor if you can be referred to a suitable allergist for this treatment. Otherwise you can be treated privately and your family doctor should be able to refer you to a suitable practitioner.

This desensitization method relies on the ability of an enzyme called beta-glucuronidase to enhance the desensitizing effect of an allergen when mixed with the allergen extract and injected into the skin. Alternatively, the skin can be scratched and the allergen extract plus enzyme applied to the area in a small plastic cup. This latter method is safer for people with violent allergic reactions because the extract is not injected into the skin and should not therefore provoke an anaphylactic reaction. (It has never yet done so, despite years of use with some very sensitive patients.) The scratch method of enzyme-potentiated desensitization (EPD) is also suitable for children who are afraid of injections, and in the hands of an expert the method is safe for quite small children.

Approximately 80 per cent of patients are helped by EPD, with about 40–65 per cent being a great deal better than before. When compared directly with conventional hyposensitization, using the same assessment methods, the two techniques produce equally good results, with EPD having no serious adverse reactions and therefore being safer. It is also much less time-consuming, needing just one or two injections a year in most cases, compared to a series of ten to 15 injections for hyposensitization.

EPD works particularly well for allergy to house-dust mite and grass pollen, but is not so good for mould allergy. It can sometimes help those who are allergic to pets but cannot bear to part with them.

However, the asthmatic must be entirely free from the allergen for 48 hours while the treatment is taking effect.

Those who do not benefit at all from EPD are usually helped by conventional hyposensitization, and the reverse is also true. This suggests that the two techniques work by fundamentally different mechanisms.

Doctors are often suspicious of techniques that work by unknown means, and tend to reject both EPD and neutralization therapy (see below) for this reason. Yet the conventional technique, hyposensitization, was in use for many years before anyone understood how it worked.

Neutralization Technique

This is also known as intradermal neutralization therapy, or the Miller technique, after Dr Joseph Miller of Alabama, who spent many years developing it and investigating its applications. In the USA it is widely practised by conventional allergists, and preferred to IIT by the majority of them. The treatment can be given in two ways – either using injections of allergen extracts under the skin, or giving the extracts in drops under the tongue, known as **sublingual drops**.

In both cases, the doctor must first discover which allergens are involved, by using a skin-prick test (see p. 304). Once the problem allergens have been identified, the next step is to establish the **neutralization dose**. This is the concentration of each allergen extract that is necessary to desensitize the individual patient to that allergen – different concentrations are required for different individuals.

To test for the correct dose, intradermal injections, which put allergen extracts into the skin, are used. These go deeper than the skin-prick tests, but are not especially painful. A tiny amount of the allergen extract is used.

If the concentration is too low to produce any significant reaction in the skin, the injection simply results in a small raised area, known as a wheal, which begins to go down soon afterwards. If the body does react, then the wheal grows slightly and takes on a characteristic appearance, becoming white, hard and raised, with a sharp edge. This is known as a positive wheal.

When a positive wheal is obtained, the dose is then reduced for the next injection, and repeatedly reduced, step by step, until a concentration is reached that fails to produce a positive wheal. The highest concentration of extract that fails to produce a positive wheal is the neutralizing dose.

Testing for the neutralizing dose can take one or two hours per allergen. Someone who is allergic to just a few items can have their neutralizing doses established in an afternoon, but for someone sensitive to several different allergens, a day or two of testing could be needed.

Once the neutralizing dose has been established, it can be self-injected by the patient, or taken as drops, whenever needed. Most practitioners suggest a daily injection for the first week, then every other day for a few weeks. After that, the patient can experiment to find their own dosing regime – as often as necessary to keep the symptoms under control. The drops are used two or three times a day at first, and then as often as needed.

How neutralization therapy might work is not known. It is possible that, when the neutralizing dose is used, the allergens are bound to skin cells inside the wheal for a long period of time, allowing them to exert a particular influence on the immune system.

Neutralization is much quicker than conventional hyposensitiza-tion: tests for the neutralization dose can probably be carried out in a single day, rather than involving repeated visits to a surgery. Compared to EPD, it is rather more time-consuming because of the testing process required. Furthermore, the neutralization point may change, so that the vaccine stops working as well. If this happens, you will need to go back for retesting.

Neutralization is fairly widely available, and there is at least one centre in Britain which can offer it under the National Health Service. In practice, many patients will have to obtain treatment privately. Ensure that the practitioner uses a skin test to determine the neu-tralization dose. Once the neutralization dose has been determined, the drops (or injection vaccine) are relatively inexpensive. Most practitioners retest for the neutralizing doses every year.

Doctors experienced in this technique have found that it is important to neutralize for all the allergens that give a positive skin test. If only one or two allergens are dealt with, even though these may be the major allergens for the patient, the results will be less satisfactory.

7

The air we breathe

'Things have changed a lot.'

'If I come in contact with anyone smoking – especially if I've been sensitized by something else, and I've got a bit of asthma anyway – I get this particular type of a cough and my lungs lock up. I feel that all the elasticity in my lungs suddenly vanishes. I also get sinusitis really quickly if I spend a night anywhere smoky.

'I don't go to pubs now, or smoky venues of any sort, and if people are smoking in a room I leave. Even just walking down the street behind someone who is smoking can start me off a bit.

'Nobody would light up a cigarette in a house in Australia now without asking – in fact people even say "Would you mind if I go outside and have a cigarette?" They don't like to smoke in the garden unless they've asked you. Things have changed a lot.'

AIR POLLUTION

This section deals primarily with *man-made* substances – such as factory
fumes and vehicle exhaust – which can act as *irritants* to sensitive
airways. Natural airborne substances that can cause allergic reactions
(such as pollen and mould spores) are dealt with in Chapter 6.

For the most part, this section deals with *outdoor* pollutants. Indoor
pollution is dealt with in full on pp. 221–6.

Can air pollution trigger asthma attacks?

In talking about asthma and pollution, it's important to remember
that not all polluted air is polluted in the same way. There are huge
differences between the sooty air of an old-fashioned industrial town,
the exhaust-laden air of a modern city, the concentrated diesel fumes
of a bus station, and the apparently clean but actually very polluted air
in the countryside close to large cities. Each has its own particular
pollutants, and each affects asthma in a different way.

Some of the ingredients in polluted air can certainly trigger asthma
attacks in people who are already asthmatic. But the effects are
relatively small – much smaller than most people imagine. For
example, a study that looked at hospital admissions in London, Paris,
Helsinki and Barcelona found that high levels of pollution only
increased hospital admissions for asthma by about 3 per cent. By
comparison, a thunderstorm in London in 1994 increased hospital
admissions to *ten times* their usual levels – that's 1000 per cent. There
was no obvious link with air pollution in this case: levels of pollutants
in London were not high on the night of the storm. So it is important
to keep air pollution in proportion.

The main culprits in triggering attacks are:

- **sulphur dioxide**, which may reach problem levels in some
  industrial areas, especially near coal-fired power stations and
  coking plants.
- **ozone**, which can reach unpleasantly high levels in country
  areas that are near large cities, but only on sunny days (see
  pp. 208–9).
- **diesel particulates**, which can become a problem in bus and
  coach stations, in many town centres, and close to main roads
  used by vans, lorries and trucks.

These pollution ingredients are described in more detail on pp. 207–11, and there is advice on avoiding them on pp. 213–5.

Is air pollution causing the asthma epidemic?

In terms of trying to understand the causes of the asthma epidemic, it is essential to bear in mind the difference between *triggering attacks* in an asthmatic and *initiating asthma* in a non-asthmatic. Just because a particular substance can trigger off asthma attacks, it does not necessarily cause asthma to develop in someone who is not asthmatic to begin with. Some pollutants do both, but others (at the concentrations normally breathed) just trigger attacks and nothing more. These pollutants are rather like cold air or exercise – taken in moderation they won't cause anyone to develop asthma, but if you already have asthma they are a hazard.

So which pollutants can increase the likelihood of susceptible people developing asthma? There is some evidence that diesel particulates and sulphur dioxide might do so, and one study also implicates ozone. This study, involving non-smokers in California, suggested that higher ozone exposure could treble the risk of asthma. But only men were affected, not women, which is puzzling, especially as women developed more asthma overall. And no other study has found such a large effect, for ozone or any other pollutant.

Most researchers have found that the effect of pollution in increasing the risk of asthma is small, and that it is only those breathing the highest levels of pollutants who are affected (for example, a child living very close to a road carrying heavy diesel traffic). What is more, those affected must have other risk factors as well. These risk factors are:

- an inherited tendency to allergies and asthma (see pp. 25–6).
- various factors linked to a Western way of life. Some of these lifestyle factors have been identified (see pp. 81–3), but it is difficult to say which are the most important for any particular region, let alone any individual.

So air pollution is not causing the asthma epidemic – it is not even a major factor. This is obvious when we look at the countries and regions that are worst affected by the epidemic. New Zealand has almost no heavy industry, very light road traffic in most parts of the country, and some brisk winds to blow away what little pollution might occur. Yet it has one of the highest rates of asthma in the world, with 17 per cent of 12-year-olds suffering from asthma.

In Australia, asthma rates are as high in the remote outback as they are in the city centres, while in Britain, rates in metropolitan areas are slightly lower than elsewhere. Within the USA, it is true, there is more asthma in inner city areas, but this is probably due to widespread cockroach allergy (see p. 123), combined with high rates of cigarette smoking and an unbalanced diet (see p. 96), rather than to air pollution.

By contrast, many people breathing very dirty air, such as Ghana's urban poor (see p. 79) have very low rates of asthma, scarcely higher than their relatives in distant villages breathing far cleaner air. The study of asthma in East and West Germany, described on p. 78, tells the same story as the Ghanaian research, except that the air in West Germany at the time was actually *cleaner* than that in the East, with about the same level of traffic pollution and far less smoke and sulphur dioxide. Researchers have continued to follow up the German study, and they find that the rates of allergy are now rising in the former East Germany, at the same time as the air has been cleaned up, the economy revives and society becomes more Westernized. Asthma rates are about the same at present, but the increase in the allergy rates may be followed by an increase in asthma.

Air pollution has become the great scapegoat for the asthma epidemic. While it is important to clean up our air – pollution is damaging in many other ways – it does no one any good to blame it as the primary cause of the asthma epidemic. By focusing on air pollution, we are failing to look for the real causes of the epidemic.

The different ingredients in air pollution

Not only is the air in different places polluted in different ways, the types of pollutants in our air have changed over time. As the asthma rates have soared over the past 40–50 years, the levels of some of the most damaging types of pollutants (e.g. sulphur dioxide) have actually been *dropping* in Britain and other Western countries, thanks to tough laws, introduced in the 1950s, curbing industrial emissions. At the same time, however, pollutants from traffic exhaust, especially diesel particulates, have increased. It is important to know about the particular ingredients that are found in polluted air, because they all affect asthma in different ways.

Sulphur dioxide
Where is it found?
Sulphur dioxide is produced by burning coal at home, and by coal-fired power stations, coking plants, and some factories. Levels of sulphur dioxide in British air peaked in 1960 and have been declining ever since, as the Clean Air Act of 1956 has taken effect. Throughout the Western world, sulphur dioxide levels are now fairly low.

Acid aerosols form when sulphur dioxide in the air combines with mist or fog to form droplets of acid suspended in the air. They are found in the same areas as sulphur dioxide and are assumed to have similar effects on asthma.

Can it trigger attacks for asthmatics?
Sulphur dioxide gas forms an acid when it enters the lungs, and acts as an irritant to the airways. In high concentrations it can make the airways constrict, triggering off attacks in asthmatics, who are far more sensitive to sulphur dioxide than healthy people. But at the sort of concentrations normally encountered, even in quite polluted air, sulphur dioxide does not have any effect on most asthmatics.

Can it encourage asthma to develop in non-asthmatics?
Some evidence suggests that sulphur dioxide may make children more likely to develop asthma, but there is disagreement among researchers about this.

Nitrogen dioxide
Several different oxides of nitrogen are produced in exhaust fumes. The one that seems to have most effect on asthmatics is nitrogen dioxide.

Where is it found?
Nitrogen dioxide is produced by all types of vehicle, and by power stations and some factories. Indoors, nitrogen dioxide comes from cigarettes, gas cookers and fires, and kerosene-burning stoves. In towns and cities with a lot of motor traffic, nitrogen dioxide can build up to high levels, especially during inversions (see p. 229).

If you cook with gas or have gas fires, you are actually more likely to encounter high levels of nitrogen dioxide at home than you are on a city street. Peak levels of nitrogen dioxide in kitchens with gas cookers are often ten times the average level on the street, and frequently exceed standards for outdoor air set by the World Health Organization.

Can it trigger attacks for asthmatics?

Nitrogen dioxide is capable of causing the most sensitive asthmatic airways to tighten, but the effect is not great and there have been major episodes of nitrogen dioxide pollution, without any substantial increase in hospital admissions for asthma.

The main problem caused by nitrogen dioxide is that for some people with allergies, it enhances their response to the allergen. So if you inhale dust-mite allergen together with nitrogen dioxide, it may have more effect than dust-mite allergen inhaled alone. Inhaling sulphur dioxide and nitrogen dioxide together boosts the response to allergen more powerfully than either gas alone.

Can it encourage asthma to develop in non-asthmatics?

For those who are not yet sensitized, the high levels of nitrogen dioxide found in some homes may make allergic reactions more likely to develop. In one Canadian study, children exposed to moderate levels of nitrogen dioxide in the home were two-and-a-half times as likely to have asthma as those breathing low levels of nitrogen dioxide, while those with the highest levels were *ten times* as likely to develop asthma. (If a dog, cat or other furry pet was kept, *and* there were high nitrogen dioxide levels, the risk of developing asthma shot up even higher, to 25 times that of children with low nitrogen dioxide and no pets.) Gas cookers were the major factor in producing these very high levels of nitrogen dioxide.

Outdoor pollution with nitrogen dioxide, being at a lower concentration, does not seem to have the same effect. For example, British towns have four times as much nitrogen dioxide as remote rural areas of Britain, yet allergies and asthma are no more common in towns. A study in Japan has confirmed that people exposed to more outdoor nitrogen dioxide do not have more asthma, nor more severe asthma.

Ozone

Where is it found?

When car exhaust fumes are exposed to sunlight, a chemical reaction occurs with oxygen in the air, which produces ozone, a highly reactive form of oxygen. Further chemical reactions then occur, involving another product of exhaust fumes, and ozone is broken down again. Because of this second reaction, there is often very little ozone in city air: it all breaks down again very quickly. But 20 miles or so outside a big city, in areas *upwind* of the city (for example, the countryside and towns just south-west of London), the ozone from the urban traffic can build up. In these more rural areas, ozone does not break down again because the pollutants are too dispersed for the second reaction to occur. So ozone, unlike other traffic pollutants, is usually at much higher levels in the country than in the town. Apart from the cities themselves, only remote country areas escape this ozone pollution.

Ozone levels tend to peak in the late afternoon and early evening. In Britain, ozone only reaches very high levels in the summer, but in hotter, sunnier climates there may be a problem with ozone pollution all year round. Once outdoor air gets indoors, ozone breaks down very quickly because of contact with other gases inside the house.

Many people are confused about ozone, because the destruction of the ozone layer is always described as a very damaging event for the Earth. But that ozone layer (which screens the Earth from harmful ultraviolet light) is thousands of feet up in the sky, well away from our lungs. At ground level, ozone is a different matter. Under natural conditions, there is very little ozone in the air we breathe.

Can it trigger attacks for asthmatics?

Asthmatics and non-asthmatics alike can be affected by ozone, with a constriction in their airways. Healthy people tend not to notice these effects, but asthmatics may have more symptoms, and may need more drugs, on days when ozone levels are high. Fortunately the effects are relatively small, and even when there are serious episodes of ozone pollution, this does not produce a huge increase in hospital admissions for asthma.

It takes 4 to 24 hours for ozone to produce its effects on the airways, so there may be a considerable time-lag between when you are exposed to ozone and when you experience symptoms.

Ozone poses another problem for some asthmatics, increasing the effects of allergen. It can heighten the reaction to pollen, for example.

Can it encourage asthma to develop in non-asthmatics?

One study in California found that ozone could increase the risk of developing asthma, but only among men (see p. 205). Many researchers are doubtful about this finding, because it does not fit in with other evidence about the distribution of asthma around the world.

Diesel exhaust particles
Where are they found?

Diesel fuel contains oil mixed in with the petrol, so when it burns it produces tiny particles. These consist of flakes of carbon (soot), coated with complex chemicals that are produced by the partial combustion of oil.

Diesel particulates, as they are known, are now the main particulates in most of the polluted air in the West. It is probably the chemicals on the surface of the particles that affect asthmatics, rather than the particles themselves.

Particulates build up when there is high barometric pressure, especially if there is an inversion (see p. 229). In Britain, the highest levels usually occur in winter.

Stricter enforcement of regulations on diesel emissions would help keep levels down and the public can assist by reporting vehicles that are belching black fumes (see pp. 458–9). Buses are often the worst offenders, and the air inside bus stations can be filthy. Don't be afraid to complain to the bus company – doing so in writing is best.

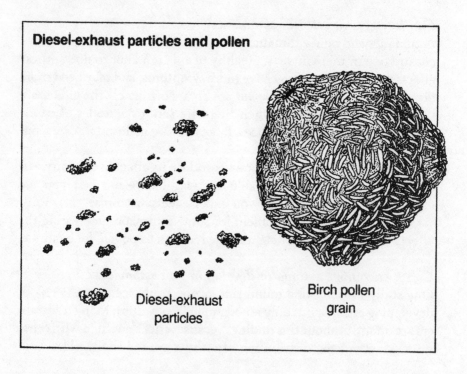

Diesel-exhaust particles and pollen

Diesel-exhaust particles

Birch pollen grain

Can they trigger attacks for asthmatics?

High levels of diesel particulates in the air tend to cause more symptoms for asthmatics, and more use of inhalers. There is a sharp increase in asthma attacks when levels rise above 50 μg per cubic metre. A study in Birmingham, England, showed that such levels were regularly reached at roadsides. (*Note that 'μg' is another way of writing microgram or mcg.*)

Can they encourage asthma to develop in non-asthmatics?

Some research suggests that diesel particulates might increase the risk of allergies and asthma developing, but this remains controversial.

Other particles and dusts

Coal- and wood-smoke particles

Burning coal or wood produces black smoke particles, but these are very different from diesel particulates. Up to the 1950s or 1960s, the particulate counts for polluted air consisted mainly of this type of particle. Since then, particulates of this kind have fallen drastically, especially in cities. However, in heavily industrialized areas such as East Germany, particulates of this type remained plentiful until quite recently.

These smoke particles do not seem to make asthma more likely to develop – in fact, quite the reverse. When researchers looked at children living in rural areas of Bavaria in southern Germany, they found that those who had coal or wood stoves in their homes were less likely to have allergies or asthma. It is possible that these children also had a more traditional kind of diet, or certain other factors that protected them from asthma. But some researchers believe that the smoke could be directly protective, and the fact that coal or wood stoves were linked with lower asthma rates in an Australian study makes this more plausible.

How could smoke possibly protect against asthma? Dr Erika von Mutius, who carried out the research in Bavaria, found that other chest diseases, such as bronchitis and pneumonia, were more common in those with wood and coal stoves. She speculates that when babies and young children suffer such infections their immune systems are stimulated in such a way that allergies are less likely to develop later (see pp. 26–7). Dr von Mutius also carried out the study that showed much lower rates of allergies and asthma in the former

East Germany (see p. 78), and she suggests that the same protective
effect could have been operating to keep asthma and allergy rates low
in the smoky eastern cities.

Latex particles
When your car tyres wear out, what happens to all that rubber? A lot
of it rubs off as tiny rubber (latex) particles which become airborne
and are inhaled. These are not irritants, they are – potentially –
allergens, but we mention them here because air that is polluted
with traffic fumes will also contain a lot of latex particles. These *might*
affect people who are severely allergic to latex (see p. 282), but there
is no evidence yet that they actually do. Latex particles will not affect
most asthmatics.

Soil dust, coal dust and mineral dust particles
In very dry areas, there may be soil or mineral dust blowing about in
the air, and some asthmatics find that this sparks off an attack.
Prolonged exposure can lead to a general worsening of asthma. Such
particles are simply acting as irritants: they do not contain the same
allergens as house dust. Coal or coke dust and the dust found in
mining areas may have a similar effect.

Wood dust, flour and bean dust
Many of the dusts found in sawmills, bakeries, food-processing
factories and food-storage facilities contain potent allergens derived
from plants. People who work with such flours and dusts are at risk of
developing asthma (see pp. 280–1) and will then remain sensitive to
the product concerned. Note that most of these dusts are allergens
rather than irritants.

Occasionally these allergenic dusts affect asthmatics in the general
public, as with several serious outbreaks of asthma in Barcelona in the
1980s, which were due to soybean dust (see p. 124).

Industrial pollution and local asthma rates
There have been several different reports of very high asthma rates in
particular areas, linked to some form of industrial pollution. Some
reports have concerned dock areas where oil is loaded into tankers,
others have claimed that asthma rates are unusually high downwind
of oil refineries and oil-burning power stations, while others have

made similar claims about cement works that are powered by burning a mix of waste solvents known as Cemfuel. None of these instances have been investigated satisfactorily, so it is impossible to say if there is a link with asthma. Little is known about which pollutants might be responsible, if there is indeed a link with asthma around these industrial sites, but it is something that should be investigated further.

Coping with air pollution

First, keep air pollution in perspective (see pp. 205–6). There are many other factors that have a much larger effect on asthma.

- If you have very severe asthma, you know that certain pollutants affect you, and you have a choice about venturing out or staying home, check on air quality before venturing outside, (see Useful Addresses).
- Summer afternoons and early evenings are the worst for ozone (see p. 209), so plan your activities accordingly, especially jogging, cycling or outdoor sports.
- When driving, if you have to pull up behind a lorry or bus, keep your distance, close the window and turn off the fan. Diesel vehicles often emit a thick cloud of particles as they set off, and this can come straight into your car through the air intakes or through open windows. Such heavy exposures set off severe attacks for some asthmatics.
- When in polluted air, breathing through your nose may reduce the amount of sulphur dioxide that reaches your lungs, and it may reduce other pollutants as well. If your nose is usually blocked, the exercises on p. 425 and p. 432 should help to unblock it.
- A mask that removes diesel particles or gases or both may also be useful (see p. 481) during periods of high pollution. Make sure that it does not restrict your breathing.
- During periods of high ozone or sulphur dioxide pollution, taking supplements of Vitamin C and Vitamin E, and eating plenty of foods that contain beta-carotene (see p. 99) will reduce the impact on your airways.
- If you live very close to a main road, you would probably reduce the chance of your children developing asthma by moving house. The message emerging from the latest research is that it is goods vehicles (lorries and trucks) which matter –

they have much more influence on asthma than cars do because of all the diesel particulates they produce. *The effects of moving will not be huge*, and it is important to take other preventive measures as well (see p. 87). For children and adults who already have asthma, and who live close to a main road, moving further away from a main road would also be beneficial, but again the effects will be limited.

- Buying a high-quality HEPA air filter to remove diesel particles from the indoor air may be a worthwhile alternative for those who live very close to a main road and cannot move house. The filter will also remove pollen and other allergens.
- When buying a new car, you can make your personal contribution to air quality by choosing a non-diesel vehicle and buying one with a catalytic converter fitted. The converter reduces the quantity of nitrogen oxides emitted. If you do need to buy a diesel vehicle, ask that it be fitted with a particle filter of the kind now fitted as standard in Germany. A car with air conditioning will reduce your exposure to diesel particulates while driving.
- If you are moving to a new area, you might want to investigate air quality levels before you choose your new home city.
- Remember that damaging levels of nitrogen dioxide are most likely to be generated *indoors*, by gas cookers and heaters (see pp. 207–8).
- Buses pumping out black smoke can be reported to your local transit authority or department of transportation. The more people complain, the more will be done to reduce this particular hazard.

Understanding pollution reports and forecasts

Pollution reports and forecasts may relate to ozone, nitrogen dioxide or particulates.

When counts are given for particulates in the air, this includes both diesel particulates and other particulates, such as those from smoky factories or domestic fires using wood or coal. But for most readers of this book, the particulates in the air will be made up almost entirely of diesel particles.

In official sources these counts will often appear as 'PM10', meaning 'Particulate Matter less than 10 microns in diameter'. This particle size is chosen because larger particles tend to settle in the nose and throat and do not reach the airways. On television, the term 'Small Particles' is used instead of PM10.

The particle counts may underestimate the quantity of particles you actually breathe, especially if you are driving, or spending much of the day beside busy roads.

'You'd think they might just be grateful . . .'

Ella first developed asthma as a child. 'My asthma wasn't so bad until we moved to Los Angeles, but now I have a lot of attacks, especially when the pollution is high. Most people understand about asthma here, but where I lived before it was different. I was told by a neighbour once that if I just controlled myself I wouldn't have any asthma. Another time, I had to tell someone at work that I had asthma, and she said "You must be anxious about something to have that." There's an attitude that says, "If you have asthma, it's your fault."

'I figure people like that are never sick themselves, and they think it's because they're doing something right, or because they are better than you. You'd think they might just be grateful for their own good health, and not want to feel all self-righteous about it as well.'

CIGARETTE SMOKING – THE LINK WITH ASTHMA

Having asthma and smoking cigarettes is about as sensible as suffering from dizzy spells and taking up tight-rope walking. Yet many people with asthma do smoke, especially in their teens and early twenties. It is something that makes doctors very depressed, because smoking is bound to make asthma worse, or to perpetuate asthma that would otherwise have gone away. For those who have 'grown out of' their asthma, it doubles the chance of it coming back (see p. 43). And smoking increases the risk of an infection that can lead to severe or 'brittle' asthma (see p. 256). Doctors often feel they are fighting a losing battle, giving asthma drugs to people who are deliberately doing something that will make their asthma worse.

If you have asthma, it is extremely important that you give up smoking. Life-long smoking can lead to chronic bronchitis or emphysema developing in middle age, and this is especially likely in anyone with asthma. This combination of breathing problems is called COPD (see p. 32) and it is usually lifelong and incurable, leading to greater and greater levels of breathlessness and disability. In the worst cases, people with COPD need a cylinder of oxygen just to be able to get up from the armchair and cross the room. Do whatever you can to avoid going down this road: and that means giving up smoking *now*.

If you already have COPD, giving up smoking will help you, however far advanced your disease. Your life expectancy increases the minute you stop smoking, and your level of disability should stabilize rather than continuing to deteriorate.

Even those who don't have asthma, but who come from families with a tendency to allergies, should not smoke. Being a smoker will greatly increase your chances of developing asthma when exposed to some other allergen or irritant in the air. To give one example, when there was an outbreak of occupational asthma at a salmon-processing plant in Scotland, none of the 230 non-smokers were affected, but of the 60 smokers, 40 per cent developed asthma. This shows how vulnerable and sensitive your airways become when you smoke.

Smoking parents and asthmatic children
Parents who smoke make their children's asthma worse, and teenagers are as badly affected as young children. Don't think, because you have been smoking around your asthmatic child for years, that there is no

point stopping now: it is definitely a case of 'better late than never'. No one living with an asthmatic child should smoke indoors, and visitors to the house who smoke should be asked to do so outside.

Should you be hoping to have another baby, giving up smoking is even more important, because smoking during pregnancy increases the risk of a woman's baby developing asthma (see p. 89). Bearing in mind that smoking also leads to more still-births and cot deaths, there are plenty of reasons for giving up.

Passive smoking

It goes without saying that those who have asthma should not be forced to breathe other people's cigarette smoke. Research shows that this can trigger asthma attacks in the short term, and makes asthmatics generally worse in the long run. If you are asthmatic and members of your family smoke, come to an agreement that they always smoke out of doors, or in a room that is especially set aside for them, with the windows open and the door closed. It is the least you can expect of your family.

Workers too have a right to breathe clean air in their workplace. An American study showed that non-smokers were more likely to develop asthma if they worked alongside a smoker. Your employer has a legal duty to provide you with clean air, and that includes ensuring that other employees do not force cigarette smoke on you. Separate areas should be created for smoking and non-smoking workers, or, if this is impossible, effective air conditioning or air filters should be installed. Insist on your rights calmly but firmly, and if you don't get anywhere ask the trade union for help.

For many people, avoiding cigarette smoke is most difficult during their leisure time. Sometimes it seems to be a choice between taking care of your health and having a social life, especially in the winter when doors and windows are closed and you cannot sit outdoors in cafés, bars or pubs. If you are determined to improve your asthma, there are ways of tackling this problem:

- Draw up a list of friends who smoke, and decide which are real friends, who you don't want to give up, and which are just acquaintances. You will probably have lost touch with the acquaintances in five years' time anyway: there is no reason to go on breathing their cigarette smoke.
- Decide to explain asthma, and the risks it entails, to the friends

who matter. It may help to get some leaflets on asthma from the Asthma and Allergy Foundation of America or a similar organization (see Useful Addresses).

- If you really want to take a strong stand on this, you could also get leaflets from ASH (Action on Smoking and Health) or a similar campaigning organization. These leaflets explain why smokers should give up for the sake of their own health (see Useful Addresses).
- Invest in some nicotine chewing-gum (available at chemists' shops) and offer your friends this when they reach for a cigarette. It will stop the craving for tobacco.
- Find out about non-smoking cafés, restaurants and pubs in your area. There are an increasing number of these (see p. 458).
- When friends come to your house, ask them to smoke outside. More and more people are doing this now, whether they have asthma or not. Your friends will soon get used to it. Have nicotine chewing-gum available as an alternative.
- If you have a favourite restaurant or pub that is particularly smoky, talk to the owner or manager about installing a good-quality air filter, or write a letter if that would be easier. Explain that it will be good for business because non-smokers and asthmatics such as yourself are currently being deterred by all the smoke.

Giving up smoking

If you yourself are the smoker, your doctor can help you give up with advice and support, and by prescribing nicotine replacements, such as chewing-gum or skin-patches, which may be cheaper on prescription than if bought over the counter. Research has shown that more smokers actually succeed in quitting if they are helped by nicotine replacements, which release nicotine into the blood and help ease withdrawal symptoms. Patches are probably the best method, with a slightly higher success rate than gum despite the fact that they sometimes cause skin irritation. Intra-nasal sprays seem to be a little less effective than the other methods.

Once you have stopped smoking altogether, you should gradually wean yourself off the nicotine replacement.

Telephone or Internet advice can provide helpful support while try-ing to give up cigarettes (see Useful Addresses).

'But a cigarette helps when I have an asthma attack ...'

Some smokers believe that reaching for a cigarette, at the same time as they reach for their inhaler, actually helps to stave off an asthma attack. What probably happens is that the thought of the cigarette calms them down and stops them from panicking.

Feelings of panic often play a large part in asthma attacks, and can make the asthma considerably worse by altering the breathing pattern to an unhealthy form of breathing known as hyperventilation (see p. 419). The soothing effects of getting a cigarette out and lighting it (a small ritual which makes many smokers feel in control of their lives) may help by stopping the panic before it starts. This does not mean that the cigarette itself is of any help – quite the reverse, because it is aggravating the inflammation in the airways. But once this illusion is established in your mind, it will be hard to break.

If you are someone who lights up when you start to wheeze, remember that the cigarette only *seems* to help, and that in the long term it is stoking up the inflammation and making another attack increasingly likely. There are other ways of learning not to panic, and these will be of long-term benefit to your airways. Yoga is one useful approach, and learning a martial art such as aikido is another. The Buteyko Method also deals with this problem. For a full range of suggestions see Useful Addresses.

Physiotherapy may be useful in shifting stubborn mucus from your airways: ask your doctor if you can be referred to a physiotherapist (see p. 298).

'. . . it's not the worst one a parent could imagine . . .'

'Danny was asthmatic as a child, and he is a smoker now. It does worry us, of course, but there's nothing really that we can do about it. I suppose, of all the risky behaviours that young males are likely to engage in, it's not the worst one a parent could imagine.'

For the parents of asthmatic children, 'letting go' is difficult but necessary. It may be better to remain philosophical, as Danny's father suggests, and to keep a good relationship going, than to try to change a teenager's behaviour by constant nagging and lecturing.

'. . . you'd get prosecuted for arson . . .'

Tim is a GP with several hundred asthmatics among his patients:
'Suppose you came home every evening, struck a few matches,
tossed them on the floor, waited until there was smoke everywhere and then rang the Fire Brigade. The first night the Fire
Brigade would come. The second night the Fire Brigade would
come. And the third night? – they'd come, and you'd get
prosecuted for arson. That's what happens if you knowingly
create "inflammation" in your house. But doctors are expected
uncomplainingly to treat patients with asthma who smoke, and
to go on treating them month after month, year after year,
calming down the inflammation in the airways that they have
caused themselves. These asthmatics are damaging themselves,
they are damaging people around them by making others
breathe their cigarette smoke, they are wasting money on cigarettes and expensive inhalers and other treatment. The fact they
are wasting my time is the least of it really. Why do asthmatics do
it? I don't understand. It is crazy for anyone to smoke, given what
we know about the health effects, but it is particularly suicidal for
asthmatics.'

'I didn't know it was asthma . . .'

Sven is 28 and has had asthma for seven years. 'I had pollen
allergy as a child, in my nose and my eyes, so I was sneezing all
the time. I was 21 when I developed asthma. I didn't know it was
asthma – I thought I had a problem with my lungs or my throat
because I used to cough badly and produce a lot of phlegm.
  'I got this first when I was in Greece for a summer. I was
smoking a lot, and all my friends there were smoking, so I
thought "Oh, something has happened with my lungs because
of the smoking." Then when I came home to Sweden this cough
went on for several weeks and didn't improve, so I went to my
doctor and he said "Basically, you've got asthma." I was really
surprised.'

INDOOR AIR POLLUTION
AND HOW TO PREVENT IT IN YOUR HOME

For many people, the air they breathe at home is much more polluted than any outdoor air. Some of the pollutants in our houses can trigger asthma attacks, or make asthma more likely to develop in young children.

Note that this section mainly deals with man-made substances in the air, not with natural substances such as mould spores which are allergens. Advice on getting rid of indoor allergens is given on pp. 127–78.

Cooking and heating

Making the right choices about cooking and heating appliances can have major benefits for those in the household who are asthmatic. The chances of young children developing asthma can also be reduced.

Choosing your cooking stove

Cooking with a gas stove substantially increases the levels of nitrogen dioxide in the house. Breathing large amounts of this gas may increase the risk of asthma developing in a child, especially if there are concentrated allergens in the house – from a pet, for example (see pp. 207–8). Adults and children who already have asthma may have some irritation of the airways from the nitrogen dioxide, and their sensitivity to allergens will be increased.

Cooking with electricity is a much better option. If you can't afford to change your existing gas stove, open the windows while you are cooking – more than one so you get a good draught blowing through – or put in a powerful extractor fan. If you are hoping to prevent asthma developing in your children, you should aim to keep them out of the kitchen while you are cooking, and close the kitchen door.

Choosing the heating in your house

Certain types of heating are linked with a greater risk of asthma:
Central heating that works by ducting hot air into rooms made wheezing four times more likely in one British study and was probably a risk factor for asthma in a Canadian study. This could be due to dust-mite allergens or some other allergens or irritants being blown into the rooms – no one has investigated further.

Enclosed glass-fronted fires burning solid fuel have been linked to a greater chance of asthma developing in British children, for reasons that are not understood.

Within Britain, the highest recorded rates of asthma are found in the Isle of Skye. Rates for asthma among 12-year-olds are 17 per cent in Skye, compared to 10–12 per cent in most of mainland Britain. Recent research suggests that the high rates in Skye and other Scottish islands are linked to the traditional method of heating local houses: burning peat. Factors linked with modern life, such as dietary changes (see pp. 81–3), could be making modern children more susceptible to the peat smoke than previous generations.
Other types of heating are linked with a reduced risk of asthma:
Open fires seemed to reduce the risk of asthma developing by about half in one English study. Better ventilation probably explains this (see p. 148). However, open fires may not be good for everyone: some asthmatics find that attacks are triggered by coal and wood smoke. If you do decide to have an open fire, it is very important that the chimney is clear and there is good circulation of air around the fire.

Researchers in Germany and Australia have found that coal or wood stoves are linked with a reduced risk of asthma (see p. 211).

Housework
Air fresheners provoke asthma attacks in some people. If you are ventilating your house well, you won't need an air freshener as the air will smell naturally fresh. Incidentally, air fresheners don't actually do anything to the air except add perfume to it. The way they cover up bad odours is by giving off a chemical that partially disables your sense of smell. For some people, this chemical has quite severe and far-reaching effects on health. In such cases, eliminating air fresheners can get rid of a whole range of puzzling symptoms, not just asthma.

Furniture polish and oven cleaner were never intended to go into the airways, but when you spray them from an aerosol can, inevitably that is what happens. Avoid using aerosols as much as you can. There have been no research studies about their effects on asthma, but it makes sense to avoid inhaling foreign substances which could irritate the airways. Most of the products now sold in aerosol form can be bought in non-aerosol forms which work just as well and are cheaper. It makes sense to avoid deodorant in aerosol form too – this can be extremely irritating to the airways. The Irish Medical Organization has recently called for a ban on aerosols in school gyms and sports centres because they have triggered asthma attacks.

Don't use fly spray or other insecticides if you can help it. A study from Ethiopia showed that people who used the insecticide Malathion in the home were twice as likely to develop allergy to dust mite. Most other insecticides have not been tested, but a study of Canadian farmers suggested that asthma might be linked with the use of carbamate insecticides (e.g. carbofuran).

Take care with bleach and other chlorine-based cleaning products, such as toilet cleaner and scouring powder. Misuse of these can lead to chlorine gas being released in unusually large amounts, and this can irritate the airways of asthmatics. Never allow bleach or toilet cleaner to become mixed with any other product. Take care with any product containing hypochlorite, chloramine, ammonia, acids or morpholine. Be careful also with the chemicals used for swimming-pool water.

Check all new products carefully before you use them. It is not just what is in them that matters, but what gases they might give off when used. An American asthmatic died within minutes when the de-rusting agent she was using to clean her dishwasher produced a cloud of sulphur dioxide (see p. 207) fumes: her airways tightened up so much that her family could do nothing to save her, despite having inhalers to hand. So read labels carefully. The words 'sulphuric', 'suphate' or 'sulphite' in the list of ingredients should alert you to the possibility that sulphur dioxide will be given off by this product. If in any doubt, find another way to do the job, or get someone else to do it for you (open the windows wide first, and leave the room while it's being done).

One of the worst irritants in indoor air is, of course, tobacco smoke. Do whatever you can to eliminate it from your home and workplace (see p. 217).

Home improvements and DIY

Formaldehyde is a commonly used chemical that can provoke asthma attacks in some people. Those most at risk are people who have worked with formaldehyde resin or formaldehyde gas (see p. 285) and acquired a sensitivity in this way. Formaldehyde is given off by injected foam cavity wall insulation. There is a type of insulation known as Micafil which is free from formaldehyde.

MDF (medium-density fibreboard), which is often used for shelving and other DIY projects, gives off a small amount of formaldehyde when sawn. It also produces very fine dust particles which should not be inhaled. Current government advice is to work outside, or in a very well-ventilated area, and to wear a high-grade dust mask.

Be careful to ventilate the work area well, and to wear a dust mask, when installing loft insulation. The MMMFs (man-made mineral fibres) used produce a fine dust which may be responsible for various diseases, including asthma.

When it comes to redecorating, it may be wise to use low-odour paints. The smell of fresh paint is due to the solvents used to make the paint, and these may act as irritants to the airways. Quite a few asthmatics are made worse by wet paint. Most DIY shops now sell low-odour water-based gloss paint, but some of the best low-odour paints, formulated specifically for those with medical problems, are only available by mail order. Tests with paint-sensitive asthmatics show that they do not wheeze with these paints.

If you are told that your house needs to be sprayed with insecticide for woodworm, ask some searching questions before you agree. Builders and surveyors often recommend spraying as a matter of course, without really thinking whether it is necessary. Ask what will happen if you don't have the house sprayed – and how quickly it will happen. There are some very old houses still standing with wood-worm holes all over them. Unless you have a heavy infestation that is threatening the structure of the house, you may be better off not having the house sprayed. All the insecticides used are toxic to some extent. Dieldrin is the worst, and should be avoided at all costs. Pyrethroid insecticides are the least likely to cause problems but can produce allergic reactions.

Polyurethane foam has caused problems for some asthmatics, because it is made using isocyanates, probably the most potent of all asthma-causing chemicals (see pp. 284–5). This foam is used in car seats, foam mattresses and furniture, and cutting or drilling it can affect the airways of people already sensitized to isocyanates at work. More worryingly, there are now 'instant foam' kits sold for DIY insulation, where mixing two different liquids together, or combining the contents of two separate aerosols, creates polyurethane foam. During the mixing process, levels of isocyanate are released that can breach the safety limit set for factories. It is not just those who have been sensitized to isocyanates at work who could be affected by such products: other asthmatics could also react very badly. In two cases from Massachusetts, DIY foam kits produced serious asthma attacks the second time they were used.

In the garage and garden
Petrol can affect some people with asthma and bring on their symptoms. Kerosene and paraffin may have the same effect. These fuels should always be in airtight containers, and any appliances that emit the smell of the fuel should be disposed of (they are probably dangerous in other ways too). Get someone else to do jobs which might involve inhalation of fumes, such as filling the car or a petrol-driven lawnmower.

Breathing a high dose of exhaust fumes, especially those from diesel cars, can inflame the airways. Try not to be in the garage with the car engine running for any length of time.

In the garden, avoid using pesticides as much as possible (see p. 223). Smoke from bonfires and barbecues may act as irritants and trigger asthma attacks for some people.

Paints sold for cars are likely to contain isocyanates, one of the most troublesome causes of work-related asthma (see pp. 284–5). If you have been sensitized to isocyanates at work, you should certainly not use such paint. Other asthmatics can probably use such paint safely but should make sure the area is well ventilated, and avoid prolonged or repeated exposure to the paint.

Choosing a place to live
A study in Canada found that children whose first home was a newer house (built after 1970) were 50 per cent more likely to develop asthma than children living in older houses. It seems plausible that this is due to the chemicals used in the construction and fitting of new houses, especially the plastics, preservatives and insulation materials. Gases are still being given off by these substances some years later.

Chemical sensitivity
Generally speaking, the hazards described so far are likely to affect most asthmatics, or a large proportion of asthmatics. But there are also some hazards that only affect a tiny minority of asthmatics – people who are especially sensitive to man-made chemicals and react very badly to a wide range of items.

This problem is often described as an 'allergy' to chemicals, but it is not an allergy in the strict sense of the word. It seems to be caused by a failure of some of the detoxification mechanisms which normally protect us by breaking down toxic chemicals which get into the body. People who have chemical sensitivity often have food intolerance (see p. 181) as well, including intolerance to food additives. They are likely to have a multitude of puzzling symptoms, in addition to their asthma, and to be greeted with despairing or disbelieving looks by their doctor, since chemical sensitivity is not yet recognized by conventional medicine.

If you suffer from chemical sensitivity, you will almost certainly have noticed the connection because the reactions are fairly immediate in most cases. The sort of things that may cause problems include perfumes and after-shave, petrol fumes, newspaper ink, pesticides, plastics and synthetic fibres. Avoidance of everything that provokes symptoms is the best treatment, but may be difficult, especially if you are away from home. There are specialist suppliers (see p. 470) who sell bedding, paints and other items designed for those with chemical sensitivity. Diagnosis and treatment in an 'environmentally controlled unit' can be valuable for some people with multiple sensitivities. Some forms of desensitization may reduce symptoms: neutralization (see p. 201) is particularly useful and EPD (see p. 200) is also worth trying.

'I was using a face mask some of the time . . .'

Richard developed asthma in his 50s. 'I started getting the asthma two years ago, when I was doing up the house. I had to cut up a lot of plasterboard and I was using a face mask some of the time, but not consistently. When you're doing lots of little jobs it's not always easy, you don't bother. The mask doesn't fit over my moustache properly anyway, it always leaks.

'I'd actually been doing up the house for a couple of years then, and breathing lots of brick dust and so on, but it seemed to be the plasterboard that did it. Funnily enough, I've got a friend who's a builder – he's using plasterboard all the time, and he's got terrible asthma. It's a really fine dust, it gets everywhere.'

WHY DOES THE WEATHER AFFECT ASTHMA?

Many asthmatics notice that the weather affects their asthma. The reasons for this vary enormously: sometimes it is the weather itself, and sometimes the effect of the weather on allergens or irritants in the air. Understanding exactly why certain weather conditions have this effect may allow you to control your asthma symptoms more effectively.

Cold weather

Asthmatics are often badly affected by cold air, especially when they go outdoors from a warm room. Their airways tighten very suddenly, as a result of airway-muscle contraction (see p. 22).

Everyone has always assumed that this was a direct effect of cold air on the airways. But new research from Finland has shown that this is wrong.

The Finnish researchers found, much to their surprise, that as long as the face is kept warm, even breathing sub-freezing air will not make the airway muscles contract. On the other hands, exposing the face to sub-freezing temperatures, while breathing warm air, will produce airway contraction.

The research shows clearly that what makes the airways contract is cold air hitting the skin of the face. Nerves in the face that sense cold communicate directly with the muscles surrounding the airways and tell them to contract. Non-asthmatics show exactly the same reaction, although they suffer no obvious symptoms as a result.

This is an extremely useful piece of research, because it shows that there is an easy way to overcome the effects of cold air on asthma: simply keep the face warm. Either wear a scarf around your face, or invest in a balaclava helmet (camping shops, outdoor shops and cycling shops should stock these).

Note that this only overcomes the immediate effect of cold air on the airway muscles. In the long term, breathing cold air while you exercise may have a damaging effect on the airway linings, making them inflamed and sensitive, leading to asthma symptoms (see pp. 295–6).

Damp weather

Asthmatics who get worse in damp weather usually find that they are allergic to mould spores. These are more numerous on damp days, especially in autumn and early winter when moulds are growing rapidly on fallen leaves and fruit.

Check the list on p. 117 to see if mould allergy is likely. Skin-prick tests may be useful in confirming this (see p. 126). Advice on avoiding moulds is given on pp. 165–70. If avoidance is not effective, desensitization might prove useful (see pp. 197–202).

Damp weather also favours house dust mites (see p. 116) but because our houses are generally rather moist all year round, you are unlikely to experience a sudden increase in symptoms during a damp spell.

Rain after drought

In some regions, rain after a long dry spell can affect those allergic to pollen. Moisture causes a sudden release of allergenic particles from the pollen grains that have been accumulating during the dry spell. This problem is common in some areas of Australia, and the culprit pollen is usually rye grass.

Hot, dry weather

During periods of very hot weather in summer, there is often a sudden surge in the number of people arriving in hospital emergency departments with asthma attacks. This may be due to two factors: pollen and air pollution.

Grasses flower in early summer in Britain, as in other countries with a sharply seasonal climate. The flowers (which are green and inconspicuous – don't expect to see a welter of colourful blooms) generally wait for hot dry days to release their pollen. Millions of grass plants, all releasing pollen at once, can create very difficult conditions for those allergic to grasses.

To make matters worse, air pollution often peaks on hot, dry and windless days in summer, particularly ozone (see pp. 208–9) which usually reaches the highest levels in the countryside just outside cities – exactly the sort of grassy places people visit for picnics and days out.

If you suffer more asthma on hot, dry days, it is worth finding out which of these two factors is playing the greater part. Note that only some asthmatics are allergic to grass, whereas almost all asthmatics are affected by ozone (but the extent to which people are affected can vary).

You may already know that you are allergic to grass pollen, but if you are at all unsure, check the list on pp. 121–3, and consider having skin-prick tests (see p. 125). Ideas for avoiding grass pollen are given on pp. 171–8. Desensitization treatment could prove helpful (see p. 197).

There are various ways in which you can have advance warning of high pollution levels, and either avoid them or protect yourself from the pollutants (see pp. 213–4).

Inversions

Warm air rises, which is fortunate as the upward air currents normally carry pollen, mould spores and air pollutants away from our noses and into the sky. At certain times of year, however, some places that are surrounded by hills suffer from inversions: the air at ground level cannot rise because there is a layer of much colder air above. This layer of cold air sits there like a saucepan lid, keeping everything trapped at ground level.

Many asthmatics suffer badly during inversions. The basic causes are much the same as those described above for hot, dry, windless days: nitrogen dioxide, ozone, pollen and other allergens (e.g. mould spores), all building up in the air.

Los Angeles and Mexico City suffer notorious inversions, when the pollution levels are so bad that they affect everybody, not just asthmatics. Rural valleys can also suffer inversions, in which pollen and spores get trapped, but the effects on asthmatics are less drastic because air-pollution levels are low.

The first step to tackling this problem is to identify your allergic reactions more precisely. If mould spores are the culprits, reducing the levels of mould within your home (see p. 166) may be helpful in reducing your asthma symptoms generally, so that you can cope better with inversions. Whichever allergens are at fault, desensitization may be beneficial (see pp. 197–202).

Escaping from inversions is difficult, unless you are free to leave town completely for several days. Air filters, masks and air conditioning can help to protect you from both pollutants and allergens (see pp. 213–4).

Thunderstorms

On the night of 24 June 1994, hospitals all over London were crowded with people suffering from asthma attacks. Some patients had to be given nebulizer treatment while sitting in the corridors, because all the cubicles were doubly occupied. Doctors working in emergency departments were astonished to see ten times the usual number of asthmatics, and some thought there must have been a chemical spill that was affecting people's breathing. As the *British Medical Journal* later observed, 'The number of additional patients in some accident and emergency departments was as great as might be expected from an accident causing mass casualties.'

Detailed investigations later found that there had been no chemical spill and no significant air pollution that night. The culprit was a huge thunderstorm which began earlier that evening. The flood of asthma sufferers began about three hours after the storm had started and continued all through the night.

This is not the first time that thunderstorms have been linked to mass outbreaks of asthma. In some parts of Australia, particularly Melbourne, thunderstorm-related epidemics occur whenever there is a very dry summer.

Many researchers have tried to establish the exact cause of these attacks. Often the pollen count is very high for a day or two before the storm, as it was in the London outbreak. One theory is that rising humidity just before the storm caused a massive release of tiny allergenic particles from the plentiful grass pollen grains in the air, which had a devastating effect on people allergic to grass pollen. In other thunderstorm-related epidemics there have been very high counts of mould spores, as well as pollen, and these too could be responsible.

This alone probably cannot explain the dramatic effects of the thunderstorm. The presence of electrically charged particles in the air may also be crucial because there is a distinct association between lightning strikes and asthma attacks. Perhaps an electrical charge makes the allergens more potent, or the airways more sensitive. Another theory is that, under these unusual conditions, the allergens bind to diesel particulates in the air, and these carry them deep into the lungs where they do not normally go. The sudden fall in temperature that occurred during the London storm could have added to the problems for asthmatic airways.

Most of those who succumbed during the London thunderstorm were young adults with hayfever but relatively mild asthma (or no previous asthma in 44 per cent of cases). They seemed to be a distinct group from the sort of asthmatics who normally finish up in hospital emergency departments.

From a practical point of view, this means that you need only be concerned about thunderstorms if you have reacted badly to one in the past. Should this be the case, watch the weather reports during the summer months, and if a thunderstorm is forecast, double your dose of preventer for the next two days, or until the storm is well past. Stay indoors if possible, or wear a high-quality mask (see p. 480) if you do need to go out. The anti-allergy preventer drug, sodium cromoglycate (see p. 338), can be useful to some people in stopping allergic reactions before they start: talk to your doctor about having this drug available for such occasions, and take it well in advance of the storm.

'. . . he had two little pink patches on his cheeks . . .'

When Sam was a toddler, and he had asthma, the thing I noticed was this cough – a little cough high in the throat with nothing behind it, a very light dry cough. We got tuned in so that the least bit of this would wake us up. Often it would go on for a while and then it would settle down, but once it got into a particular repetitive pattern, you had to get up and do something about it.

'Another thing we noticed – sometimes in the evening if he had two little pink patches on his cheeks, and his eyes were a bit bright, then when you listened to his breathing, you'd usually find it was shallower. That tended to alert me that his asthma was getting worse. It was often like this on evenings when it was really frosty and he'd been playing outside. He'd come in and I'd look at him and think, "Oh dear . . ." When he looked like that it often meant a really bad asthma attack was going to come on in the night.

'In the end, we got so that we could tell it was that kind of evening from the temperature outside, and we'd get him in a bit early. Then he'd be OK.'

CAN ASTHMA ATTACKS BE BROUGHT ON BY SMELLS?

Many asthmatics find that strong smells will bring on an asthma attack. One survey in New York found that smells had a bad effect on 95 per cent of asthmatics. The smells most frequently identified as causing problems were insecticide sprays, household cleaning agents especially those containing ammonia, cigarette smoke, perfume and cologne, fresh paint, traffic exhaust fumes and cooking smells. Sweetly scented flowers such as hyacinths, lilac, lavender and honeysuckle are also a problem for many asthmatics, whereas other quite unpleasant smells may produce no reaction.

A survey of asthma patients in Sweden (where allergy to birch pollen is common) found that a great many were badly affected by the smell of birch twigs as well as the scent of flowers. The doctors conducting this research recommended that strongly scented flowers should be avoided in hospital wards, and that medical staff should not wear strong perfume, or smell of tobacco.

Smell or irritant?

In the case of cigarette smoke, fresh paint and exhaust fumes, the smell accompanies the presence of various irritants in the air, such as tobacco smoke particles, solvents in the case of paint, and nitrogen dioxide in the case of exhaust fumes. These irritants have a direct effect on the airways, so the smell may not be the actual trigger for the asthma attack. For some people, however, a reaction to the smell may be adding to the damaging effect of the irritants.

In the case of perfume, cologne and scented flowers, it is the smell itself, and the smell alone, that is affecting the asthmatic. Tests on asthmatics have shown that there is a reflex reaction between the nose and the airways: the impact of the smell in the nose sends a message along a nerve pathway to the airways, making them contract. The effects can be quite severe, and many asthmatics find they have to get off trains or buses if someone near them is wearing strong perfume. A strong smell can sometimes produce a severe asthma attack, needing hospital treatment.

Surprisingly, people who have completely lost their sense of smell can still be affected by perfume. Such people notice that their asthma has suddenly got much worse and, when they ask others, discover that someone in the room is wearing very heavy perfume. Their symptoms clear up when they avoid this person. How this reaction might occur is not known.

Patterns of reaction

There are different patterns of reaction to smells. For some asthmatics, the reactions only occur when the asthma is poorly controlled, but for others these reactions are a constant problem.

Most people react immediately to the smell and then recover fairly promptly when the air clears, but some have a delayed reaction which continues for one or two nights after exposure to the smell.

Psychological reactions to smells

If you believe that something will bring on asthma, it often does, through a psychological reaction known as conditioning (see p. 35). Once you have experienced an asthmatic reaction to a smell a few times, you may well have a conditioned reaction to that same smell. It is very difficult, for you or anyone else, to tell the difference between a psychological reaction and a physical reaction to the same smell.

Obviously, it makes sense to try to avoid developing conditioned reactions: you have enough to cope with with your existing reactions to the smell. We can only repeat our general advice about coping with conditioned reactions to asthma triggers (see p. 36).

Coping with reactions to smells

If you react to smells with a worsening of your asthma, the obvious treatment is to avoid the smell as much as possible:

- Explain the problem to friends and colleagues who wear heavy perfume, and ask them to go without it when they are around you. If they seem to think that you are making an unnecessary fuss, show them this book, and emphasize that smells can produce dangerous asthma attacks in susceptible people.
- Do not use air fresheners at home. Far from 'neutralizing odours' as the advertisements claim, they can actually trigger off asthma attacks.
- Use unperfumed cosmetics, soaps and shampoos. The 'Simple' brand, available in most chemists' shops, can be useful: all their products are unperfumed.
- Avoid using insecticide sprays if these affect you. The best way to get rid of flies is to open several windows and swipe about

energetically with a newspaper – you will undoubtedly miss every fly, but they soon get the message and go outdoors. For house dust mites and other carpet-dwellers, try a powerful dehumidifier or the steam cleaner described on p. 479. Ants can be killed with special ant-bait sold in garden centres and hardware shops.

- Buy unperfumed household products only. Even without perfume, however, some products may have a smell that affects you. Experiment with different products to find ones that are safe. Most household jobs can actually be done with unperfumed washing-up liquid, aided by scouring pads and the occasional spot of bleach where necessary (but take care with bleach too – see p. 223).
- Be careful at the hairdresser's. Many products used in hair dressing have a strong smell that can affect asthmatics.
- When choosing plants for the garden or greenhouse, or buying cut flowers, avoid heavily scented flowers. The most common offenders are hyacinths, marguerites, lily-of-the-valley, broom, mimosa, stocks, marigolds, pelargoniums, freesias, narcissus and daffodils, chrysanthemums, honeysuckle, lavender, carnations, pinks, sweet williams, lilies, jasmine, wisteria, daphne, privet, mock orange, lilac, buddleia, sweet peas, wallflowers and elder. Some asthmatics are only affected by one plant, but others react to all or most scented flowers. Note that this is not an allergic reaction to pollen: scented flowers produce very little airborne pollen and cause allergic reactions only rarely – see p. 120.
- If you are sensitive to aspirin (see p. 257), be very cautious about menthol and mint aromas, such as those in toothpaste, cough sweets or indigestion remedies. Menthol and mint are chemically similar to aspirin, and may provoke a bad reaction in aspirin-sensitive asthmatics. (For other asthmatics, inhaling menthol regularly twice a day can actually open up the airways a little, according to some recent research from Japan.)
- Approach aromatherapy oils with extreme caution. If any seem to make your asthma worse, stop using them immediately, and wash off any oil that is already on your body.

The list above deals with smells that are simply smells, not associated with any irritant or allergen. For advice on avoiding irritants such as paint fumes in the air at home, see pp. 221–6. Exhaust fumes are dealt with on pp. 206–12, and cigarette smoke on p. 217.

Some smells are hard to avoid. If, at times, you simply have to put up with a particular smell, you may be able to stave off an asthma attack in various ways:

- A minority of asthmatics find that holding their nose stops the smell from affecting them.
- The anti-allergy drug sodium cromoglycate will prevent the reaction to smells in some asthmatics. Ask your doctor if this could be prescribed as an experiment.
- Research shows that the drug atropine, which blocks the nerve impulse from the nose to the airways, will prevent the reaction to smells in most asthmatics. Unfortunately, this drug has a lot of side-effects, and could not be used regularly for this purpose. However, the group of reliever drugs known as anticholinergics (see p. 345) have a similar action to atropine, and they may help block the reaction. Your doctor should be able to prescribe an inhaler of this type to see if it is helpful to you.
- If none of these treatments works, and you cannot avoid the problem smell, just use your ordinary B-2 reliever inhaler before each exposure. This will not tackle the root of the problem and block the reaction before it starts (as cromoglycate or an anti-cholinergic would do), but it will make your symptoms much less severe.

Did you know?

Asthmatics are often overcharged for life-insurance premiums. A survey of different insurance companies found large differences in the size of the extra premium charged to people with asthma, even when the medical history of the applicants was the same. So it pays to shop around.

When taking out holiday insurance, read the small print carefully. Some companies will not pay out for treatment for asthma attacks.

8

Diseases and drugs that make asthma worse

'As soon as I stopped using the drops I began feeling better.'

Alice has suffered from mild asthma all her life. Now in her early seventies, she recently found that she was far more breathless and wheezy than usual. 'It was a couple of months ago that I saw the optician, just to have my glasses checked, and he told me something was up with my eyes and I should go to the doctor. I couldn't feel anything wrong, but the optician said it was glaucoma and you can go blind if you don't do something about it. I was a bit worried of course, but the doctor I saw said it was just my age, and if I used these drops twice a day I'd be alright.

'It was just after that my asthma started playing up, only it never dawned on me that it was anything to do with these drops. Well, you wouldn't think something going in your eyes could affect your chest would you? I went out shopping for the day with two of my friends, and I had to keep stopping to get my breath, which isn't like me. My chest was really hurting.

'After a week or two of this I was getting worried, and I went back to the surgery. This time it was a different doctor, and she looked at my notes and said "Oh dear, you shouldn't really have been given those . . ." As soon as I stopped using the drops I began feeling better. Now I've got some different ones which the doctor says are just as good. It's a relief to find that the asthma is alright again. I wouldn't have liked to have gone on like that.'

The eye drops that affected Alice's asthma contain a drug called a beta-blocker (see p. 262).

COLDS, FLU AND CHEST INFECTIONS

Many asthmatics find that their symptoms get much worse when they have a cold, especially if it 'goes down on to the chest'. Influenza (flu) may also trigger attacks for some people.

Researchers have recently found an explanation for this effect. Asthmatics tend to react to the viruses that cause colds in a different way from non-asthmatics, with immune responses that favour inflammation and allergy.

Often the very beginning of a person's asthma dates from a bad cold, a bout of flu or a chest infection. Some viral infections that affect babies can also make them more likely to develop asthma later (see p. 93).

If colds are a trigger for your asthma, try the following measures:
- Take a Vitamin C supplement daily (see p. 103), as this may help to reduce the number of colds, or at least their severity.
- As long as you are not allergic to pollen, you could try taking bee propolis, available from health food shops. It is said to have a protective effect against viral infections, but there is no scientific evidence yet to support this. Fresh garlic, eaten every day, can be useful in stopping a cold from 'going down on to your chest'.
- Eat well, with plenty of fresh fruit and vegetables, plus some meat and fish or other rich sources of protein, to strengthen your defences against infection. Get lots of sleep, and generally look after yourself, as this will increase your resistance to colds.
- Avoid breathing cold air, especially if foggy or polluted, as this may make you more susceptible to colds and chest infections. Stay home, or wear a scarf over your face if you have to go out.
- Keep away from smoky rooms during the winter, as anything which irritates your airways will add to your problems.
- If flu triggers your asthma attacks, have an influenza vaccination each autumn: this reduces the chance of getting flu during the winter. Ask your GP about this—flu shots are often available at low cost.

Are antibiotics useful?
Many asthmatics who are affected badly by chest infections ask their doctors for antibiotics, but in fact these are of no value. It is very

largely *viral* infections that make asthma worse, not bacterial infections, and antibiotics do not work against viruses.

There is no cure for the common cold or for influenza. Although there are a few anti-viral drugs these have unpleasant side-effects and are very expensive. They are only used for very serious viral diseases such as hepatitis.

Cold remedies: could they make asthma worse?

The non-prescription medicines for colds and flu, which are widely advertised on television during the winter, are not cures in any sense. All they do is to reduce the symptoms a little. For most people they will probably have little effect on the asthma symptoms that accompany or follow the infection. But anyone who is sensitive to aspirin or aspirin-like drugs (see p. 258) would be made worse by these medicines.

Someone who rarely took aspirin normally might not have noticed their sensitivity to these drugs: in this case it might seem as though colds and flu are a trigger for the asthma, when in fact it is aspirin and aspirin-like drugs. If you always take these potions for your cold or flu, try getting through without them next time, and see if you still get asthma as badly.

Menthol, used in inhalation oils, cough sweets and in many non-prescription medicines for colds and coughs, can also affect people with aspirin sensitivity (see p. 234).

Avoiding infections

Asthmatics can reduce the number of infections they pick up by keeping their distance from people who have colds or flu, and not hugging or kissing when greeting people during the winter months. Most friends and relatives will be understanding about this if you explain that your asthma can be triggered by infections. Remember that people who have a cold coming on may be infectious before they are actually suffering many symptoms themselves.

Steroids and colds

If your asthma is triggered by infections, you will probably be advised to double your dose of inhaled steroids as soon as a cold or flu begins. This is very sound advice, and doubling the dose promptly can give you much more control over your asthma in the long term.

You may be aware that steroids tend to reduce resistance to infections, which raises the obvious question – could steroid treatment make matters worse? This question has been investigated, and the evidence is reassuring: *inhaled* steroids do not make you more susceptible to chest infections. However, long courses of steroid tablets do reduce your resistance (see p. 360). One way you can avoid having to take steroid tablets is to use your inhaled steroids religiously, which will keep the inflammation of your airways under control. Other measures such as allergen avoidance and reducing exposure to irritants are also useful (see pp. 2–3).

Those who suffer severe asthma attacks in response to colds, bad enough to end up in hospital, may do much better if they are given a short treatment with steroid tablets as soon as each cold begins. One study showed that this strategy kept them out of hospital, and drastically reduced the number of days on which they wheezed. Overall, they took about the same amount of steroid as they would have done if admitted to hospital with severe attacks. Clearly the benefits of steroid tablets can outweigh the disadvantages.

'You've really got to be a bit more sensible . . .'

'I was in my early thirties, and trying to do too much. My doctor had actually been warning me that I was being really foolish, because I was getting quite run-down. He said "You've really got to be a bit more sensible about what you're doing." I was going to him a lot for sinus trouble and for bronchitis, and in the end I got really sick with this bronchitis which didn't go away as it should have done. The doctor said "Well, what you've got now is asthma."

'The other thing that I think might have started it off was that I was doing some teaching, and breathing in a lot of chalk dust. I've never been sure if that did it, but I was aware of that dust irritating my lungs.'

SINUSITIS

Many people with asthma have sinusitis as well, and the sinusitis can make the asthma considerably worse, for reasons that are not well understood. Some recent research suggests that there may be an allergic reaction to the microbes that are infecting the sinuses, and this contributes to the asthma symptoms. Among people with severe asthma, sinusitis is sometimes a large part of the problem.

If the sinusitis is treated, the asthma often improves and may clear up completely. In one study of a group of children with asthma and sinusitis, only 20 per cent still needed their inhalers after the sinusitis had been treated, and only 15 per cent still wheezed.

Unfortunately, sinusitis can be very difficult to treat, especially if it has been going on for a long time. But with persistence, most people's sinusitis can be treated successfully. It is worth going through with this treatment, even if it is lengthy and time-consuming, because you could find that you have far less troublesome asthma afterwards.

The symptoms of sinusitis
The main symptoms of sinusitis are:
- a blocked and stuffy nose
- a persistent cough, especially at night (but this can also be a symptom of asthma – see p. 308)
- post-nasal drip (mucus running down the back of the nose into the throat)
- pain in the face, around the cheeks or over the eyes (it may be worse when you bend forward)
- a sore throat, especially in the morning
- bad-smelling breath
- feverishness
- loss of senses of smell and taste
- headache, earache and/or pain around the teeth

All these symptoms can be caused in other ways. Even though you have several of these symptoms, you may not necessarily have sinusitis, so it is important to see your doctor for a proper diagnosis. Some cases of sinusitis are not particularly easy to diagnose, and special tests and scans may be needed. You may be referred to an Ear Nose and Throat Clinic for an expert opinion.

The two kinds of sinusitis

Sinusitis may come on suddenly after a cold or other infection and last for a few weeks: doctors call this 'acute sinusitis'. This usually clears up on its own, but you will probably be offered some treatment by your doctor.

If sinusitis lasts for longer than six weeks, it is called 'chronic sinusitis'. (In medical terms acute just means short-lived, while chronic means a lingering illness: note that acute symptoms are not necessarily more severe than chronic ones.)

Some doctors believe that chronic sinusitis is a different disease altogether from acute sinusitis. It is certainly much harder to treat.

What causes chronic sinusitis?

Chronic sinusitis usually starts with inflammation of the nose and sinus cavities, often caused by an allergy or a cold. The inflammation is severe and causes the sinuses to become blocked. This means that the mucus cannot drain away, so it sits in the sinus cavities in a puddle. Eventually this mucus becomes infected with bacteria. The infection causes more inflammation and this makes the membranes which line the sinus cavities swell up, causing more blockage. At this point the sinusitis becomes a vicious circle, making it very difficult to treat.

Occasionally, chronic sinusitis is caused by a fungal infection, rather than a bacterial one. This can be particularly difficult to diagnose. Repeated tissue sampling (tissue biopsy) may be needed to establish that a fungus is responsible. The fungi involved can, in rare cases, be invasive and spread from the sinuses to the surrounding bone, so this problem needs prompt and thorough treatment with anti-fungal drugs.

The wrong treatment can make chronic sinusitis worse

Many people with chronic sinusitis have been treated repeatedly with antibiotics. Some of the bacteria have been killed each time, but because the sinus cavity is so congested there is always some little hideaway where a few bacteria survive. The bacteria that survive are, not surprisingly, those that are least sensitive to the antibiotic. This process, repeated many times, eventually breeds a race of bacteria which is resistant to one or more of the antibiotics that have been taken. (Fortunately, the bacteria involved are not invasive; that is, they do not spread beyond the sinus cavities.)

For anyone who has got to this point with their sinusitis, treatment is extremely difficult. *Fortunately very few people reading this will have developed such a severe problem – yet.* But there is always that risk, especially if you have had lots of courses of antibiotics. This is why it is so important to treat chronic sinusitis really thoroughly, and, if possible, get rid of it once and for all.

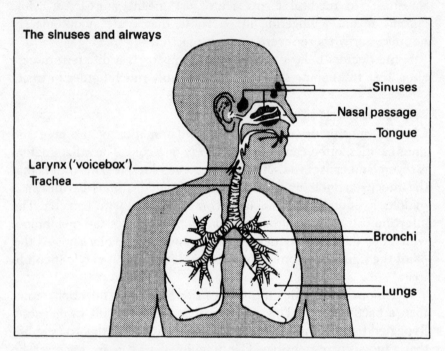

The sinuses and airways

Sinuses

Nasal passage

Tongue

Larynx ('voicebox')

Trachea

Bronchi

Lungs

You need proper medical help for this. Too many people try to treat chronic sinusitis with non-prescription medicines. Some of these can actually make the problem worse. The biggest problems come with decongestant nose drops: after a week or so the nose gets 'addicted' to these drops, and as soon as you stop taking them the congestion comes back with a vengeance. This is called 'rebound congestion'. Some people who experience it just keep on taking the drops, and in time they need more and more of them.

The correct treatment for chronic sinusitis

Chronic sinusitis is a big nut and you need a big hammer to crack it. The following treatment is generally recommended by doctors who are experts in this field.

You should have all six of these treatments at the same time:
1. A three-week course of antibiotics to treat the infection
2. Steroid drops in the nose to calm the inflammation
3. Washing out the nose daily with salt water (saline)
4. A course of tablets that reduce the congestion in the nose
5. For three days *only* (see above), nose drops that reduce congestion
6. Steam inhalations

You may also be given other drugs, such as steroid tablets, anti-cholinergics (see p. 345), anti-histamines to treat any allergic reactions, and drugs that help to clear mucus or dry up the membranes in the nose and sinuses. Some doctors also suggest breathing hot dry air as a treatment.

At the end of three weeks, if the sinusitis has not cleared up, another three-week course of a different antibiotic is given. The idea is that if there are any bacteria resistant to the first antibiotic lurking in your sinus cavities, the new antibiotic will kill them off.

If, after another three weeks, you still have sinusitis, you will be given yet another antibiotic, different from the previous two. This strategy of changing the antibiotic is the best method of avoiding antibiotic-resistance developing in the bacteria. *Whatever you do, don't give up at this stage*. It is vitally important that you take all the courses of antibiotics in full, and that you always see the doctor promptly at the end of each course, so that there is no gap between the courses of antibiotics. There's absolutely no point in going at this treatment half-heartedly, skipping the treatment some days because you are in two minds about it, or giving up halfway through. Indeed, this is positively harmful.

Long courses of antibiotics kill off the beneficial bacteria in the intestine, and may cause long-term bowel problems. It is a good idea, after the antibiotics, to take a bacterial replacer (see p. 483), which puts back the beneficial bacteria in the gut.

Helping yourself during this treatment
There are several things you can do for yourself at the same time as embarking on the medical treatment described above. Eating very spicy food can help to clear the congestion, so try a hot curry or chilli each evening. An osteopath may also be able to improve the drainage from the sinus cavities by gently manipulating parts of your face.

Try to work out if an allergen, or an irritant in the air, is at the source of your sinusitis: a little detective work (see pp. 2–3) may be needed to identify such problems. Think about any changes in your life that happened before the sinusitis began, such as getting a new pet, moving house, starting a new job, changing the heating in your home or installing humidifiers. (Bear in mind that allergies to newly encountered allergens may not develop immediately – it can take up to two years.) You may need skin-prick tests to identify your allergen (see p. 125).

Coming into regular contact with any irritant chemical can also cause chronic sinusitis, and you should think about anything you have begun using at work or at home. Cigarette smoke can also act as an irritant and help to cause sinusitis.

If you find that an allergen or irritant is at the root of the problem, do whatever you can to reduce your exposure to the offending item. In the case of allergy, desensitization treatments may be an option worth trying (see pp. 197–202).

A few people who have chronic sinusitis are sensitive to aspirin, and some are not aware of this problem (see p. 257). It is worth looking into this because, if you discover that you are affected, avoiding aspirin *and all other aspirin-like drugs* (see p. 258) may substantially improve the sinusitis.

Food intolerance can also make sinusitis much worse. If you think you might have food intolerance (see p. 182) you could try an elimination diet to identify the culprit food.

'But I hate the idea of taking all those antibiotics'

Many people are reluctant to take antibiotics, especially for long periods of time. If you feel strongly about this, you could try all the self-help measures described immediately above *before* starting on an antibiotic-based treatment programme. They may be sufficient, especially if you find you have an allergy underlying the chronic sinusitis.

Some people also recommend alternative therapies, such as homeopathy or Chinese herbal medicines, for chronic sinusitis. There is no evidence to support these claims, as no research has been done, but there is no harm in trying these treatments if you want to.

If there is no improvement, you could then go on to the antibiotic programme: delaying this treatment for a few months will do no harm. What is potentially harmful is starting the antibiotic programme and then stopping halfway through.

Surgery for sinusitis

The last resort, for anyone whose sinusitis does not respond to treatment, is a surgical operation. The aim of this is to increase the size of the drainage channels leading out of the sinus cavities, so that the mucus drains away more easily.

The most modern and successful form of operation can be done under local anaesthetic and you do not need to stay overnight in hospital. This operation is much less drastic than the old-fashioned forms of surgery: it simply enlarges the natural drainage holes rather than creating new ones.

However, any operation is very much a last resort, and should not be done unless absolutely necessary.

Inherited diseases that can lead to sinusitis

A minority of people with chronic sinusitis have some underlying inherited problem, such as cystic fibrosis or a defect in the tiny hairs (cilia) that push debris and mucus out of the sinuses and airways. People with these problems need specialist treatment. Occasionally, if children have cystic fibrosis but it is not particularly severe, the doctor may not be able to diagnose the problem immediately. Such children may also wheeze (see p. 313).

'Whenever I get run down . . . it comes back.'

'Fortunately, my asthma is getting less and less as I get older, but whenever I get run down, through working too hard and not getting enough sleep, it comes back – first the sinusitis and then the asthma. It's like I'm a sitting duck. Sometimes it starts with a bit of hayfever, then the sinuses start off really quickly.

'I've been tested and they've discovered that I'm allergic to the sinusitis bug. I've found now that if I get onto the sinusitis really quickly, and take a course of antibiotics, I can short-circuit everything. That might mean I've got five days of antibiotics and that's it, instead of being on antibiotics for two months or so to clear it up.'

ATHLETE'S FOOT, RINGWORM, *CANDIDA* AND OTHER FUNGAL INFECTIONS

Doctors have long recognized that people with asthma have a tendency to get certain fungal infections of the lung. An allergic reaction to the fungus may develop, which in turn makes the asthma worse.

Until recently, this was thought to be the only connection between fungal infections and asthma. But new research has shown that there is also a link between asthma and fungal infections elsewhere in the body, such as athlete's foot and intertrigo (a rash on areas of skin that rub together, such as in the armpits or between the thighs). Again, there is an allergic reaction to the fungus which either causes the asthma or makes it much worse.

More controversially, there are also claims for a link between asthma and 'Candida' (yeast) infection.

Fungal infections of the lung

A fungus or mould known as *Aspergillus fumigatus* can infect the lungs of some asthmatics and make their asthma worse. This fungus is normally found in compost heaps, mouldy straw, animal droppings (it is especially plentiful in chicken houses and aviaries), wood chips and other decomposing material. Thousands of invisible spores, which are like microscopic seeds, are floating about everywhere in the air around us, so they are very easily inhaled into the lungs. Most people are not affected by these spores – the immune system easily defeats them – but in some people, especially those with asthma, they begin to grow in the lungs, which become infected by the fungus.

The main reason that the *Aspergillus* infection causes serious problems is that the asthmatic then has an allergic reaction to the fungus. It is the allergy to the fungus that makes the asthma so much worse.

The correct name for this condition is allergic bronchopulmonary aspergillosis. Asthmatics are vulnerable to it because they have a lot of mucus in the lungs, and this gives the fungus a foothold – something to begin growing on. (People with cystic fibrosis, those who have had tuberculosis, or those taking immunosuppressive drugs for cancer are also vulnerable to infection by *Aspergillus*.) There are three main signs that should lead your doctor to suspect this problem:

- Your asthma continues to deteriorate, despite treatment, and you need more and more steroids to control it.
- You are coughing up rubbery plugs of phlegm, either golden-brown or green in colour.
- When your asthma gets worse, you usually feel feverish at the same time.

Talk to your doctor if you have these symptoms. A proper diagnosis can only be made by carrying out skin-prick tests for allergy to *Aspergillus*, and examining your sputum under a microscope.

Allergic bronchopulmonary aspergillosis is treated with steroids to control the allergic reaction, and physiotherapy to clear the mucus from the lungs. Anti-fungal drugs might also be tried, but your doctor may be reluctant to try them as they have not proved very effective in the past. A new drug, itraconazole, is thought to be of some help.

Athlete's foot (tinea pedis)

This is another fungal infection, but because the feet are a very long way from the lungs, the connection with asthma was not noticed until recently. Dr Tom Platts-Mills and other researchers at the University of Virginia discovered that some people with athlete's foot become allergic to the fungus that is infecting their feet and toenails. This allergic reaction to the fungus can produce symptoms of asthma, or make asthma worse in someone who is already asthmatic.

Your family doctor is unlikely to know about this new research, so you need to be well informed before talking to your doctor about this possibility. You may well be greeted with puzzlement and disbelief, so go armed with the facts and be prepared to persist.

There are at least three different fungi that can cause athlete's foot, but the two principal ones both belong to the group called *Tricho-phyton*. Researchers have shown that there is definitely an immediate allergic reaction to *Trichophyton* in some asthmatics with athlete's foot, and that inhaling very small amounts of the fungus can produce asthma symptoms. When the athlete's foot is treated successfully, using anti-fungal drugs, there is often a great improvement in the asthma. (Your doctor may want the reference for this research: it is *The Lancet*, 22 April 1989, pp. 859–62.)

Once your doctor has confirmed that you have athlete's foot, you should be given anti-fungal creams, or an anti-fungal drug which you

swallow in capsule form and which works its way through your
system to the feet. There are some very good modern drugs, which
are much more effective than the older treatments for athlete's foot.

It is important to treat the infection thoroughly, because the fungus
penetrates deep into the skin and can quickly reappear if not completely destroyed. You should also be careful not to re-infect yourself,
by following these guidelines:

- Wash all your towels and bath mats in a high-temperature
  wash when you start the course of treatment, and again when
  you complete it.
- Do not share towels or bath mats with other people, and never
  borrow their socks, sandals or shoes.
- Wear plastic sandals or flipflops when walking around swimming pools, and in public showers and changing-rooms.
- If any member of your family also has athlete's foot, take the
  same precautions in the bathroom at home – and ask them to
  go for treatment too.
- Dry your feet very thoroughly every time you wash them,
  especially between the toes; kitchen roll does a better job than
  most towels, and you can throw it away afterwards, which
  reduces the risk of re-infection.
- Wear cotton socks, rather than nylon or other synthetic
  fabrics, and try to wear shoes made of leather or canvas,
  which will allow sweat to evaporate from your feet.
- Only wear trainers or gumboots when you really need to.
- If your feet get wet, change your socks and shoes promptly.

Intertrigo and onychomycosis

These too are fungal infections: in fact, like athlete's foot (see above),
they are often caused by types of *Trichophyton* fungus.

Intertrigo is an itchy and scaly rash which develops wherever skin
rubs against skin: between the thighs, in the armpits, below the breasts,
in folds of skin on the stomach, and between the fingers and toes. Those
who are overweight are much more susceptible to intertrigo.

Onychomycosis (also called 'ringworm of the nails' or tinea un-
guium) affects the fingernails and/or toenails, which develop white
patches at first, then pits on the surface, and finally become thick,
crumbly and whitish-yellow (or even green) in colour. Infection of the
toenails often goes with athlete's foot.

The way in which these infections cause asthma is exactly the same as for athlete's foot, and the diagnosis and treatment are identical. If your doctor needs a reference for this research, it is the same as the one above for athlete's foot. Keeping your skin dry in the infected area, and losing weight if you need to, will help to prevent the problem coming back.

Candida infection

Candida is a yeast that lives naturally in the gut, usually causing no trouble. However, it can sometimes spread and cause infections in other parts of the body. A yeast is a type of microscopic fungus, so *Candida* infections can be treated with anti-fungal drugs.

So far so good: everyone would agree on what is written above. But after this, there are two different versions of the *Candida* story: the one that conventional medicine accepts, and the one that is popular with alternative practitioners and with some doctors who think the conventional view of *Candida* is too limited.

The conventional view

The main problems caused by *Candida* are thrush infections in the throat and vagina, and sometimes on the penis. These have well-defined symptoms and are easily treated with anti-fungal drugs. A few patients with damaged immune systems, caused by anti-cancer drugs or AIDS, may develop more widespread *Candida* infections, but this *never* happens to people with a normal immune system. Using inhaled steroids, without rinsing out the mouth afterwards, can make asthma sufferers more susceptible to thrush infections in the throat (see p. 352). But that is the only link with asthma – there is no evidence that *Candida* can cause asthma or make it worse.

The alternative view

It is quite easy for *Candida* to get out of control and cause widespread problems throughout the body. This condition is known as candidiasis. Several aspects of modern life make candidiasis more likely, including repeated courses of antibiotics, eating a sugary diet, and taking the contraceptive Pill. *Candida* grows in a mould-like form (that is, it spreads and branches like a mould) as well as in a yeast form (single cells). It is when the mould-like form develops in the intestine that it causes so much trouble. There is often an allergic reaction to the *Candida* which produces some of the symptoms. Because there is a cross-reaction between *Candida* and yeast in the diet, eating yeast products will produce further symptoms. The symptoms caused by candidiasis are very varied, and may include diarrhoea or constipation, wind and bloating, itchy anus, fatigue, poor concentration, irritability, depression, confusion, headache or migraine, pre-menstrual problems, recurrent cystitis, recurrent thrush, skin rashes and aching muscles. Occasionally the symptoms include asthma.

So what is the truth about Candida?
As often happens, the truth is probably somewhere between these two extreme positions. There are certainly a number of patients with mystery illnesses, including the sort of symptoms listed above for candidiasis, who respond very well to a diet that is low in sugar and yeast, and/or treatment with anti-fungal drugs. But researchers have failed to find any evidence of *Candida* overgrowth in their bodies. The conclusion is that some kind of yeast or other fungus is causing the symptoms, but that is not *Candida*. This is why we refer to the condition treated by alternative practitioners as 'candidiasis', and the culprit as '*Candida*'. So far the real culprit has not been identified.

As regards the number of people affected by candidiasis, the alternative position is probably too extreme. There has been something of a craze for '*Candida*' in the complementary health field, and the number of sufferers has been exaggerated.

However, there are certainly a few people with asthma who do experience a marked improvement in their symptoms if they are treated for 'candidiasis'. It is only worth trying this treatment if you have quite a number of the symptoms listed above (under 'The alternative view'). Bowel problems and an itchy anus are characteristic, and if you have neither of these it is unlikely the 'candidiasis' treatment will help your asthma.

Treating 'candidiasis'
We recommend the following four-step treatment:

Stage 1:
If you are taking the contraceptive Pill, change to another form of contraception.

Take all kinds of sugar out of your diet: this includes honey, syrup,

jam, chutney, pickles, cakes and biscuits, soft drinks, fruit squash –
indeed, anything that tastes sweet. Do not eat baked beans or peanut
butter (except sugar-free brands). Also avoid dried fruits, and change
any medicines taken as syrups to tablet form.

By not eating any sugar, you are giving the yeast/fungus far less to
feed on in the gut. Stay on this stage for a month or more. If you are no
better, go on to Stage 2.

Stage 2:
Continue with all the restrictions of Stage 1.

In addition, cut fruit out of your diet completely, except for fresh
lemon juice. Eat plenty of fresh vegetables, in salads or lightly cooked,
to get enough Vitamin C. You can also have rosehip tea which is rich
in Vitamin C.

Do not eat white bread or anything made with white flour (e.g.
pastry, pasta). Small portions of wholemeal bread or potatoes are fine,
but aim to eat mostly vegetables and high-protein foods such as meat,
fish and eggs. Avoid cheese, pickles and anything fermented. Eat lots
of herbs, spinach and freshly crushed garlic, as these are believed to
combat yeast in the gut.

Cutting out fruit and white flour reduces the food supply to the
yeast even further. Stay on this diet for at least a month, and longer if
you begin to feel partially better. If you get substantially better on this
diet, fruits and other excluded foods can be gradually re-introduced
later, but not sugar.

Stage 3:
Continue with all the restrictions above, and cut out foods containing
yeast as well. There are more of them than you might imagine: see the
list on p. 194. By not eating any yeast, you will avoid provoking
allergic cross-reactions.

If there is a partial response to this diet, that is a good sign, and you
should think about going on to Stage 4.

Stage 4:
*You must talk to your doctor before trying this stage, as it is quite a drastic
diet, and may not be safe for everyone.*

Cut out all starchy foods: potatoes, bread, flour, rice, pasta, sweetcorn, parsnips, lentils, beans, etc. Nuts other than cashew nuts can be
eaten, but only in small quantities.

This extreme diet gives the yeast almost nothing to live on, as no sugar and almost no starch are eaten. You cannot stay on a diet of this kind for long, but it may be helpful in getting the problem under control.

If you feel you are on the right track, because there is some improvement with this diet, try to find a doctor who is knowledgeable about 'candidiasis' to help you: you may have to go privately, unless you are lucky enough to have a very open-minded GP. (If you are choosing a doctor or an alternative therapist, avoid those who are part of the 'Candida' craze and think that 'candidiasis' explains all the ills of the world. You may not have 'candidiasis' at all, so you need someone who can keep an open mind.) A doctor will be able to give you additional help in the form of anti-fungal drugs, which you may well need.

'So we tried treating them with anti-fungal drugs . . .'

Professor Tom Platts-Mills and his research team at the University of Virginia in Charlottesville have carried out pioneering work on fungal infections and asthma. He describes how this work began: 'When I first arrived in Charlottesville in 1982, the senior allergist here was Professor John Guerrant. He said "I've got to warn you that here in Virginia we have people who have very severe fungal infection of their feet, and they also have urticaria. If you treat their feet, their urticaria gets better."

'I followed his advice, and then I started noticing asthmatics in our allergy clinic who also had fungal infections of their feet. They were mostly men with severe adult-onset asthma. We gave them skin-prick tests with the fungus and these were positive – showing they had an allergic reaction to it. So we tried treating them with anti-fungal drugs and in many of the cases their asthma got much better."

'Like so many things in medicine, this had in fact been noticed before. I've since discovered that a Dr Sulzberger suggested a link between athlete's foot and some cases of asthma in 1936.'

OTHER MEDICAL PROBLEMS
THAT CAN MAKE ASTHMA WORSE

Apart from fungal infections (see p. 246) there are several other illnesses and medical conditions that tend to make asthma symptoms worse. In some cases, dealing with these may be the key to improving your asthma.

Hayfever and other allergic symptoms in the nose

If you have hayfever or some other kind of allergy affecting the nose (for example, to house dust mites, pets or moulds), it is a good idea to get this treated, because your asthma may well improve as a result. The nose affects the lower airways in several ways. If it is blocked with mucus, you will breathe through your mouth instead of your nose, and the air inhaled will not be warmed and filtered before it reaches your lungs. This makes the air more irritating to the airways. There may also be a nerve reflex connecting the nose to the airways, which could have a direct effect, making the airway muscles contract when allergens aggravate the nose. Finally, the mucus from the nose can run down into the airways, especially at night, causing additional blockage. (Sometimes this is the fundamental problem and the 'asthma' goes away when the runny nose is treated – see p. 313.)

There are four main treatments for these nasal allergies:
- Steroid drops – far less risky than most people imagine because the drops are going straight to where they are needed, which allows a very low dose to be used. Little of the drug enters the bloodstream and side-effects are therefore minimal. Don't hesitate to try steroid drops for your nose, because the beneficial effect on your asthma could be huge.
- Cromoglycate drops – not effective for everyone, but an extremely safe drug, so worth a try. These can be used in place of steroids, if they work for you.
- Anti-histamines, either as tablets or drops – these are used mainly for hayfever and other seasonal allergies, not for year-round symptoms.
- Decongestants – used for short periods of time only (see p. 242).

Heartburn

The proper medical name for this is **gastro-oesophageal reflux** or **GER**. It is a type of indigestion, caused by the contents of the stomach welling upwards into the oesophagus, the tube that connects the mouth to the stomach. Normally a valve-like constriction at the bottom end of the oesophagus (a sphincter) stops this happening.

The stomach acid burns the lining of the oesophagus, causing inflammation. Because there are some nerves linking the oesophagus with the airways, this can make the airways tighten up a little and bring on asthma symptoms. To make matters worse, if stomach acid comes up into the throat during the night, tiny droplets of it may be inhaled and irritate the airways directly.

Unfortunately, people with asthma are more likely to suffer GER than others, probably because the over-inflated lungs exert pressure on the stomach.

Heartburn – a burning sensation in the centre of the chest, sometimes extending up to the throat – is the most typical symptom of GER. Other symptoms include:

- regurgitation of stomach contents into the mouth
- pain in the chest
- frequent choking
- difficulty in swallowing
- burping and general indigestion

It is important to realize that *not everyone with GER has heartburn* as a symptom, although they may have some of the other symptoms listed above. If there is no heartburn, their problem often goes undiagnosed, and the link with their asthma is not recognized.

You should talk to your doctor if you have any of the following:

- heartburn, acid regurgitation, choking or other symptoms listed above
- asthma attacks that often occur just after meals
- night-time symptoms, particularly coughing, which are worse if you eat your evening meal very late
- asthma attacks that regularly coincide with bouts of indigestion
- a bitter or sour taste in your mouth when you wake up in the morning

Treatment for GER includes antacids and other drugs. You can also help yourself by not eating late in the evening and by raising the head of your bed above the feet using 10-cm (4-inch) blocks, so that you sleep with your head higher than your stomach. (Raising the head with pillows does not work.)

Certain foods make GER worse, and you should avoid these, especially in the evening:

- alcohol
- chocolate
- tea and coffee
- peppermint and spearmint
- very fatty foods
- milk

Hot spices and very acid foods, such as grapefruit, will irritate the oesophagus on the way down, making the inflammation worse. These should be avoided until your symptoms subside.

One group of drugs used to treat asthma, the theophylline-type drugs, can make GER worse. These drugs are given in tablet form only, so if you are taking any tablets for your asthma, check if they belong to this group (see pp. 374–5). *You must talk to your doctor before changing the dose or stopping these drugs.* Certain drugs given for conditions other than asthma can also make GER worse; check with your doctor that nothing you are taking could have this effect.

Sometimes the only effective treatment for GER is a surgical operation to tighten the sphincter between the oesophagus and the stomach. This reduces heartburn in 90 per cent of cases, and improves asthma symptoms in 75 per cent of cases.

Obesity

Being overweight can make asthma worse. The burden of fat around the rib-cage makes it more difficult for the lungs to expand fully, and the diaphragm (see p. 416), which moves downwards during the in-breath, has to fight against the extra layers of fat that surround the internal organs of the belly. At the same time a heavier body requires more effort simply to move around, and this demands more oxygen. So the breathing system is expected to work harder, but more obstacles are put in its way. All this can make asthma much more troublesome.

Obesity can also make asthma more likely to develop in those who are not yet asthmatic.

Sleep problems

Asthma can disturb sleep, as many asthmatics know, but one form of sleep disturbance can itself cause asthma-like symptoms. The problem is called obstructive sleep apnoea syndrome. Apnoea simply means 'not breathing' – people with this problem repeatedly stop breathing while they are asleep. They will not usually be aware of this, but they will find themselves waking up regularly during the night and being very tired during the day. Loud snoring is often part of the picture, and some people also feel they are choking during the night.

It has only recently been realized that obstructive sleep apnoea syndrome can actually cause wheezing as well. Unfortunately, there is no easy way to diagnose this problem apart from a sleep study, which involves spending a night in hospital. If your GP can arrange such a test it might well be worthwhile: there is effective treatment for the sleep problem which will also eliminate the wheezing.

Other diseases

Chronic bronchitis and emphysema can coexist with asthma and make it worse, in COPD (see p. 32).

Infections with a type of pneumonia caused by a microbe called *Chlamydia pneumoniae* may play a part in causing very severe forms of asthma including 'brittle asthma', but the severe asthma persists long after the infection has cleared up. This discovery has not, so far, led to any improved form of treatment for brittle asthma. Smokers are much more vulnerable to *Chlamydia pneumoniae* infection – another good reason why asthmatics should not smoke.

Stress and panic attacks can play a part in asthma, often a very large part (see pp. 34–9). Hyperventilation is often part of the picture in these cases (see p. 419).

Food intolerance can be a major unidentified factor for some asthmatics (see p. 181).

Some women find their asthma gets worse when they are pregnant (see p. 288), while others improve. Monthly periods, or the premenstrual period, can also bring on more severe asthma symptoms (see p. 66).

It may not be the disease itself that is making your asthma worse, but the drugs prescribed for it (see p. 262).

ASPIRIN AND ASPIRIN-LIKE DRUGS

The majority of people with asthma are not affected by aspirin. But a minority of asthmatics have a very bad reaction to aspirin: for them, it can bring on a severe asthma attack, which is sometimes fatal. The symptoms associated with aspirin sensitivity are described on pp. 47–8: if you are suffering symptoms of this kind, *don't delay in getting medical help*.

Recent estimates put the number with aspirin sensitivity at about 10 per cent of all asthmatics. There are also a few asthmatics who actually find their asthma *improves* if they take a small amount of aspirin each day. Why this is, no one knows.

Aspirin sensitivity is not an allergic reaction. It is due to a difference in the way the body produces and processes a group of messenger chemicals called prostaglandins. Because it is not an allergic reaction, it cannot be tested for reliably with skin-prick tests. Taking a small dose of aspirin and seeing what happens is fraught with hazards, and time-consuming for the doctor, so is now out of favour. The quickest and safest way to test for aspirin sensitivity is to inhale a tiny amount, but very few doctors actually carry out this test. (Note that after you have had a reaction to aspirin, you will be immune to its effects for up to five days, so the test will not work. High doses of steroids will also prevent the test from working.)

Most people who develop aspirin sensitivity do so in their teens or twenties. Aspirin sensitivity often, but not always, begins after a viral infection. This problem is very rare in children, although aspirin is risky for children in other ways.

Most people who develop aspirin sensitivity have other symptoms already, besides asthma. The main symptom is the repeated growth of nasal polyps (small, soft lumps, which are completely harmless, inside the nose). Other symptoms are a runny or blocked nose all year round (chronic rhinitis), sinusitis, and little or no sense of smell. If you have these symptoms in combination with asthma (or without asthma as yet) you may well develop aspirin sensitivity at some stage.

It may take anything from a couple of months to 20 years from when you have the first symptoms in the nose (polyps and/or rhinitis) to when you begin reacting badly to aspirin. So the timescale varies enormously, but aspirin sensitivity is likely to arrive eventually for most polyp sufferers. Only a very small number of people have asthma, nasal polyps and chronic rhinitis but never develop aspirin sensitivity.

The order in which the symptoms develop can also vary to some extent. For example, some people have the polyps and rhinitis, but no asthma until they actually develop aspirin sensitivity. The first reaction to aspirin is also their first asthma attack.

Avoiding aspirin-like drugs

If it was only aspirin that caused these reactions it would be simple enough to deal with. Unfortunately there are a lot of other drugs that are similar to aspirin and have the same effect. If you suffer from aspirin sensitivity you need to know which ones they are, and must be very careful about avoiding them. Every year, a number of people die because a busy doctor momentarily forgets that other drugs have a similar action to aspirin.

All the aspirin-like drugs that need to be avoided are known as non-steroidal anti-inflammatory drugs (NSAIDs). Like aspirin these are used for pain relief (for example, in headache and backache remedies such as Nurofen), for the treatment of arthritis, and for several other inflammatory diseases. (Note that aspirin itself has an additional use, as a treatment for heart disease.) *Unfortunately, you will not see the words non-steroidal anti-inflammatory drug on the packet.*

At the time of going to press, there are 25 or more distinct drugs to be avoided, and many of these are sold under several different brand-names, creating a list of hundreds of names. This list grows each year, as new drugs or new brands are launched. Rather than list all these names – such a list would soon be out of date – we suggest that you stick to the following guidelines:

- Whenever you are prescribed any new drug by any doctor or consultant, mention that you are sensitive to aspirin (or, if you only have nasal polyps at present, mention this). If you are at all concerned about what you have been given, double-check with the pharmacist when the prescription is filled.
- Whenever you buy any painkillers, headache or migraine tablets, or cold and flu remedies, always buy them at a chemist's shop and check with the pharmacist that they do not contain aspirin or aspirin-like drugs. Never take any drugs of this kind unless you have bought them yourself.

You should also be cautious about anything flavoured with peppermint, mint or menthol (see p. 234). Cough sweets, cold remedies, inhalations, and 'heat rub' creams sold for aching muscles, are all likely to contain menthol, so take care with these.

Is acetaminophen safe?

Painkillers that do not contain aspirin generally contain acetaminophen. While most will be able to tolerate this, about 5 per cent of people who are sensitive to aspirin also react to acetaminophen. If you are taking acetaminophen for the first time, we suggest that you start with a very small amount (half a tablet) and wait for two to three hours to see what happens. Make sure that you have a way of getting to a hospital should anything serious happen.

The outlook for asthmatics with aspirin sensitivity

Avoiding aspirin and aspirin-like drugs will prevent you having sudden and devastating attacks of asthma. Unfortunately, your asthma will probably not go away, however careful you are about avoiding aspirin, unless it came on very recently in direct response to taking an aspirin-like drug. Sadly, most people with aspirin sensitivity have quite severe asthma.

What other options are there?

- Try the new leukotriene-antagonist drugs (see p. 340). Until recently aspirin-sensitive patients got the same general treatment as other asthmatics. But that has changed with the introduction of drugs such as zafirlukast, which act by blocking the action of substances called leukotrienes. There is good reason to believe that these drugs will be particularly useful for asthmatics with aspirin sensitivity (because leukotrienes and prostaglandins – see p. 257 – are part of the same complicated messenger system). One of these new drugs, zileuton, has proved valuable in treating the nasal symptoms of those sensitive to aspirin. We suggest that you ask your doctor about the possibility of trying these drugs.
- Avoid salicylates in food. Many foods contain substances that are similar to aspirin, called salicylates. New evidence suggests that the salicylates in food do not actually produce the same reaction in the body as aspirin, so this diet (which is a parti-

cularly difficult one to follow) is rarely used now. But if you are searching for solutions, and want to give it a try, we suggest that *for two weeks only* you simply avoid all fruits, vegetables, herbs and spices, nuts, yeast (see p. 194), coffee, tea, cola drinks, honey, peppermint, liquorice, processed foods, bottled sauces and alcoholic drinks. Basically, you can eat meat, fish, milk, cheese, eggs, cereals and oil/fat. *You must take a good multivitamin and mineral supplement.* If there is a substantial improvement in your asthma, ask your doctor to refer you to a dietitian for advice on a long-term low-salicylate diet.

- Consider sensitivity to food additives. In the past some doctors have suggested avoiding food additives such as tartrazine and benzoates, as these were thought to cause problems for some people with aspirin sensitivity. Recent studies suggest that asthmatics who react to aspirin are no more or less likely than anyone else to react to these additives. However, it is worth considering the possible role of these additives.

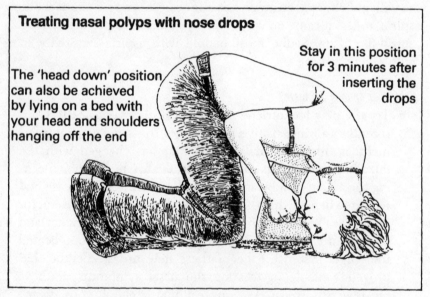

Treating nasal polyps with nose drops

The 'head down' position can also be achieved by lying on a bed with your head and shoulders hanging off the end

Stay in this position for 3 minutes after inserting the drops

There are also treatments to be cautious about:
- If you have lost your sense of smell because of nasal polyps, you may be offered surgery to remove them. Sometimes surgery on the nose can make asthma much worse, or bring it back when there has been no sign of it for years, so we would

suggest that you get expert advice on all the advantages and disadvantages of an operation for your polyps. Make sure you have tried all other treatments (for example, steroid drops, properly inserted – see above) before you opt for surgery.

- Some doctors offer a course of desensitization treatment for aspirin sensitivity. This does not improve the asthma, so the only value in doing this is to allow people to take aspirin or aspirin-like drugs, if they have severe arthritis, for example. Given the safety record of these drugs when taken long-term at high doses, and the doubtful benefits to many arthritis sufferers, particularly those with osteoarthritis, it may be best to avoid going down this road. Talk it over with your doctor and get a second opinion if in doubt.
- Do not take omega-3 fish oil supplements (see p. 103).

'When I have an attack, I need space so bad . . .'

Donna developed asthma in her forties, when she and her family moved from New Mexico to Florida. Despite good medical treatment, she still has regular asthma attacks.

'A lot of things bring on attacks for me. The worst is aspirin, and I have to be real careful to keep away from that. Sometimes, I don't know what brings on the attacks – they just seem to come out of nowhere.

'When I have an attack, I need space so bad, but my family are just all over me. I hate that. I need to concentrate on breathing, and they keep asking questions – "Are you OK?" – "Do you want another pillow?" – "Have you got your medication?" Of course I've got my medication. I'm a responsible adult, not a kid.

'They hover around me and I feel a whole lot worse as a result. I can't concentrate on breathing if I keep having to answer all these questions, and I get even more breathless.'

OTHER DRUGS THAT CAN AFFECT ASTHMA

The drugs that pose the greatest threat to asthma sufferers are aspirin
and aspirin-like drugs, which are dealt with on p. 257. Unlike aspirin
and its relatives, all the drugs listed here are prescription drugs, and
your doctor should be alert to the problems they can pose for
asthmatics. But doctors are overworked and can easily forget about
your asthma when prescribing these drugs, so it is as well to be aware
of the dangers yourself.

Beta-blockers

No one with asthma should be taking beta-blockers as they make the
airways contract and can bring on a serious asthma attack. Beta-
blockers affect beta-receptors in the airways and have the opposite
effect to a B-2 reliever drug.

Beta-blockers are sometimes prescribed for:
- high blood pressure
- angina
- prevention of heart attacks, after a first attack
- irregular heartbeat and other heart problems
- migraine
- thyroid problems
- anxiety (including short-term stress: they are sometimes given
  to help people get through a driving test if they keep failing
  through being nervous)

There are alternative drugs for all these disorders. If you think that one
of your drugs might be a beta-blocker, the simplest way to check is to
go to any chemist's shop and ask the pharmacist.

Asthma sometimes develops in people who have been taking beta-
blockers for years. The beta-blockers do not seem to be responsible for
this, but once asthma has begun, they will make symptoms worse, so a
new drug should be found.

Eye-drops for glaucoma

Some of the eye-drops given for glaucoma contain beta-blockers.
Even the very small amounts absorbed from the eye into the bloodstream can have a bad effect. If you have glaucoma, there are other
drops you can use.

Drugs containing female hormones

The female hormones affect asthma, which is why, as adults, more women suffer from asthma than men, and why asthma often gets worse just before a woman's monthly period (see p. 66).

The contraceptive Pill

Taking the contraceptive Pill, which contains the hormone oestrogen, may make asthma worse. There are progesterone-only pills which may cause fewer problems. Ask your doctor about these.

Those who have never suffered from asthma are also at slightly increased risk of developing asthma, as a result of taking the contraceptive Pill. This risk continues even after the Pill has been stopped.

For a few women, taking the Pill seems to reduce their asthma symptoms.

Hormone Replacement Therapy (HRT)

HRT contains oestrogen, so taking this may cause asthma to worsen in some women. However, there are others, often women with severe asthma, who find they get substantially better when they begin taking HRT.

HRT also increases (by about 50 per cent) the chances of women developing asthma for the first time. To put it another way: after women have gone through the menopause, their risk of developing asthma is smaller, but taking HRT cancels this out. (If you are trying to decide whether to take HRT or not, this disadvantage should be set against the important advantages, especially in protecting against osteoporosis.)

This increased risk of asthma with HRT only applies to women who have gone through a natural menopause. For some unknown reason, those who have had their ovaries removed by surgery (as part of a full hysterectomy, for example) have no extra risk of asthma if they take HRT.

Other drugs that can make asthma worse
Drugs for heart disease

The drug digoxin (brand-name, Lanoxin) is used for some forms of heart disease. It is thought to make asthma symptoms slightly worse. Beta-blockers (see above) also make asthma worse.

Drugs for diabetes
For those who find that alcohol brings on an asthma attack (see p. 265), the drug chlorpropamide (brand-name, Diabinese), prescribed for some diabetics, may aggravate the effects of alcohol.

Drugs for acne
A drug prescribed for acne, isotretinoin, has been recorded as causing an asthma attack.

Non-steroidal anti-inflammatory drugs
These are the aspirin-like drugs, used as painkillers and for arthritis. They can have serious and immediate effects on aspirin-sensitive asthmatics (see p. 258).

They may also have more subtle, long-term effects on other asthmatics, when taken very regularly, because they block the effects of Vitamin C. This prevents it fulfilling its role as a protector of the airways (see pp. 98–9). This effect is likely to be small. Taking a regular Vitamin C supplement would probably offset this, but there is no evidence on this point. Finally, these drugs can cause problems for those with exercise-induced asthma (see p. 73).

Omega-3 fish oil supplements
These supplements, taken for arthritis and other conditions, can make asthma symptoms worse for some people (see p. 103).

Drugs (for other diseases) that can improve asthma
All the drugs so far listed make asthma worse. One drug used for other diseases does actually improve asthma.

Frusemide (also called furosemide) is given to treat water retention (oedema) and kidney failure. It is a type of diuretic. This drug often produces an improvement in asthma, probably by reducing the level of sodium in the blood. The level of sodium in the blood is influenced by the amount of salt eaten in food, so if frusemide has proved beneficial for your asthma, you should try a low-salt diet and see if your asthma improves. Frusemide is not prescribed for asthma because it is a strong diuretic and potentially dangerous if taken long-term.

'Social drugs'
Both alcohol and caffeine are drugs, and both can have drug-like effects on the airways.

Caffeine

Caffeine tends to open up the airways, and it has this effect on most asthmatics. The amounts needed to have any noticeable effect are several cups of strong coffee. Taking in this much caffeine will probably produce some quite unpleasant side-effects, such as a pounding heart or shaky hands. There are also long-term problems with taking in high doses of caffeine, such as persistent insomnia, headaches, nervousness and 'restless legs', so you would be best advised to use your reliever inhaler instead. The reliever drugs have been chemically tailored to have the maximum therapeutic benefit for the minimum of side-effects. Many people feel less frightened of coffee and tea because they are familiar and people assume them to be harmless. Familiarity is very reassuring, but sometimes misleading. People who drink excessive amounts of tea or coffee can make themselves quite seriously ill, or mentally disturbed.

One group of drugs used for asthma, the theophylline-type drugs, are chemically very similar to caffeine, but target the airways more precisely. In fact, tea contains theophylline itself as well as caffeine, but only in very small amounts, far too little to have any effect on asthmatic airways.

Alcohol

Not every asthmatic is affected by alcohol. Of those who are, some experience bronchodilation (opening up of the airways), while others experience bronchoconstriction (tightening of the airways). You probably already know which group you fall into, but if you are not sure, careful experimentation should tell you.

If you are among those whose airways open up with alcohol, there is probably no harm in sometimes having a small drink to relieve your asthma symptoms, with or without your reliever inhaler, but obviously you should not make a daily habit of this.

For those whose airways tighten up with alcohol, the good news is that it may not be alcohol itself, but something else in the drink. Each different kind of alcoholic drink contains a variety of other chemical ingredients besides alcohol, which give it its special taste and aroma. These additional ingredients are called 'congeners'. Wine contains different congeners from beer, and whisky has different congeners from sherry or vodka. So you may find that although your usual tipple has a bad effect, another kind of alcoholic drink is perfectly safe for you.

If it is alcohol itself that affects you, anti-histamines may be useful in preventing this reaction (see p. 332).

Drugs that interact with asthma drugs

Several drugs interact with the drugs given for asthma. A drug of this kind could make your asthma worse, by weakening the power of your asthma drugs, or it could make the asthma drugs more toxic. Your doctor should be aware of these interactions, and avoid giving drugs that don't mix. But oversights do occur, so it is as well to be aware of these interactions yourself. This is particularly important if you are taking a theophylline-type drug (e.g. Theodur, Uniphyllin, Phyllocontin) as the level in the blood can rise dangerously when other drugs are taken.

The major interactions for each type of asthma drug are listed, in the appropriate section for that drug, on pp. 350–69.

Remember too that alcohol, nicotine and other recreational drugs can affect asthma drugs – see pp. 350–69 for details.

'I sounded like a raven with bronchitis . . .'

Side-effects from asthma drugs (see pp. 350–69) can be quite individual. Elisabeth Butler is a retired nurse with asthma. 'I got a very odd reaction from taking steroids tablets recently. I was on quite a high dose, and it affected my voice so that I sounded like a raven with bronchitis for a month. My doctors sent me off to an ear-nose-and-throat specialist, who passed me onto a speech therapist. She said I'd been misusing my voice all my life, which at sixty-five was quite a shock. She showed me what I was doing wrong, and how to put things right, and to my amazement I came out speaking normally. It seems that I'd got into some bad habits of tensing certain muscles around my vocal chords. But it was definitely the steroid tablets that made it worse, so that I could hardly speak at anything above a croak.'

Very few other people are likely to get this side-effect from steroid tablets, but it is worth remembering that unusual reactions do occur occasionally. This case also shows that some side-effects are due to the combination of the drug and some other cause: it is worth treating the other cause.

9

Special situations

'. . . my lungs just seemed to get stronger . . .'

Dean is now 28. He has suffered from asthma since he was seven years old. 'When I first started doing cross-country running, when I was 13 or so, I just couldn't do it because I'd always get an asthma attack and be sucking on my inhaler while everyone else raced past. But by the end of secondary school I was the fastest person in my year. I found that by getting fit, the asthma became much less of a problem. I often got an attack from the exercise itself, but I used to take my Ventolin inhaler if I needed it. Gradually I needed it less and less, because my lungs just seemed to get stronger. I used to play four rugby matches a weekend sometimes, and I did a lot of swimming as well. I was really fit then. Later, after I left school, I used to play rugby for the county team, but my back got injured in a tackle, and I've had to stop. I've got much less fit now, and my asthma's a bit worse again.

'I know I should take up some other sport. I keep meaning to do something, but we're really busy at work and I haven't got round to it. I know if I started sport again, it would be difficult with my asthma at first, but once I'd got through that I'd feel better.'

WORK AND ASTHMA – WHICH JOBS ARE RISKY?

Asthma brought on by substances inhaled at work (known as occupational asthma) is a serious problem. Surveys in the USA and Japan suggest that 5–15 per cent of all asthma is work-related, while in Britain the figure is at least 5 per cent. These cases of asthma are almost certainly preventable.

The number of people suffering from occupational asthma is steadily growing, and for 60–90 per cent of them, the asthma does not go away, even though they stop breathing the offending substance. In the early stages, occupational asthma *is* reversible as long as exposure stops completely, but it is very likely to become irreversible in time.

Occupational asthma can come on after a few weeks in a new job, or it may take months or even years to develop. Most cases occur within the first two years of being exposed to the substance concerned.

Doctors and trade unionists are concerned that occupational asthma is still not recognized in many cases, or not recognized soon enough. If you think you may have occupational asthma, it is very important to act quickly, before your health is permanently damaged. Nearly half of those with irreversible occupational asthma get out of breath while simply walking, never mind running or playing sport. Some are seriously disabled by their asthma. One in three people with work-related asthma eventually has to give up their job because of their asthma. In health terms it is far better to give up the job, if you have to, or accept a transfer (see p. 276), *in the early stages* of the disease, while you can still regain your health.

The different types of asthmagen

Substances that are known to provoke asthma are called *asthmagens* or *respiratory sensitizers*. There are two basic kinds of asthmagen:
- Some asthmagens act as allergens. In other words, they provoke an allergic reaction by the immune system in the same way that pollen or house dust mites can produce an allergic reaction (see p. 110). Allergens in the workplace are mostly produced by plants or animals, and they are particularly common in food-processing industries. The same potentially allergenic substances – such as flour – are used in millions

of homes without any problem, because the amount in the air is so much less. It is the high concentration of allergens in the air that sparks off occupational asthma.

- Other asthmagens act as haptens. This means that they cannot act as allergens in their own right, but become attached to proteins in the human body, which are then changed chemically and can act as allergens.
- Other asthmagens provoke asthma without causing any allergic reaction – they are acting as irritants to the airways. These are all man-made chemicals.

Other terms used to describe asthmagens are *high-molecular weight substances* (meaning substances that act as allergens) and *low-molecular weight substances* (meaning haptens and irritants).

The different kinds of workplace asthma
Terminology is very important here because of the legal implications of workplace asthma. If you are trying to get a job transfer or compensation, you need to be clear about what these different terms mean.

Occupational asthma
In Britain, this term refers to asthma that is directly caused by an asthmagen at work. It is a specific reaction to that asthmagen. Once the person is sensitized to the particular asthmagen, they will probably always react to it, even in very tiny amounts.

Most of those with occupational asthma did not have asthma before being exposed to an asthmagen at work. But there are also people who had asthma beforehand, and who then develop occupational asthma as well. In other words, they develop a specific sensitivity to something inhaled at work, on top of their pre-existing asthma.

Work-aggravated asthma
People who already have asthma, not caused by their work, may be made worse, from time to time, by exposure to high levels of irritant substances at work. This is a *non-specific* reaction to the irritant, which makes it different from true occupational asthma. The level of exposure to the asthmagen which will cause this to happen may be very different from the level needed to initiate occupational asthma.

In Britain, employers are legally required to take steps to prevent this problem occurring, as well as to prevent occupational asthma.

RADS

RADS stands for Reactive Airways Dysfunction Syndrome. It refers to asthma that develops after a *single* exposure to very high doses of an irritant chemical such as chlorine, sulphur dioxide or ammonia. The kind of high-dose exposures that bring on RADS only occur during a chemical spill. In one incident, there were 20 cases of RADS among local people after a train carrying pesticides crashed into the Sacramento River. RADS is still controversial, but many medical experts do now accept that it exists. Among those at risk of RADS are firefighters and pulp mill workers.

The term IIA (Irritant-Induced Asthma) is sometimes used when people have developed asthma after being exposed to *two or more* high doses of irritants (but not exposed continuously). It is probably very similar to RADS in terms of its underlying mechanism.

RADS and IIA seem to be different from other forms of occupational asthma in various ways. The symptoms are somewhat different, and they do not respond very well to B-2 reliever drugs.

Workplace asthma or work-related asthma

These are umbrella terms which refer to all the conditions listed above.

Diagnosing occupational asthma

The symptoms of occupational asthma are the same as for ordinary asthma (see pp. 23–4). You should suspect occupational asthma if the symptoms began within a year or two of:
- beginning a new job
- moving to a different part of your existing workplace
- taking on a new task at your existing workplace
- changes in the procedures, substances or equipment used
- the breakdown/deterioration of sealed processing units (fume cupboards, spray booths etc.) or extractor fans
- damage causing leakage from machines

Asthma that clears up during your annual holiday is very likely to be occupational asthma, although this can sometimes be a symptom of stress at work. In the early stages, occupational asthma may also clear up at weekends, or in the evenings. Later on in the course of the disease it will not improve, even though you are away from work for months or years.

Skin-prick tests (see p. 304) can help in the diagnosis, but only if the asthmagen concerned is an allergen or hapten (see p. 269).

For more information on getting a medical diagnosis see p. 275.

Workplace asthma and the law

In Britain, the 1997 Disability Discrimination Act ensures that no one can be dismissed from their job because of asthma. If you have been dismissed, you may be entitled to compensation.

Prevention of asthma is based on the COSHH (Control of Substances Hazardous to Health) Regulations, which are rather vague and general in places, and often misunderstood by employers. The main points are listed p. 272.

If employers have failed in their duties to prevent asthma, and if a person can be proved to have occupational asthma, compensation is payable. In order to prove that you have occupational asthma, you may be required to take a challenge test where you inhale the asthmagen in a clinic or hospital, after a period of not breathing it at all for some months. Or you may simply be monitored while you have time off, and again when you go back to normal workplace exposure.

The employer has a right to ensure that your asthma has definitely been caused by something inhaled at work. Even those working in high-risk jobs may develop asthma for other reasons – asthma that is not directly caused by anything at work and would probably have come on anyway, regardless of their job. In addition, there may be conditions at work which make asthma worse, such as breathing cold air, or strenuous physical exertion, but this is not occupational asthma.

Some countries still rely on a list of known asthmagens, and only accept cases as occupational asthma if they involve one of these substances. This system has been abandoned in Britain and many other countries, because it fails to identify cases where the asthmagen is a newly used chemical, not linked with asthma before.

Preventing workplace asthma

What employers should do

Employers could prevent most cases of asthma by keeping asthmagens out of the air. In Britain, the COSHH regulations require employers to:

- assess the risks of asthma
- carry out health checks on people exposed to known asthmagens
- where possible, substitute less harmful chemicals for potent asthmagens
- if substitution is not possible, reduce levels of exposure by creating enclosed units (e.g. fume cupboards, ventilated spray booths, glove boxes) for all hazardous processes
- check these enclosed units for leaks regularly
- in addition to enclosing asthmagens, provide good ventilation and extraction systems that make the air in the workplace safe to breathe
- *as a last resort*, provide personal respiratory protective equipment (masks, powered respirator helmets, etc.) where necessary

There are also guidelines on asthma prevention published by the Health and Safety Executive, but these are not legally binding, unlike the COSHH regulations.

New asthmagens are being identified in industry all the time, and employers are expected to act promptly to prevent outbreaks of asthma from these substances. If any member of the workforce develops occupational asthma, the employer is legally obliged to report this to the Health and Safety Executive or the Department of Environmental Health, depending on the type of workplace. The employer should also organize medical checks on all other members of the workforce, identify the asthmagen concerned, have the amount in the air measured, and introduce enclosure and ventilation systems that substantially reduce this amount. When this is done promptly and thoroughly, most of those who have already developed asthma should recover, and no new cases should occur.

In industries where asthma risks are already known, there should be regular medical check-ups, especially on new employees. A responsible employer should ensure that new workers are given a check-up after one month, three months and six months, and then at six- to twelve-month intervals thereafter.

What workers should do
When thinking about taking up a new job
Those who have allergic diseases such as hayfever (whether they have asthma or not) should avoid working with laboratory animals or in bakeries, or in other high-risk jobs involving allergens (see pp. 280–3 for a full list). Their chance of developing asthma in these jobs is much greater than normal.

If you come from an allergy-prone family, even though you do not have allergies or asthma yourself as yet, you should also think twice about such jobs.

Those with asthma *but no allergies* have a slightly higher chance of developing occupational asthma if they go into a risky job, but the difference in risk between them and healthy people is not that large. The same applies to asthmatics who have allergies and who are contemplating jobs with asthma risks *not* caused by allergens. For both these groups, the greatest danger is that they will not notice if they begin to develop occupational asthma, and may continue working there when they should stop. They may then develop irreversible occupational asthma, and find that they are much less healthy than before they began work.

The Health and Safety Executive's information line (see p. 274) can advise on the risks associated with particular types of work, and the National Asthma Campaign helpline may also be useful (see p. 452).

In addition to finding out about the risks of a particular type of job, you need to look into the safety record of the employer in question. This is more difficult. Generally speaking, larger companies are more careful about safety procedures than smaller ones. Talk to your doctor or specialist who may well know if this workplace has a good or bad reputation locally. Other people who already work there may also be a good source of information. Ask them if there are any cases of occupational asthma already, how the company deals with these cases, if the company has a good record on safety generally, and if there is a trade union Safety Representative.

If you find you need more information about occupational asthma, the Internet can be useful; most public libraries now offer Internet access and can help with searches. Some good websites dealing with occupational asthma are listed on pp. 456–7.

Incidentally, these choices about employment are ones for *the individual employees* to make for their own protection – an employer cannot refuse to take anyone on because they have asthma already or are prone to allergies. The reasoning behind this is that the workplace should be safe for everyone, as far as possible. With one in three of the population susceptible to allergies, it is quite unacceptable to exclude such a large number of people from major industries. Furthermore, although those who are already prone to allergies may be rather more likely to get asthma in certain occupations, they are not the only ones affected. There are many other victims of occupational asthma who are not allergy-prone and could not be identified in advance. So the focus should be on getting asthmagens out of the air, not keeping the more vulnerable workers out of the workplace.

Starting a job where there is a known asthma risk
If you take the job, observe all the safety procedures that are in place, and if you smoke cigarettes, give up now. Smoking greatly increases the risk of developing asthma, particularly from allergens at work: the risk is five times higher than for non-smokers.

Where you have the option of turning on extractor fans, or wearing protective gear, always do so. In the case of small workplaces, such as hairdressers, simply opening doors and windows to improve ventilation will be helpful.

If you feel that safety procedures are inadequate, talk to your trade union Safety Representative. If you do not have one, contact the local Health and Safety Executive (for manufacturing industries, farming, mining, docks, etc.) or the Environmental Health Department (for service sector workplaces such as shops and offices, and for concerns about the exposure of the general public to workplace emissions). The numbers for both these departments can be found in your local telephone book. The Environmental Health Department will be listed under the city council or the district council.

These agencies can run a check on safety procedures in your workplace, without revealing the identity of the person who made a complaint. It will be presented to the employer as a routine check, so they need never know that a complaint has been made. In any case, if you make a complaint about safety procedures, you are protected by law from being dismissed for doing so. (However, it is still better for the union Safety Representative to request these checks.)

There may be mild symptoms which start before occupational asthma begins. These can include sneezing, a blocked or runny nose, itchy eyes, glazed or watery eyes, a dry cough, sweating and a feverish feeling. A skin rash or swelling from direct skin contact with an allergen (e.g. latex, laboratory animals) is also possible. Watch out for any of these symptoms and see your doctor should they appear. If you are working with an allergen, skin-prick tests (see p. 304) could be used at this stage to see if you have developed an allergy to the substance concerned.

At the first signs of occupational asthma

Acting promptly gives you the best possible chance of recovery. If exposure to the asthmagen stops immediately, your asthma should disappear completely.

See your GP as soon as possible. Make it clear that you think the problem may be work-related and provide full details of your symptoms, their timing, and how they relate to work exposures. Ask to be referred to a chest specialist as quickly as possible, so that a definite diagnosis can be made. This is essential if you are going to make a claim for compensation. You could also be referred to the local Employment Medical Advisor of the Health and Safety Executive.

Too many people with occupational asthma are just sent off with a reliever inhaler when they first see their GP. The delay in identifying work as the source of the problem, and ending the exposure to the asthmagen, is often responsible for the asthma becoming a lifelong problem.

Your GP may not know much about occupational asthma, and may be more inclined to attribute the asthma to other causes, so it is useful to be well informed before you go. Try to find out about the substances that could be in the air in your workplace – are isocyanates or platinum salts used, for example?

If the GP is reasonably convinced that your asthma is related to your work, he or she should be able to give you a sickness certificate, so that you can have a period of time away from the workplace, to see if you recover.

Once your GP is sure you have occupational asthma, he or she is legally obliged to report this, either to your employer or to the

Employment Medical Advisor of the local Health and Safety Executive. This is to ensure that the workplace is checked for safety, so that other workers do not develop asthma. Your GP must ask your permission before contacting your employer, and you have a right to withhold that permission.

The occupational nurse or doctor at the workplace may also be a good source of medical advice and support. (In particular, they are better placed to diagnose occupational asthma, because they see far more cases than the average GP.) In some workplaces they are truly independent of the management and can offer confidential advice and treatment. But in some workplaces, workers showing the early signs of occupational asthma may be targets for dismissal on other grounds, or find themselves in the next round of redundancies, to save the company from a possible compensation pay-out. All occupational health services will, of course, *claim* to be independent, but the problem of divided loyalties does indeed exist. Claiming to be independent is easy: each occupational health service has actually to demonstrate its independence over a period of years. Ask your colleagues for their views, especially those who have worked with the company for a long time, and talk to your union representative.

Once it is clear that you have occupational asthma, your employer should offer you another job where there is no exposure to the asthmagen. Ideally, this should be in a completely different building and on a separate site. If you are in a building nearby, the air can be contaminated by fumes from the original workplace, or the asthmagen may be brought in (in tiny amounts, but enough to affect a sensitized person) on manufactured objects, packing materials or the clothing of other workers.

If you have caught the problem early, and if you are completely free from exposure to the asthmagen, your asthma should start to get better within a few days or weeks. The symptoms may disappear completely, but remember that you are probably still highly sensitive to the original asthmagen, even years afterwards, so be careful to avoid inhaling it again, even in tiny amounts. If another member of your family works in the same place, they may bring home trace amounts of the asthmagen in their clothes and hair: if you notice continuing symptoms, ask them to leave their workclothes somewhere outside the house and shower as soon as they get home.

Where the employer cannot offer you any other job free of the asthmagen, there may be a stark choice between becoming unemployed or carrying on in the same workplace, staying as far away as possible from the asthmagen and using respiratory equipment (see below). This is a tough decision, because if you stay on, even with all possible precautions, there is a risk of the asthma continuing or getting worse, and of it becoming incurable. If you are accidentally exposed to a very high dose of the asthmagen, you could even have a fatal asthma attack.

For those with irreversible occupational asthma, compensation should be paid. Make sure that you have a definite diagnosis of occupational asthma, based on monitoring during a return to work, or a specific challenge test with the work asthmagen. You should be assessed for permanent disability two years after exposure to the asthmagen ends. The Citizens' Advice Bureau can refer you to a solicitor for legal advice about seeking compensation. You may also be entitled to Industrial Injuries Benefit, which is based on your level of disability. Talk to the Benefits Agency about this.

Respirators and breathing apparatus
If you are employed and need respiratory equipment, your employer is responsible for providing it, but it is very important that you should be well informed yourself about this equipment.

There are two types of respiratory equipment:
- Those that filter the surrounding air to remove asthmagens. These are called *respirators* in Britain (but in other countries this term is used more loosely to describe all kinds of respiratory equipment). Respirators may rely on the strength of the in-breath to pull the air through the filter, which can be a problem for some asthmatics because they cannot breathe in strongly enough. Other respirators have a battery-powered unit to assist with pulling in the air.
- Those that give you a completely separate supply of air, either from a compressed-air cylinder, or via an air-hose (airline) supplied with air from outside the work area. These are called *breathing apparatus* in Britain.

The respiratory equipment must be right for the job. For example, a device intended for filtering out dusts will be no use whatever against paint spray or solder fumes. There are tough regulations governing the type of equipment and the type of filter required for each type of asthmagen. Large companies are likely to know about these regulations and stick to them, but small outfits, such as local car-repainting workshops, electronic repair shops or joineries, may well be ignorant of the regulations.

If respiratory equipment has a face mask, it must form a tight seal with your face to be effective. A beard will interfere with this, and stubble can be just as bad, so shave carefully. Faces vary enormously in shape, and it is a mistake to think that one type of respiratory equipment will automatically fit every worker in the workplace. Make sure your face mask fits, and if it doesn't, ask for a different type of mask or a different type of respiratory equipment. Keep asking until you get one that's right for you.

Go through a 'fit check' every time you put the mask on. For example, with respirators, you can check the fit by covering the air intake and breathing in sharply: if the mask fits properly, the mask should collapse on to the face, and stay stuck to the face for several seconds. A different fit check may be specified by the manufacturer: follow the instructions.

In Britain, if you have doubts about the respiratory equipment you have been given, or the way it is being used, you can ring the Health and Safety Executive's information line (see p. 274) for free and confidential advice.

If there is any difficulty in breathing through the respiratory equipment, or if you can smell the substance being handled, the replaceable filter cartridge or the whole equipment should be replaced. However, you should not rely on smelling the asthmagen to warn you of leaks – by the time you can smell it, you may already have been exposed to damaging levels.

You should be trained in the use of your respiratory equipment by someone who is familiar with its use. The equipment should be inspected, tested, cleaned and repaired after each use, and it should be stored properly in a sealed container. Filters should be replaced regularly. Your employer is responsible for all this, but it makes sense to check for yourself that it is being done, and to give the mask a visual inspection before you put it on.

Keep your mask on throughout the work period. Taking it off, even for just a few minutes, is potentially risky, especially with the most powerful asthmagens. If you find it impossible to keep the mask on, talk to your employer or line manager about this. Another type of respiratory equipment might be the answer – a powered device, for example, which assists with pulling in the air, making the equipment less tiring to wear for long periods.

Bear in mind that no form of respiratory equipment provides complete protection against asthmagens: there is always the chance of some small amount getting through. This is why respiratory equipment is not the answer for someone who has already developed occupational asthma but wishes to remain in their job.

Those who are self-employed and really cannot change jobs (for example farmers) are sometimes able to use a powered respirator helmet, which allows them to go on working despite the presence of their allergen. The helmet itself is fairly light and comfortable. The air filter, powered by a battery, is carried on the back. Air is taken in, filtered and pumped up a flexible tube into the back of the helmet. Channels inside the helmet carry it over the head and pump it out at the front. A plastic face shield extends downwards from the helmet. Although it is open at the bottom, the outside air is prevented from entering by the constant downward flow of filtered air. You should ask for advice from your local Health and Safety Executive (see p. 274) on the suitability of this equipment for your particular circumstances.

Drug treatment for occupational asthma

Treatment is essentially the same as for other forms of asthma. You will almost certainly be given a B-2 reliever inhaler. If you have a severe attack you can take a large number of puffs without coming to any harm – indeed, it is vital that you use it as much as necessary in an emergency (see p. 51). But on a day-to-day basis, make sure you don't use the B-2 reliever too often as it can make matters worse when used excessively (see p. 323).

If you are offered inhaled steroids, it would be sensible to take these, as they will calm the inflammation and may improve the chances of your making a complete recovery.

Where the asthma has been caused by an allergen, cromoglycate-type drugs (see p. 338) may be helpful in reducing the reaction until such time as you can leave the workplace. Ask your doctor about prescribing this in addition to other asthma drugs.

Drug treatment should not be seen as a way of allowing you to go on working with the offending asthmagen. Getting away from the asthmagen is the only sensible way to treat occupational asthma.

'I would give every penny back to get good lungs again . . .'

After working in an electronics factory for three years, Violette Hutchins developed asthma. She can no longer do any sort of work, is in constant pain, and has to take six different drugs for her asthma. Although her trade union obtained £500,000 for her in compensation, Violette feels this cannot replace her health. 'I am existing, not living. I'm very grateful to the union, but I would give every penny back to get good lungs again. The money just gives me a better standard of misery.'

The soldering fumes that made Violette ill were known to be a cause of asthma ten years before she began her job, but her employers never told her of the risks. This is not uncommon. A survey at a clinic for occupational lung disease found that 91 per cent of affected workers had never been warned about the risks of getting asthma at work.

Which jobs are risky?
The list of workplace asthmagens is a long one – over 200 different substances – and it continues to grow. So the number of different workplaces with a risk of asthma is also very large. The list below is just a very brief guide to the most notorious offenders, *not* a comprehensive list.

Workplaces with high-allergen risks
If you have any tendency to allergies (or if you come from an allergy-prone family) these workplaces are best avoided. Smoking cigarettes substantially increases the risk of developing asthma in these jobs.

Bakeries, flour mills and other food-processing plants
In bakeries and flour mills, the allergens concerned may be wheat proteins found in the flour, or enzymes added to the flour mix, some of which are derived from fungi. 'Baker's asthma', as it is known, can be very slow to develop and only come on many years after starting work.

Tea importers and packers are at risk because tea dust is a potent asthmagen. So too is the dust from soybeans and others beans, including gram flour.

The risks of occupational asthma are particularly high where fish and shellfish are processed, especially if automated gutting machines are used without adequate ventilation, as these fill the workplace with a fine spray containing allergenic proteins. Outbreaks of asthma have been linked to the processing of salmon, crab, snow-crab, prawns, sea squirts and trout.

With all these allergies, it is possible that the affected person will react to the same substance when it is eaten. You should experiment very carefully with eating any food that has been a cause of occupational asthma. Note that the bad reaction may persist long after the job has ended. In one case, doctors found that a French woman who had developed asthma while working briefly in a bakery as a teenager, was still allergic to the enzyme additive in bread 20 years later, and suffered asthma when she ate bread.

Farms, saw mills, docks and cotton mills
Any workplace where dust from plant products is swirling around in the air can, potentially, produce occupational asthma.

In the case of farms, it is the dust from grain and hay that is often responsible, although mould spores (see p. 117) can also be the culprit. Where moulds are identified as the cause, keeping harvested crops dry and the storage area well ventilated may solve the problem.

In saw mills and joineries, wood dust can be a potent cause of asthma, especially dust from hardwoods, and from red cedar (*Thuja plicata*).

Where soybeans or other beans are being loaded for transport and storage, or unloaded at docks, there is a risk of asthma from the dust. Prevention measures should include lids on the storage silos to keep in the dust during transfer of the beans.

In cotton mills, high levels of cotton dust in the air can bring on occupational asthma. Studies in the USA show that smokers are affected by levels that are legally defined as 'safe', while non-smokers remain unaffected.

In all these situations, dust masks may be necessary, but it is important that they are up to the job (see p. 480). Simple types of dust mask, called 'nuisance dust masks', do not give reliable protection.

Detergent and pharmaceutical factories

The enzymes added to 'biological' washing powders are potential allergens and can cause asthma in some workers, especially if used in powder form rather than as granules.

The pharmaceutical industry also uses some enzymes, which can act as allergens and cause asthma. People working in factories processing natural products such as psyllium or ispaghula (for use as laxatives) are also susceptible to asthma. They should subsequently avoid taking medicines containing the offending substance.

There are many other drugs that are not allergens but can cause asthma.

Hospitals and clinics

The major allergen in hospitals is latex, used in gloves and other equipment. Although nursing staff and surgeons are those most likely to develop latex allergy, there is at least one case of a hospital administrative worker being affected.

Hospital workers are expected to protect themselves against this problem which almost always begins with an allergic rash on the hands. Turning the gloves inside out (to relieve the skin irritation from the powdered surface) puffs powder into the air and hastens the development of asthma.

Powdered latex gloves release 15,000 times as much allergen into the air as unpowdered gloves. Unpowdered, low-allergen gloves greatly reduce the risk of latex allergy developing, and vinyl gloves are even more effective. Some people are able to tolerate one brand of latex glove, but not another. These preventive measures should be taken when the skin rash starts, before there is any sign of asthma.

Someone who is allergic to latex will probably react to other rubber items (e.g. rubber gloves, condoms, balloons, elastic bands) at home. A few people *might* also react to latex particles in the air on city streets although there are no documented cases of this (see p. 212).

There is a cross-reaction between latex and certain foods, notably bananas, chestnuts, avocados, kiwi fruit and figs: you may react to these foods, so proceed cautiously. A reaction to traces of latex in food, derived from latex gloves worn by food-processing workers, has also occurred but is rare.

For anyone with severe latex allergy, wearing a Medic-Alert bracelet (see p. 459) is advisable. A car crash or other accident could land you in a hospital operating theatre, and the medical staff need to know that you are allergic to latex. Cases of anaphylactic shock (see p. 111) have occurred in these circumstances.

Chiropody and podiatry clinics
Chiropodists and podiatrists may develop an allergic reaction to the fungus that causes athlete's foot, inhaled on skin flakes, and this can cause occupational asthma.

Laboratories where animals are kept
Asthma can develop in people working with laboratory mice, rats and other rodents. The allergen originates in the animals' urine, and becomes airborne as the urine dries. Mink urine can have the same allergenic effect.

Laboratories that keep insects, and production plants where mass rearing of insects or spiders occurs (for biological pest control, for example), are also a potential problem, due to small airborne particles from the insects' bodies.

Factories making or using rubber items
There is a risk of latex allergy (see above, under 'Hospitals and clinics') in factories producing rubber gloves, rubber dolls and other items made of latex. Anyone who regularly wears latex gloves for factory work is also at risk.

Workplaces with asthma risks caused by haptens or irritants
In some of these workplaces, four people in every 100 are likely to develop asthma during their working lives. The risk of occupational asthma persisting after the exposure stops is higher with these asthmagens, so it is even more important to stop exposure promptly if asthma symptoms develop.

Most of the new industrial asthmagens come into this category. New chemical substances are being introduced all the time, and any of these might carry an asthma risk, which may not become apparent for many years.

Always ask to see Safety Data Sheets for all the chemicals you are using, and read labels on all containers.

Platinum-refining works and steel-welding works
Platinum refining produces salts of platinum or hexachloroplatinates.

These act as haptens (see p. 269) and are among the most powerful asthmagens known. Some studies suggest that if workers are exposed to high enough concentrations of platinum salts, they will *all* develop asthma in time.

Welding steel, using either electric arc or gas metal arc welding, is associated with a risk of asthma.

Electronics factories
Soldering electronics components releases colophony fumes which are powerful asthmagens. Colophony fumes come from pine resin (colophony flux), and contain abietic acid: it is this which irritates the airways. Sealed units, such as fume cupboards and glove boxes, are required to contain the fumes.

Car-painting, aircraft-painting and boat-painting workshops
The offending substances here are isocyanates (see below) used as hardeners in spray paints. They are only found in two-pack paints, usually in part B.

A ventilated spray booth should be used. The best type is a down-draught booth, where the air comes down through the roof of the booth and is extracted through the floor.

In addition, if you are paint-spraying, a respirator unit that covers the face *completely* is the minimum safety requirement in Britain – don't settle for less. In other countries, such as Australia, even this is considered inadequate because it relies on filters to take the isocyanate out of the air. Filters can fail, so in these countries paint-sprayers must wear breathing apparatus that supplies air from a cylinder or from a fresh air intake outside the spray booth. For more information on using respiratory equipment, see pp. 277–9.

Isocyanate-based paints and varnishes are used for many other purposes within industry. Occupational health officers encourage the use of safer paints and varnishes wherever possible, because isocyanates are so dangerous.

Chemical works and plastics, foam and rubber factories
Isocyanates, some of the most potent asthmagens known, are also widely used in the production of waterproofing agents, polyurethane varnishes, polyurethane plastics and foams (used for insulation and other purposes), and some forms of rubber. The isocyanate used for these purposes is also referred to as TDI (toluene di-isocyanate).

Cement and sealing activators also contain isocyanates in the form of MDI or MBI. Respirators for use with MDI must meet certain regulations – air-purifying respirators are not sufficient. Fibreglass manufacturing is also linked with asthma.

Formaldehyde resins are asthmagenic, as is formaldehyde gas released in their manufacture. The manufacture and use of acid anhydrides to make resins is also a potential cause of occupational asthma. The chemicals concerned include phthalic anhydride, maleic anhydride, trimellitic anhydride and pyromellitic anhydride.

Hospitals and dental surgeries
In addition to latex (see p. 282) there are other asthmagens in hospitals, including glutaraldehyde (used to sterilize endoscopes, respiratory therapy equipment and dental instruments), hexachlor-ophene, formaldehyde and ethylene oxide. The developing process for X-rays uses glutaraldehyde, sulphur dioxide and acetic acid, and should be carried out within an enclosed unit to avoid causing asthma.

One study in the USA showed that respiratory therapists, whose job is to give nebulizer treatments, were twice as likely to develop asthma as comparable hospital workers. This finding has not been explained. It seems unlikely that it is caused by exposure to asthma drugs or to virus infections. Glutaraldehyde sensitivity may explain some cases.

Hairdressers
The asthmagens here include several chemical substances in hair preparations which can act as irritants, notably persulphate, and a few plant-derived items (e.g. henna and black henna) which can act as allergens.

Offices
These are not generally high-risk places, but some office workers are affected by photocopier toner.

Did you know?

The number of people with occupational asthma is growing. The Trades Union Congress estimates that a new case of occupational asthma develops in Britain every 75 minutes.

'Some people do try to cover up their symptoms . . .'

Gina is an occupational health nurse in an industrial area of England. She deals with a whole range of health problems, including asthma and chronic obstructive pulmonary disease (COPD).

'I work for a company that supplies occupational nurses to different industries. Most companies can't afford to have their own occupational nurse, so they employ one of us for a day a week. I go into lots of different workplaces: car plants, shipyards, big bakeries, tea companies. All these places have an asthma risk. With the cars and the ship-building, it's the welding and the paint-spraying that's the problem, the isocyanate paints especially. That's one of the biggest asthma risks, but breathing in flour or tea dust can be almost as dangerous. I try to get the workers to see that I'm on their side, that I'm trying to help them. Some of them think that if they talk to me about their symptoms, I'm just going to "tell on them" to the management, but it's not like that. A lot of my work is about gaining their confidence. Some people do try to cover up their symptoms at the regular check-ups that we give them when they've been working in a dangerous area for three months or six months or a year. They're afraid of losing their jobs. I try to get them to see that there is absolutely no point in doing this, because if you get severe asthma you're going to have to give up your job anyway, and you've probably got a lifelong health problem into the bargain. The sooner you get out of that dangerous area the more chance you have of recovering.

'On the whole I think workers are getting more health-conscious. When I carry out the tests on the older men, the ones who've been smoking for 20 years and never wear a mask because they think it's cissy to wear mask, their lung function results are dreadful, even if they don't have asthma or COPD yet. The younger guys are less bothered about wearing the masks, they just accept them. And mostly they don't smoke which makes an enormous difference. Their lung function results are in a different league altogether.'

PREGNANCY, BIRTH AND BREAST-FEEDING

There has been a lot of research into the effects of asthma on pregnancy and on the unborn child. The effects of asthma drugs have also been studied intensively. The overall conclusion is that there is not a great deal to worry about, although severe uncontrolled asthma can be bad for both mother and child.

Are asthma drugs dangerous to the unborn child?

This is the major question for most asthmatic women. It is also a major concern for doctors, and great care is taken in prescribing asthma drugs during pregnancy.

As long as your doctor is aware that you are pregnant, there should be absolutely no danger. In many other areas of asthma treatment there is some controversy (as will be clear if you read other sections of this book), but on the question of asthma and pregnancy there is remarkable unanimity among doctors and medical researchers: what is dangerous to the baby is severe uncontrolled asthma, *not* the drugs needed to treat asthma. This conclusion is not based on any complacency about drugs: there has been a lot of very careful research to see if any asthma drugs might harm the foetus. Since the Thalidomide tragedy, this is something that doctors are extremely careful about.

Ideally, the doctor should be told *before* you become pregnant, at the time you decide to try for a baby, so that your prescription can be changed if the drugs you are currently taking pose any threat, however small, to the unborn child. By talking to the doctor at this early stage, you can be sure of being established on the safest asthma drugs, with your asthma well controlled, from the moment of conception. This is important because the foetus is at its most vulnerable to damage by drugs during the first three months, and *especially the first few weeks after conception*.

All the asthma drugs that are recommended for use by pregnant women have been very carefully screened for any possible damage that they might do to the unborn child.

'But I'm already pregnant . . .'

Don't panic. *None* of the asthma drugs poses any special risk to the unborn child, although some anti-histamines (used to treat hayfever and other nasal allergies) do. There is probably nothing to worry about, but see your doctor as soon as possible. If you can't get an appointment straight away, talk to your pharmacist in the meantime. Don't stop taking your asthma medication, unless advised to do so by the doctor or pharmacist, as a severe attack is the most dangerous thing for the baby.

Which asthma drugs can be taken during pregnancy?

Although none of the asthma drugs poses any special risk during pregnancy, your doctor will probably want to play safe by putting you on a drug that has been very rigorously tested for possible damage to the foetus. Certain asthma drugs have been rigorously tested in this way, and if you are taking these you can have absolute peace of mind. It may take a little while for you to adjust to these drugs, if you have been taking something else previously. Don't be afraid to go back to the doctor if you feel your asthma is not under proper control.

If at all possible, drugs taken by mouth should be avoided during the first three months of pregnancy. Inhaled drugs are far safer as little enters the bloodstream.

Does asthma get worse or better during pregnancy?

About one-third of women with asthma have fewer symptoms while they are pregnant. This is not as surprising as it might seem. Some other diseases involving an over-active immune system, such as rheumatoid arthritis, also tend to subside during pregnancy, because the body reduces immune activity to prevent attacks against the baby (whose genes are different from those of the mother, making it a potential target for immune attacks).

For another third of women, their asthma stays about the same when they are pregnant.

Unfortunately, one-third of female asthmatics have much more severe symptoms during their pregnancy. For these women, careful monitoring and increased doses of asthma medicines are essential. The deterioration usually occurs between week 24 and week 36 of the pregnancy: the last four weeks are generally much better.

Very occasionally, asthma appears for the first time during pregnancy, and can be quite severe.

Most women get back to normal, as regards their asthma, by about 3 months after the birth.

In general, women with severe asthma are more likely to deteriorate during pregnancy, while those with mild asthma are more likely to improve. Recent research also shows that a baby girl is more likely to produce worsening symptoms than a baby boy. However, it is impossible to predict exactly how pregnancy will affect asthma for any particular person. Not only is there huge variation from one woman to another, but some women may have a different response to different pregnancies.

Effects on breathing

There are also some straightforward effects on breathing due to the greatly increased size of the womb. In the last few months of pregnancy (after the fifth or sixth month) the baby's head pushes upwards against the diaphragm (see pp. 414–6), which restricts its downward movement, and thus the expansion of the lungs, during the in-breath. The ribs move outwards to compensate, so that the chest is wider, and often this completely offsets the loss of space below. However, some women do find it more difficult to take deep breaths in the late stages of pregnancy, and lying down can make the problem worse because this pushes the diaphragm up even further.

Breathing exercises that strengthen the breathing muscles and establish a healthy pattern of breathing (see pp. 421–45) may be helpful in preventing this problem. They should be started in the early stages of pregnancy, or before conception if possible.

In addition to this difficulty, higher levels of the hormone progesterone occur during pregnancy, and these can trigger hyperventilation (over-breathing). One of the strange symptoms of hyperventilation is a feeling of 'air hunger', which can be confused with the breathless sensation of an asthma attack (see p. 419). Anxiety and panic may also lead to hyperventilation, especially during labour, so it helps to learn some relaxation techniques early on (see pp. 446–51).

Hormone changes during pregnancy also affect the nose, making it blocked and causing some women to snore for the first time in their lives. If you have this problem, try the nose-clearing exercises on p. 425 and p. 432.

Can asthma attacks occur during labour?

It is very rare for a severe asthma attack to occur during labour. Most asthmatics get through the delivery without any troublesome asthma symptoms. However, it is important that the midwife and other staff are aware of your asthma, just in case, and know what drugs you are taking.

If you have taken steroid tablets at any time during the previous two years, make sure the midwife and doctors know this. If you have taken long courses of steroids, or repeated short courses, you may need some low doses of steroid to see you through the stress of labour (see p. 359). Details of how long the courses were, and when you took them, will be useful.

What effect can a mother's asthma have on the baby?

If asthma is not well controlled during pregnancy, there is an increased risk of the baby being born prematurely, or being smaller than average. Unfortunately, premature babies are more likely to develop asthma themselves, compared to babies born at the right time. This will add to their risk of asthma later in life, a risk which is already higher for a child with an asthmatic mother.

The death rate for newborn babies is also slightly higher than average if the mother has poorly controlled asthma. This is probably due to the unborn child suffering from a shortage of oxygen when the mother has a really bad asthma attack.

However, if you have suffered an asthma attack during your pregnancy you should not worry unduly. One study of 47 pregnant Finnish women who had been admitted to hospital with a severe attack of asthma found that there were no serious long-term effects on the baby or mother. The fact that the attacks were treated promptly probably helped to prevent damage to the baby.

So if you do feel a severe attack coming on while pregnant, *call an ambulance without delay*. The ambulance will be carrying oxygen which is particularly important for helping the baby through the attack. Make sure the ambulance crew and doctors realize you are pregnant.

Any woman who has suffered a severe attack while pregnant should ask her doctor if it would be a good idea to increase her dose of inhaled corticosteroids to prevent another attack. For patients who are not already taking inhaled corticosteroids, it would probably be a good idea to start taking these regularly.

Asthma can also have unpleasant consequences for the expectant mother, if not well controlled. If severe, asthma can increase the risks of high blood pressure and pre-eclampsia during pregnancy.

The precautions that pregnant asthmatics should take

1. Talk to your doctor, before you conceive, about the drugs you are taking. Some of the prescriptions may need to be changed.

2. If you use any non-prescription medicines, such as anti-histamines or expectorants, talk to your pharmacist, before you conceive, about the safety of these.

3. You should not reduce the dose of the drugs at this time. It is particularly important to keep asthma under control during pregnancy. Your doctor may want to add other drugs, such as inhaled corticosteroids, to give you better control over the asthma.

4. If you have severe asthma normally, or if your asthma gets much worse during your pregnancy, it would be useful to monitor your peak flow twice a day (see p. 315) so that you can have some advance warning of serious attacks. Avoid allergens and asthma triggers as much as possible (see pp. 2–3) to minimize the risk of serious attacks.

5. In the unlikely event that you are a smoker, make every possible attempt to give up cigarettes before becoming pregnant. Smoking while pregnant aggravates your asthma, and increases the risk of having a small or premature baby. Your child will also run a greater risk of developing asthma if you smoke while pregnant (see pp. 88–9).

6. If you have sometimes suffered a major allergic reaction, to food or bee stings for example, you may have been issued with an adrenaline (epinephrine) self-injection kit. Using adrenaline (epinephrine) during the first three months of pregnancy may carry some risks to the baby: talk to your doctor now about what you should do in an emergency. Be extra vigilant about avoiding your allergen.

7. If you are already undergoing immunotherapy (see pp. 197–200), this can be continued at a steady 'maintenance dose', but the dose should not be increased. This is because there is a small risk of a major allergic reaction (anaphylaxis – see p. 111) during immunotherapy, especially when the dose is increased. Anaphylaxis can lead to a spontaneous abortion of the baby.

8. Skin-prick tests for allergy are not recommended during pregnancy, as these also carry a very small risk of anaphylaxis.

9. Many mothers-to-be are anxious to avoid passing their asthma on to their children. This is something to think about even before the child is conceived (see p. 87).

Asthma and breast-feeding

The drug theophylline (see pp. 374–5) can go through into breast-milk, and may make babies restless and irritable. Some mothers find they can reduce the problem by always taking the drug just after a feed, so that the amount in the milk is minimized. Alternatively, ask your doctor about changing to another drug. All other asthma drugs are considered safe during breast-feeding.

'relaxing is the most important thing . . .'

'As a child, I remember a school nurse telling me what to do about my asthma. I'd walk to school, about a mile along this very clogged, polluted road, and that always seemed to trigger it, especially when it was hot and sunny. So I'd arrive at school and go straight to the sick bay. She'd get me to sit down, lean forwards, put my head down and make "tummy balloons". That was extremely helpful. I realise now why leaning forwards helps so much – it raises your rib cage away from your spine, so you've got some space. And of course the "tummy balloons" are about breathing with your diaphragm.

'Later, as a teenager, I took up singing, and that helped because it trained me in deep lung breathing. The asthma has always made me more aware of my breathing, how you have to breathe past that constriction and breathe deeply and relax – relaxing is the most important thing. You've got to get over that panicky reaction which makes the asthma so much worse.'

SPORT AND ASTHMA

There is no reason why asthma should stop you from playing sport. Exercise is good for everyone, and especially good for asthmatics as it improves their lung capacity, strengthens the breathing muscles and keeps their airways elastic and flexible. Children and teenagers with asthma gain great benefits from sport because it makes them stronger physically, and helps build up confidence.

Taking part in games is good for asthmatic children in other ways too. If they are always excused games, they tend to become the sedentary, sickly 'outsider', and are less accepted by other children, whereas playing sports helps them feel more healthy and normal. Social acceptance is very important, and may make it easier for children to manage their asthma, simply because they are happier and better adjusted.

Many top athletes and sportsmen are asthmatic, including runners Steve Ovett and Jackee Joyner Kersee, cricketer Ian Botham and swimmer Liz Hobbs. American athletes taking part in the 1984 Summer Olympics were tested for asthma, and 11 per cent showed symptoms, although only one in four of these had realized that they were asthmatic. Between them, these asthmatics won 15 gold medals, and 26 silver and bronze medals. Their success shows that asthma need not stop asthmatics from taking part in sports.

'But exercise makes me wheeze . . .'
Many asthmatics are deterred from sports because they find that an asthma attack is always, or often, triggered by strenuous exercise. This is known as exercise-induced asthma or EIA (see pp. 68–73).

You should not let EIA stop you from playing sport. The important thing to realize is that once you get fit, you will have far less trouble with EIA, because you won't pant at the least exertion, so your airways will not dry out so easily (see pp. 68–9).

In one study, where 26 asthmatics went through an intense physical training programme, the number suffering from EIA dropped from 17 before the training to only three afterwards. Those who took part were much less worried about exercising after the programme, and their asthma was better overall.

When you first begin exercising, EIA may well be a problem but it is one that can be overcome in various ways:

- Short-acting B-2 reliever drugs (see pp. 371–2) can be taken 15–20 minutes before starting to exercise. They can be taken again during the game or race, as necessary, but if you always need a second dose at half-time this is a bad sign (see p. 71).
- If you need to stay active for more than four hours, and it is difficult to stop and take a second dose, a long-acting reliever (see pp. 344–5) may be useful: ask your doctor about prescribing this.
- Other drugs may be added if necessary: the cromoglycate-type drugs (see p. 338) work in a different way from reliever drugs and together they make a good team. These must be taken at least 30 minutes before exercise begins.
- Keeping asthma well controlled with regular use of preventer drugs – usually steroids (see p. 336) – will allow the other drugs to have maximum benefit.
- Warm-up exercises (see pp. 72–3) before strenuous activity begins can be helpful, in allowing the airways to adjust gradually to the extra flow of air.
- The body's own natural adrenaline will help keep the airways open. This can be stimulated in many different ways. Some long-distance runners with asthma do a few short sharp sprints before the race to stimulate their adrenaline. Excitement or anger will also do the trick.

Choose your sport carefully

Breathing cold, dry air tends to bring on asthma attacks, so skiing, ice-skating and mountaineering are more likely to cause problems. If you do want to go skiing, down-hill skiing is more asthma-friendly than cross-country because it is less strenuous – assuming there are ski-lifts!

Running (especially over long distances), cycling, and basketball all tend to induce asthmatic attacks more than other sports. Football, in which there are short bursts of strenuous activity, with lulls of more relaxed play in between, is often easier for the asthmatic to cope with. Like other team sports, it also allows the asthmatic to play in a position that requires less running around, such as goalkeeper.

Indoor sports may be less troublesome, especially in winter, because the air is warmer. Gymnastics and aerobics have both proved beneficial for asthmatics. Judo and other martial arts are particularly good, for both adults and children, because they encourage calm and regular breathing (see p. 429).

Swimming is generally thought to be the best exercise for those with severe asthma, because the warm moist air of an indoor pool prevents drying-out of the airways. However, a few asthmatics are affected by the chlorine fumes from the disinfected water. Swimming outdoors may be possible: ask around locally for suitable pools or other swimming places, such as rivers, lakes or the sea. You should always go with a friend who is a strong swimmer in case you get into difficulties, and take a dose of your reliever before going into the water.

If you are very unfit, gentle swimming may be a good way to start regaining your strength. It is particularly good for strengthening the muscles involved in breathing, and for teaching steady, calm, controlled breathing patterns which are beneficial to asthmatics. Most swimming pools hold classes for children, and for adults who have never learned to swim. Sometimes there are special swimming groups for young people with asthma.

Some sporting activities are risky for asthmatics

The use of pressurized oxygen, as in scuba diving (see p. 445) and sky-diving, could be dangerous for those with asthma. Make sure you have a trainer with specialized knowledge of working with asthmatics, and talk to your doctor first.

Very high altitudes (above 1540 metres – 5000 feet), where there is less oxygen in the air, can cause 'altitude sickness' if the ascent is too rapid and the body does not have sufficient time to adjust. The symptoms are headaches, nausea, lightheadedness and disorientation. Altitude sickness affects everyone who normally lives near sea level, but it might be slightly more problematic for someone with asthma than for an entirely healthy person. If affected, stop the ascent, descend to a lower altitude for a day or two if possible, and rest as much as you can. Extra asthma medication may be needed.

On the plus side, house dust mites do not live at high altitudes, so if dust allergy plays a role in your asthma, the mountains may be the best place to go.

Could intensive athletic training cause asthma?

Intensive training, especially in cold air, or air that contains high levels of allergens or irritants, may make athletes more likely to develop asthma. This conclusion comes from research in Finland which found that elite athletes were three to six times more likely to have asthma than the average person. The risk was higher for long-distance runners (800 metres and marathon) than for sprinters, jumpers, throwers and decathletes, probably because they are breathing heavily for longer periods of time.

Cold air is thought to be the primary cause: among competition-standard figure-skaters, 30 per cent suffer from asthma. Repeated drying of the airways, from prolonged training in the cold, seems to make them increasingly sensitive.

Are asthma drugs allowed in competitive sports?

When people ask this question they are usually worried about steroids. But the steroids used to treat asthma (corticosteroids) are completely different from the anabolic steroids that are used illegally in weight-lifting, athletics and some other sports, to build up muscle mass and reduce body fat. Several types of inhaled corticosteroid are officially permitted in international events. Corticosteroids in tablet or injection form are not allowed, however.

Some of the reliever drugs (see p. 341) used for asthma are said to have a mild anabolic effect – that is, they build up muscle in the same way as anabolic steroids. One of these, Clenbuterol, was at the centre of a dispute involving two British weightlifters in the Barcelona Olympics in 1992. There is still controversy over whether this drug really does have an anabolic effect or not, but it is officially banned. However, as Clenbuterol is not one of the widely used reliever drugs, this is not really a problem for asthmatics. Several other reliever drugs are permitted, including popular ones such as Ventolin, and so are the cromoglycate-type drugs (see p. 371). There is no reason why any asthmatic should be prevented from competing, as asthma can be well controlled using the permitted drugs.

10

Getting medical help

> '. . . there's a lot we can do,
> but I wouldn't claim that we have all the answers.'

Duncan is a young GP with many asthmatics in his care. 'You've got to accept that there is no such thing as perfection in medicine. It's always evolving, and getting better – and that's its strength really. The problems come when patients expect us to know absolutely everything and get everything right first time. Of course we can't: that's just a totally unrealistic expectation.

'Asthma is a particularly difficult thing to treat unless the patient has realistic expectations of the doctor, and is prepared to take responsibility for their own health. When someone will do that, and you feel like you're working together with them as a team, then the asthma is much more manageable.

'I think the modern asthma drugs are amazingly good, and if you talk to the older doctors, who remember what awful lives asthmatics used to lead in the past, there's no doubt that things have improved. So there's a lot we can do, as doctors, but I wouldn't claim that we have all the answers. I've seen some patients improve dramatically when they try an alternative therapy. Sometimes I can explain it, because they were twitchy and anxious about the asthma before, and it's calmed them down, but sometimes it's a mystery why it's worked.'

DOCTORS, ASTHMA NURSES AND SPECIALISTS

If you or your child have wheezing, breathlessness, recurrent cough-ing or other symptoms (see pp. 23–4) that might be due to asthma, the first step in getting medical help is to see your GP or family doctor. He or she decides if it is really asthma or not, by asking you about the symptoms and carrying out certain tests. The diagnosis of asthma is easy in some cases, but more difficult in others (see p. 306).

The GP will almost certainly prescribe drugs in the first instance, and then hand you over to the asthma nurse if there is one in the practice.

The role of the asthma nurse

Most GP practices in Britain now have an asthma nurse, who has taken a special training course in asthma. Her job is to show you how to use your inhaler correctly, to teach you what to do with a peak-flow meter (see p. 315), to discuss any concerns you may have, and to see you regularly, over the coming months and years, to check if the drugs are working well and keep an eye on your progress.

The asthma nurse knows as much about asthma drugs and the orthodox medical treatment of asthma as the doctor – possibly even more, because she has more time to specialize in asthma and to keep up-to-date with the new drugs and inhaler devices. She also has far more time to spend with you, so she can explain everything in detail. If she thinks that you need to see the doctor again, because there is something else going on besides asthma, because the diagnosis may have been wrong, or because the drugs aren't working well, she will tell you. If *you* feel that you would like see the doctor again, you only have to say so.

Seeing a physiotherapist

Some GP clinics now have a physiotherapist available, who you may be able to see. The role of the physiotherapist is to show you how to drain mucus from your lungs.

It is important to clear mucus for a variety of reasons. First, if it is sitting in your airways, it narrows them even further, making asthma attacks worse. Parts of the lung can even become blocked off com-pletely by mucus. Second, having a lot of mucus in the airways can make you more susceptible to infection of the lungs by a fungus known as *Aspergillus* (see p. 246).

A hospital consultant (see below) may also be able to refer you for physiotherapy at the hospital.

Referral to a specialist (consultant)

Specialists (consultants) treating asthma include paediatricians, chest physicians and allergists. Only some asthmatics will be referred to a specialist.

You or your child are likely to be referred if:
- the asthma seems difficult to control, or is unstable
- the diagnosis is uncertain
- there are complications, such as bronchitis, emphysema or a heart condition
- there are other medical problems besides asthma, which are either linked to the asthma (e.g. allergic eczema), or which make the asthma more difficult to manage

Patients under 18 will be referred to the paediatrician, while those over 18 will be referred to a chest physician. A few patients – including both children and adults – will be referred to an allergist.

The main reasons for referral to an allergist are:
- Asthma that occurs when there is a very severe allergic reaction causing general collapse (anaphylactic shock), usually after insect stings, or eating a particular food (see p. 111).
- Asthma in association with severe eczema or other allergic problems.
- Asthma which seems to be caused by an allergen, and where it is important to know if the allergen has been identified correctly (for example, a girl who wants to go riding, and who may be allergic to horses, but who cannot be sure because other allergies – for example to mould spores – or simply nervousness at being in a new situation, might be responsible for the wheezing she often gets at the stables).

What to expect if you see a paediatrician

Paediatricians generally treat *all* the different kinds of diseases that affect children, although some specialize in particular diseases.

A paediatrician will give your child a very thorough examination and look for any other kinds of illness besides asthma. Then there may be lung-function tests (see p. 303) and other investigations that relate specifically to asthma.

Some paediatricians also do skin-prick tests (see p. 304) and you may be given advice on avoiding allergens. In some clinics there is a specialist allergy nurse who deals with this. It is advisable to read Chapter 6 of this book as well, as there have been a lot of recent advances in allergen avoidance and it is now quite a complex field: many of the newer techniques and products are a great improvement on what was available formerly.

The paediatrician will also arrange regular lung-function tests to check on the effects of treatment and will deal with any associated symptoms such as a runny nose, sinusitis (see p. 240) or post-nasal drip (see p. 33).

What to expect if you see a chest physician

Chest physicians treat all the different kinds of lung diseases, including bronchitis, pneumonia, emphysema, and chronic obstructive pulmonary disease (see p. 32).

You will be given a very thorough physical examination, including lung-function tests (see p. 303). Although most chest physicians are not specifically trained in allergy, some chest physicians also carry out skin-prick tests (see p. 304). They can give some advice on avoiding allergens, but you would do well to read Chapter 6 of this book as well.

What to expect if you see an allergist

Allergists are specifically trained in treating the allergic diseases, such as anaphylaxis (see p. 111), true food allergy, hayfever and contact dermatitis. They also treat diseases such as asthma, eczema or urticaria where these are caused, or partly caused, by allergies. Some allergists can also offer diagnosis and treatment of food intolerance.

In order to confirm that allergies are present, and identify the allergens accurately, an allergist may carry out various tests for allergic reactions, such as skin-prick tests and RAST (see pp. 304–5).

Should more asthmatics be referred to a specialist?

In Britain, most patients with asthma are not referred to a specialist. Referral to an allergist (rather than a paediatrician or chest specialist) is an even rarer event, because there are so few allergists available. This is not a problem in the USA, however, where allergists are more common.

GPs can manage the vast majority of asthma cases perfectly well on their own, but referral to a paediatrician or chest specialist is a good idea for those whose asthma is unstable or difficult to manage, and for anyone who is getting steadily worse despite treatment. A specialist can also be of value to anyone who has doubts about the diagnosis of asthma. If you feel that you would like to be referred, talk to your GP about your concerns and ask if referral is possible.

The question of referral to an allergist is more difficult, because the resources are simply not available. Even if your GP believes it might be of benefit to you, a referral may not be possible, because there are no NHS allergists at all in large areas of Britain. Where there are consultant allergists, the waiting list may be unbelievably long. For example, in many parts of the country there is a waiting list of two years for non-urgent appointments – and unless you have very severe life-threatening asthma which is clearly allergic, or you have an anaphylactic reaction to food or insect stings (see p. 111) you will be regarded as non-urgent. Even those who have experienced these frightening reactions may wait four to seven months for an appointment.

If you or your child have ever suffered anaphylactic shock (see p. 48), you must be referred to an allergist. Don't take 'no' for an answer in this case because anaphylactic shock is particularly dangerous for asthmatics. You should be given injectable adrenaline (epinephrine) for emergency treatment (see p. 348).

Some GPs and asthma nurses have undergone training in skin-prick tests (see pp. 304–5), but the cost of buying all the different allergen extracts that are needed for thorough skin-testing deters most GPs from doing skin-prick tests in their own offices. Instead they tend to rely on a rough-and-ready system for identifying allergens and giving advice about their avoidance: anyone with year-round asthma is assumed to be allergic to house dust mites, anyone with asthma in the spring or summer only is assumed to be sensitive to pollen, and anyone who has attacks mainly in response to infections is assumed not to have allergies playing an important part in their asthma.

These rough rules-of-thumb may work in some cases, but they will give the wrong answer for a great many others. Not everyone with

summer asthma is allergic to pollen – some are reacting to summer
moulds (see p. 122) or cockroaches or even to foods eaten only in
summer. An asthmatic with year-round asthma may be allergic to
household moulds or pets, or affected by irritants in the air at home or
at work. Many have multiple allergies. People with infection-related
allergy may be allergic to house dust mites as well, and part of their
problem is that staying in bed with a bad cold boosts their intake of
mite allergen dramatically because the bedding is infested with mites.
So making guesses can be very misleading. If asthmatics know exactly
what affects them, they can take appropriate avoidance measures.

By using the checklists on pp. 114–25, you can probably pinpoint
your allergies fairly accurately. If you are still unsure, and think you
need skin-prick tests, ask your GP again, and if that fails, consider
getting them done privately (see p. 125).

'. . . she's never wheezed again . . .'

'Our eight-year-old has hayfever, and a couple of years back she
suffered a really bad bout of it. One evening the sneezing and
runny nose got worse and then it led on to wheezing and being sick.
It was very worrying. She seemed unable to breathe, so we called
the doctor. He gave her drugs and after a few hours she recovered.

'The doctor contacted us the next day, to say we should bring
Lucy into the surgery. He wanted her to start on inhalers – two
different kinds. I was inclined to think that he must know what
he's doing, but my wife was against it altogether. She said "Let's
just see what happens first."

'Lucy has been taking the anti-histamines for her hayfever
much more regularly since then, so the hayfever isn't so bad, and
she's never wheezed since that day. I feel pleased that we didn't
just accept her taking asthma drugs, because it's obvious she
doesn't need them.'

In this case, the diagnosis of asthma was clearly premature and
Lucy's parents were right to 'wait and see'. But for children who
do have asthma, it is a mistake to refuse treatment, especially
steroids, because untreated asthma can cause long-term damage
to the airways (see p. 327).

MEDICAL TESTS USED FOR ASTHMA

Lung-function tests

These are tests carried out with a spirometer, a machine that can measure how much air is breathed out and how much is left in the lungs, as well as the speed at which the air flows through the airways. Measuring lung function with a spirometer is described as spirometry.

The standard lung-function tests include:

- **Forced expiratory volume (in one second)**: This measures the amount of air which can be forced out of the lungs during the first second of the out-breath. It will be lower in asthmatics than in non-asthmatics because of the narrower airways. FEV1 mainly measures the narrowing in the small airways of the lung (the bronchioles), whereas peak flow measures the narrowing of the larger airways. Sometimes asthmatics show a distinct reduction in FEV1 without there being much change in peak flow, so it can be useful to do this test.

- **Forced vital capacity**: This is also known simply as 'vital capacity'. If you breathe in as far as you can, and then breathe out as far as you can, the amount of air breathed out is the forced vital capacity. There will still be some air left in the lungs, and this is known as the residual volume. Owing to the narrow airways, many asthmatics have difficulty expelling the air, so there is more left in the lungs at the end of the out-breath than there should be. The residual volume is higher than normal, so the forced vital capacity is lower.

- **Residual volume**: The air left in the lungs at the end of an out-breath. This is measured with a plethysmograph. See 'Forced vital capacity' above.

- **Peak flow**: This is the maximum speed at which the air leaves your lungs during the out-breath. It is also known as peak expiratory flow rate. Asthmatics have a lower peak flow than normal, unless their asthma is well controlled. Peak flow can be measured with a simple portable machine called a peak-flow meter. Many asthmatics now have their own peak-flow meter and use it to help improve the management of their asthma (see p. 315). A spirometer can also measure peak flow, and it gives more accurate readings.

Exercise test

This is a test that shows if the airways get narrower after exercise. The peak flow or the forced expiratory volume (see above) is measured before exercise and just afterwards. Many asthmatics have much lower readings after exercise because their airways have narrowed. This shows that they have exercise-induced asthma (see p. 68).

Reversibility test

For this test, peak flow is measured before and after inhaling a dose of a B-2 reliever drug such as Ventolin (see p. 342). If the peak flow improves by 15 per cent or more after taking the drug, this suggests a diagnosis of asthma.

Tests for allergic reactions

Skin-prick tests

These tests can show if you have allergic reactions or not. A small drop of liquid containing an allergen, such as house dust mite or cat saliva protein, is placed on your arm. A small prick is made in the skin under the drop of liquid, so that a tiny amount of the allergen gets into the skin. If you are allergic to the substance concerned, a small red bump develops soon afterwards. This test is reasonably accurate, but a few people get a bump even though they are not allergic to the substance

The skin-prick test

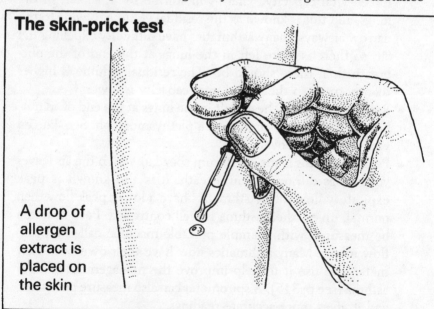

A drop of allergen extract is placed on the skin

(a false positive), and others have no reaction even though they *are* allergic (a false negative). Despite these limitations, skin-prick tests are often useful in identifying allergies (see pp. 125–6).

Provocation tests
If allergy is suspected as a trigger for asthma, a provocation test may be used. This involves inhaling a small amount of the suspected allergen, and observing the effect on the airways. This test should only be done in hospital as there can be a severe reaction.

Patch tests
These tests are used for contact dermatitis, a different type of allergic reaction from that which affects asthma.

RAST and ELISA
Both these tests require blood samples, which are then screened for their reaction to particular allergens.

X-rays
Chest X-rays may be taken to rule out the possibility of bronchitis or other diseases. Most asthmatics have normal chest X-rays. Sometimes the X-rays show that the lungs are over-inflated because of the asthma, or that there is a mucus plug which has caused one part of the lung to collapse.

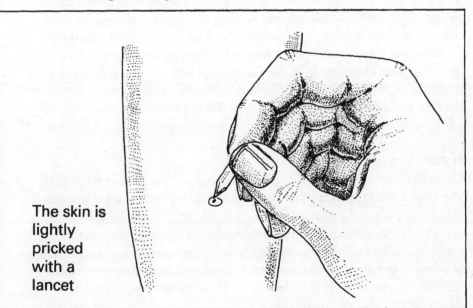

The skin is lightly pricked with a lancet

CAN THE DOCTOR BE SURE IT'S ASTHMA?

For the majority of patients, the simple answer to this question is 'Yes'. Although there is no straightforward definition of asthma, and no tests that can diagnose asthma with absolute certainty, most doctors feel that they 'know it when they see it'. The average, uncomplicated case of asthma in adults is fairly easy to diagnose, and the same is true for children over the age of five.

However, it is also true that patients now diagnosed as asthmatic would have been given a different diagnosis (for example wheezy bronchitis) 30 years ago. To some extent, this is because asthma was under-diagnosed in the past: doctors were reluctant to give a diagnosis of asthma, because being asthmatic was seen as a stigma (see p. 34). Now that asthma is no longer thought of as a psychological problem, and there is no stigma attached to the disease the pendulum has swung the other way.

Some doctors believe that the pendulum may now have swung too far in the opposite direction, and that certain patients get the label asthma when it is not really appropriate. This section should help you decide if this might be the case for you or your child.

It is important to remember that, for every person who is labelled asthmatic when they do not have asthma, there are probably two or three people who have asthma without it being recognized as such by their doctor. So there is both over-diagnosis and under-diagnosis of asthma. The situation varies from one country to another, and from one district to another: over-diagnosis may be more common in one area, under-diagnosis in another. But overall, the situation is steadily getting better: doctors and researchers are constantly trying to improve the ways in which asthma is diagnosed, so that more patients get the right diagnosis.

Essential tests

Unfortunately, there is no single test that can show for certain that you have asthma. Much of the diagnosis will depend on what doctors call 'taking a good history': this means asking you about the actual symptoms, their timing, what brings the symptoms on, when the problem began and other such details. It is important to be as accurate as possible in telling the doctor about these, and to include everything that seems relevant. It may be useful to write the important points down before you go to the clinic.

Once your 'history' has been taken, the doctor will carry out certain tests. These are the essential tests that should be carried out before you are given a diagnosis of asthma:
- peak flow
- reversibility test

These tests are described on pp. 303–4. If there is any doubt about the diagnosis of asthma, the doctor may ask you to check your own peak flow at home every morning and evening for a week or two, and record the results on a chart. The pattern of the results can help in deciding if you have asthma or not.

Some patients may also be given further tests:
- Lung-function tests (see p. 303), also called spirometry, if the symptoms are severe, or if there is also some bronchitis or emphysema, as in chronic obstructive pulmonary disease (COPD) – see below. Few GPs or family doctors have a spirometer in their surgeries, so you will probably be referred to a hospital specialist for these tests.
- Skin-prick testing (see p. 304), if allergies are suspected, and cannot be identified accurately by other means, such as noticing what brings on the symptoms. A small number of GPs can do skin-prick tests in the surgery, but most do not have this facility, so you would be referred to a hospital allergist.

When asthma is difficult to diagnose
There are certain situations in which it is difficult for a doctor to say whether someone has asthma or not. These are the main ones:

In very young children
Lots of babies wheeze, especially when they have colds or chest infections. About 30 per cent of infants wheeze at some time or another. Baby boys are particularly likely to wheeze because their airways are less well developed at birth. Infant wheezing often clears up of its own accord, and is not necessarily going to develop into asthma. There is great debate among doctors about whether wheezy babies should be labelled 'asthmatic' or not, and how bad the wheezing should be before they are given asthma drugs.

Opinions vary, so if you are concerned about the treatment given, you may want to talk it over with another GP in your practice: there is no harm in asking to see a different doctor for your next appointment.

One useful thing you can do, if your baby wheezes, is to minimize the chance of this turning into asthma at a later stage. Cigarette smoke and high levels of allergens (house dust mites, pets, etc.) increase the risk of infant wheezing developing into true asthma. Useful measures for reducing allergen exposure are described on pp. 89–93 under 'Improving the baby's environment'.

When the main symptom is coughing

It is only relatively recently that doctors have recognized 'cough-variant asthma'. In this form of asthma, coughing is the main symptom, rather than wheezing. People with this symptom are still less likely to be diagnosed as having asthma.

For children with recurrent coughing (usually defined as two or more episodes per year of coughing without a cold) it may take a long time before the doctor thinks of the possibility of asthma. But this is only true of some doctors. Others may label a coughing child as 'asthmatic' all too readily, without doing enough tests.

Recent studies suggest that children who have a recurrent cough but who *never* wheeze should not be diagnosed as asthmatic, because they generally show no signs of allergy and they differ in several other important respects from asthmatic children. By contrast, children who have both recurrent coughing and wheezing are similar to children with 'classical' asthma. Many children with recurrent cough and no wheeze are simply suffering the effects of smoking by their parents.

When a child wheezes with chest infections

Children often develop wheezing when they get chest infections, but do not wheeze at other times. Thirty years ago, this would have been called 'wheezy bronchitis'. Today it is frequently called asthma. There is some debate about which label is more accurate, and more useful in terms of treatment, but most doctors feel that it is valuable to treat this condition with asthma drugs. Treatment with asthma drugs does not 'turn wheezing into asthma' as is sometimes claimed.

When older patients have another lung disease as well

Among older people, especially those who have smoked for many years, asthma may be part of a larger picture of inflammation and damage to the air sacs of the lung (emphysema) and/or to the airways (bronchitis). This combination of problems is known as chronic obstructive pulmonary disease (COPD) or chronic obstructive airways disease (COAD). It may be difficult or impossible for the doctor to tell if there is asthma present, or how much it is contributing to the overall problem. Since many patients with COPD are helped by asthma drugs, doctors tend to try these out for a while, even if they are not sure how big a role the asthma is playing in the disease. If the drugs help, it is reasonable to assume that there is some asthma. Trying out the drugs for a while does no harm, so there is nothing to be lost.

Older people are often very frightened of the diagnosis of asthma, and feel there should be some definite proof that they have asthma before taking asthma drugs. Unfortunately, if you have COPD, the only way to tell if asthma is part of the problem is to take the drugs and see if they help. We would recommend that you try them. If you are frightened about the label 'asthma', talk over your fears with the doctor: you will probably find that you have got the risks out of proportion.

When asthma occurs only at night

A tiny minority of asthmatics have asthma only at night, and seem to have perfectly healthy airways by day. Even sophisticated tests will not reveal any abnormality in the airways during the day, making it difficult for doctors to diagnose the condition. By using a peak-flow meter at home, morning and evening, and recording the results, patients can provide the doctor with the information needed to diagnose this problem.

Conditions that can be mistaken for asthma

The previous section deals with situations where it is difficult to say what is asthma and what is not, because there is no simple medical definition of asthma, or because a person's asthma is mixed in with other diseases. In these situations diagnosis is difficult for any doctor, and there may be no 'right answer' as regards the diagnosis.

That is quite different from the situation where someone has disease A and a doctor mistakes it for disease B. Unfortunately, this does happen occasionally for all kinds of reasons: because doctors are only human, because they are rushed off their feet, or because they may not know all the facts at the outset and it makes more sense to plump for a common diagnosis such as asthma than for something very rare that produces similar symptoms. The following diseases and conditions are quite different from asthma, but may be mistaken for it because they produce similar symptoms.

In children
A small object inhaled and stuck in the airways
Something small, like a bead, a peanut or part of a toy, can be inhaled by a small child and then get stuck in the wind-pipe, or lower down in the airways. This may produce a wheezing sound (because it restricts air flow) and be mistaken for asthma. Most of these objects (including anything made of plastic) will not show up on an X-ray. The main clue that this is the cause of 'asthma' is that the wheezing came on very suddenly. However, in some cases the wheezing only develops weeks or months after the object has been inhaled. Detecting the inhaled item requires an instrument called an endoscope – a tiny camera mounted in a long thin tube – which allows the doctor to look inside the airways. Using the endoscope for guidance, the object can also be removed. But prevention is better than cure: don't let very young children play with tiny objects that could be inhaled, and if it's impossible to keep the baby away from the older children's toys, try to count all the Lego pieces so you'll know if one goes missing!

Inhaled milk
Babies and toddlers may inhale droplets of milk while they are feeding, and these can cause wheezing or coughing which may be mistaken for asthma. If your child's asthma comes on mainly after feeding, this possibility is worth investigating, but bear in mind that there could be other explanations.

Gastro-oesophageal reflux (GER)
Children and babies can suffer from this problem, just as adults can. Indeed, it is particularly common in children under 18 months. There will usually be clues that this is the true problem, not asthma, such as frequent vomiting associated with 'asthma attacks', or symptoms that come on at night or whenever the child is lying down.

Heiner's Syndrome

This is a severe form of cow's-milk allergy leading to wheezing and frequent bouts of pneumonia. The child usually seems sickly, and growth is slow. A full diagnosis requires blood tests to check for anaemia, and examination of sputum under the microscope. The only effective treatment is to remove cow's milk from the diet completely. Needless to say, this must be done under full medical supervision.

Bronchiolitis

This is a viral infection of the lungs which affects the small airways called the bronchioles. It mainly affects babies and toddlers. The usual cause is Respiratory Synctial Virus (RSV) and there are epidemics of RSV every two or three years. Unfortunately, RSV infection is thought to make the later development of asthma rather more likely (see p. 93). In adults, RSV often causes nothing more than a cold or cough, but when passed on to a baby this can become a severe infection, with wheezing, coughing and laboured breathing. This can be mistaken for asthma, but there will usually be fever as well which should lead to the right diagnosis. Because antibiotics have no effect on viruses, bronchiolitis is usually treated with steroids to reduce the inflammation. So no great harm will be done if bronchiolitis is initially diagnosed as asthma.

In children or adults
Problems with the vocal chords

Some people get into the habit of contracting their vocal chords when they are breathing in. This makes a loud wheezing sound, which may seem to be coming from the chest and can therefore be mistaken for a severe asthma attack. They may feel very breathless as well, but the level of oxygen in the blood is normal whereas in asthma it falls during a severe attack. The underlying cause of these problems with the vocal chords is usually a psychological one, so treatment consists of psychotherapy as well as speech therapy. This problem often occurs in people who do actually have asthma as well.

Hyperventilation

Hyperventilation is another name for over-breathing: taking in more air than you need, usually by breathing very fast. One of the symptoms of hyperventilation is, surprisingly, feeling breathless.

For a complete list of symptoms see pp. 419–20. Sometimes people diagnosed as having asthma simply have hyperventilation, and if they learn to breathe properly their asthma symptoms will disappear. There are also many people with asthma who hyperventilate as well, especially when they are feeling anxious about their asthma (see p. 36). The hyperventilation makes their asthma symptoms worse.

The following clues suggest that hyperventilation is part or all of your problem:
- You do not wheeze.
- You feel hungry for air, rather than breathless.
- You often feel panicky, especially when you have an asthma attack.

The treatment for hyperventilation is to be retrained in correct breathing (see pp. 422–8). The underlying problems that led to hyperventilation may also need treatment by psychotherapy or relaxation training (see pp. 446–51).

Habitual coughing
Some people get into the habit of coughing, usually as an expression of some underlying stress or emotional problem in their lives. The cough has a characteristic honking or barking sound, and it interferes with daily activities or with sleep. This problem can be mistaken for asthma, but there will be no improvement when asthma drugs are taken. Coughing can, of course, be caused in many other ways as well, and the doctor will need to eliminate these possibilities first. The treatment for habitual coughing involves relaxation therapy, speech therapy and possibly psychotherapy.

Gastro-oesophageal reflux (GER)
Occasionally patients with what looks like asthma actually have gastro-oesophageal reflux which is the sole cause of the asthma-like symptoms. Some people do not have the typical symptoms of heartburn (see p. 254), which is why it goes undetected. In cases such as these, the main clue is asthma that does not respond to inhaled steroids at all. If gastro-oesophageal reflux is your problem, even though you do not have heartburn, you will probably have noticed some symptoms in connection with eating: talk to your doctor about these.

Low-level carbon monoxide poisoning

Carbon monoxide is a poisonous gas that may be given off by gas fires or other gas appliances which are burning badly (with a predominantly yellow flame, rather than a blue flame with yellow only at the tip). Inhaling large amounts of carbon monoxide is fatal, but inhaling small amounts day after day just produces symptoms such as breathlessness, tiredness, headaches and nausea. Occasionally people with low-level carbon monoxide poisoning have been diagnosed as having asthma.

Bronchiectasis

Diseases caught in childhood, such as pneumonia or whooping cough, can stretch the airways and damage their linings. This may produce breathlessness later in life, which can be mistaken for asthma. However, people with bronchiectasis can also develop asthma.

Mucus from the nose running into the lungs

If you have a very bad case of rhinitis (inflammation of the nose), you may be producing a lot of mucus which runs down from the back of the nose into the throat and airways, especially at night, making you cough. This is called 'post-nasal drip'. The coughing it causes can sometimes be mistaken for asthma, if proper tests of lung function (see p. 303) are not carried out. Where the rhinitis is due to an allergic reaction, treating the nose with anti-allergic drops will clear up the 'asthma' symptoms.

Bronchitis

People can develop asthma for the first time after the age of 60 or 70, and sometimes this is misdiagnosed as chronic bronchitis. If you have never smoked, nor worked in an industry with toxic fumes, you are unlikely to have chronic bronchitis and much more likely to have asthma.

Inherited diseases

There are several inherited diseases which can produce symptoms similar to asthma.

One is **cystic fibrosis**, which may not be recognized if it is relatively mild and the child grows normally. In such cases wheezing is often the most obvious sign of cystic fibrosis, and may be diagnosed as asthma.

If there is cystic fibrosis in your family, or that of your partner, discuss this possibility with your doctor.

Some people have an inherited problem with the **cilia**, the tiny hairs that line the airways and push out debris, mucus and dust. These cilia do not work as well as they should, so mucus accumulates in the airways and produces wheezing. There will also be sinusitis, congestion of the nose, and possibly problems with the ears. (These symptoms can be mistaken for the combination of symptoms which occur in people sensitive to aspirin – asthma, inflammation of the nose and nasal polyps – see p. 257.) This problem is quite difficult for the doctor to diagnose without special tests.

A third inherited disease which can be mistaken for asthma is called **alpha-1-antitrypsin** deficiency. There is now an effective treatment for this disease.

More serious diseases

Very occasionally, some types of heart disease can produce symptoms that look like asthma initially. The same is also true of certain forms of cancer affecting the lungs or nearby regions of the body. *Note that this is very unlikely to be the explanation for your asthma* – such cases are extremely rare. But it is important that you tell your doctor about any unusual symptoms you might have, such as unexplained weight loss, swollen ankles, or severe fatigue that is not due to any obvious cause such as stress or overwork.

'she had that same dry little cough . . .'

Sally is a nurse in a large college in New York State. 'There was one Asian student, and I was called to her because she had what she thought was a cold. But she had that same dry little cough that my asthmatic daughter has.

'I asked her about asthma, and she said she'd never had it, but we got the doctor, and that was it – she did have asthma. He gave her Ventolin and it made a big difference to her. The students who've come from countries where asthma is still unusual have trouble recognizing it.'

PEAK-FLOW METERS:
AN EARLY-WARNING SYSTEM FOR ASTHMA

Most patients with asthma are now given a peak-flow meter, and told to use it morning and evening, recording the result on a chart or graph. The idea is to detect narrowing of your airways – that is, the beginnings of an asthma attack – before there are any noticeable symptoms. In other words, the peak-flow meter is an early-warning system for an asthma attack.

Your doctor or asthma nurse should tell you how to interpret your peak-flow readings. As a general rule, these are the signs of worsening asthma:

- A big difference between the morning and evening readings every day. Alarm bells should ring if the morning reading is regularly less than 75 per cent (three-quarters) of the evening reading.
- Average readings falling to less than 75 per cent of your best reading. If this happens you should see your doctor soon.
- Readings falling to less than 50 per cent of your best reading. *If this happens seek immediate medical help*: this indicates a severe and possibly life-threatening attack.

The right way to use a peak-flow meter

The peak-flow meter measures the maximum speed at which you can force air out of your lungs. You breathe out as hard as you can, and this pushes the pointer up along the scale. It stops at the maximum point, which is the fastest rate at which you expelled the air.

The standard instructions for using a peak-flow meter are as follows:

1. Push the pointer back to zero.
2. Don't take any unusually deep breaths before you start.
3. Stand up and take a deep breath: breathe in quickly and don't hold your breath before you blow.
4. Hold the meter horizontally and seal your lips tightly around the mouthpiece.
5. Make sure you are not touching the scale or obstructing the movement of the pointer.
6. Blow into the meter as hard as you can, as if you were blowing out candles on a birthday cake: but make sure you do not puff out your cheeks (see below).

7. Look on the scale to see which number the pointer is at: this is the reading.

8. Repeat twice, and choose the highest reading of the three; mark this on your graph or chart.

What can go wrong when using peak-flow meters

As long as you are using the peak-flow meter properly, it is a very useful addition to your management programme. Unfortunately, it is often used wrongly, and it can then be worse than useless, because it may fail to show an oncoming asthma attack, while creating a sense of false confidence that leads you to disregard worsening symptoms.

To benefit from your peak-flow meter you should:

- Be shown how to use it by your doctor or asthma nurse, who should check your technique thoroughly.
- Have your technique checked every time you go to the asthma clinic (take your meter with you) as it is easy to get into bad habits.
- Always stand up to take your peak-flow measurement, always do it in the same way, and try to have no distractions – don't try to carry on a conversation at the same time, for example.
- Keep your peak-flow meter clean – the asthma nurse should show you how.
- Never puff out your cheeks when preparing to blow into the peak-flow meter – this will give you a reading that is too high.
- Never move your tongue while blowing into the peak-flow meter; some people push their tongue forward in an action rather like spitting, which forces more air through the meter and gives a reading that is too high.
- Always use your own peak-flow meter, not someone else's: unfortunately, the portable peak-flow meters are not precision instruments and the measurement they give will vary from one meter to another; however, this does not matter when you are using the same meter every day, because what you are interested in is how much your peak flow has *changed*, and the meter is good enough to show that.
- At every appointment, get the asthma nurse or doctor to compare the reading from your own peak-flow meter with the reading from the clinic's peak-flow meter or, preferably, the

clinic's spirometer (they are more accurate); this will give you a good idea how well the reading on your meter corresponds to your actual peak flow.

- When you replace your peak-flow meter, go on using the old one as well for the first week, so that you have some idea how the measurements relate to each other.
- Make sure that you have not had a puff of your reliever inhaler before taking your peak flow reading. At least *four hours* should elapse between your last dose of reliever and your peak-flow measurement. If you sometimes have to take your peak flow less than four hours after your reliever drug, make a note on your chart that this reading is artificially high because of the reliever.
- If travelling to a mountain region bear in mind that a change of altitude will affect the meter: if you go up to 3000 metres (10,000 feet) there will be a fall in your reading of about 17 per cent, which is due to the meter and nothing to do with your airways, (If your reading stays the same, your peak flow has actually improved, as often happens at high altitude – see p. 116).
- try always to use your peak-flow meter indoors, at about the same temperature every day, as cold air will also give an artificially low reading.
- even though you have a peak-flow meter, do not rely on this alone to show you that an asthma attack is coming on. Your symptoms are also a very good guide, and should never be ignored just because your peak-flow reading seems normal. The more sensitive you can become to small variations in your symptoms the better you will be able to control your asthma (see p. 49).

How often should peak-flow meters be replaced?

The standard advice is to replace peak-flow meters frequently, but new evidence suggests that this may not be worthwhile. A recent study showed that some peak-flow meters are still 'as good as new' after 14 years of use, but that a few deteriorate and become much less accurate after a year or so. So it is the individual meters that vary, and it is difficult to tell if you have a good one or one that is rapidly becoming inaccurate. This is why you should take your meter with you, to be checked against more accurate instruments, when you visit the asthma clinic. Only buy a new meter if your present one is becoming inaccurate.

11

Drug treatment

'**Before the modern drugs came in,
my asthma was completely crippling.**'

John, now 46, has had severe asthma all his life. 'I personally think the situation for asthmatics is much better now than in the past. I had asthma as a child, before all the modern medicines were available, and I coughed so much and so violently that I got black eyes and strained my diaphragm. When I was ten, I missed most of a year of school. I couldn't walk upstairs without someone to support me, I had so little breath. My whole life closed down and I spent hours just struggling to breathe, with no relief. Then when I was 18, in the late 1960s, the real revolution in asthma drugs started, and that just transformed my life. I still wasn't well after it, but I was so much better. Before the modern drugs came in, my asthma was completely crippling.'

'**I prefer to feel that I can control the asthma myself.**'

Rachel, now 30, has had asthma since childhood: 'I'm much happier now that I manage without the inhalers, because I don't like taking drugs of any kind, and I prefer to feel that I can control the asthma myself. When I'm doing housework, I wear a scarf round my mouth and nose to keep the dust out. I try not to get stressed out, because that makes my asthma worse, and I've found out that avoiding milk and cheese improves matters. I still get asthma attacks sometimes, but I know now to breathe slowly and stay calm, and that usually sorts it out.'

ARE ALL THESE DRUGS
REALLY NECESSARY? AND ARE THEY SAFE?

If you look at other popular books and articles on asthma, you will find that they are of two distinct kinds: either complacently in favour of drugs or vehemently against them.

The pro-drug publications seem to assume that all asthmatics will unquestioningly accept the word of their doctors that drugs are the best option.

The anti-asthma-drug pamphlets and books, on the other hand, are crusaders against the medical establishment. Most of them, unfortunately, tend to pick out the bits of scientific evidence that support their cause, while entirely ignoring the rest. Several are inaccurate and out of date (see below). They often describe harmful side-effects as if these are inevitable, without explaining that many side-effects are extremely rare, or can be avoided if you watch out for the warning signs.

Neither type of publication makes much attempt to look at the other side of the argument, or offer a balanced discussion. We will try to do better – to present both sides of the question in an unprejudiced way, so that you can make up your own mind.

Do asthma drugs work?

Some of the anti-drug publications suggest that asthma drugs do not actually work. Is there any truth in this?

Certainly, a few people will get no effects from some asthma drugs. However, in the case of steroids, B-2 relievers and most other types of drug, this is a very small minority of people. Only cromoglycate and the anti-cholinergic drugs are ineffective for a significant number of people.

Sometimes asthmatics think that certain drugs do not work for them, because they do not have an immediate effect: they think that everything should work as fast as a puff of Ventolin. This is a mistake, especially in relation to steroids and other preventers (see p. 335).

Everyone with asthma will find some drugs that are effective. And if you talk to older people, who have had asthma all their lives, most will tell you that the new drugs which have become available in the last 30 years have transformed their lives.

Can the drugs make asthma worse?

This is a frequent claim against asthma drugs. The answer is 'Generally speaking, no', but there are some important exceptions:

- Several inhaled drugs can sometimes have the opposite effect to that intended, making the airways get tighter instead of opening up. This is called 'paradoxical bronchoconstriction' and it only affects *a very small number* of people. The effect is immediately noticeable. If this happens to you, stop using the drug straight away.
- Using B-2 relievers too frequently can, in the long term, make the airways more sensitive. This is not immediately noticeable, and it is potentially dangerous, so all asthmatics should be aware of the risks. For more details see pp. 322–6.

The claim that steroid drugs can make asthma worse – a claim made by some anti-drug pamphlets – is entirely unfounded.

Are asthma drugs squeezing out other treatments?

Drugs dominate the modern treatment of asthma, and there are huge profits being made out of the asthma epidemic. In 1997, the *Financial Times* of London published a report for the business world called 'Asthma – Disease Trends and Market Opportunities.' The global market for asthma drugs is over $5.5 billion, and is expected to reach $11 billion by 2002. In other words, asthma is big business.

All this commercialism is not wholly a bad thing: competition between the companies encourages research and innovation, leading to many new drugs, some of which are more effective and have fewer side-effects. In asthma, there is also a lot of research into inhaler devices, and the competition here has led to a new generation of inhalers, such as the Diskhaler, Turbohaler and Accuhaler, which have enormous advantages over the old aerosol inhalers (see p. 376).

But the intense commercial pressure, which involves heavy promotion and advertising of drugs to the medical profession, may help to produce a pattern of treatment that is not always in the patient's best interest. Other factors conspire with this commercial pressure to favour drugs over other treatments. Many patients want to be given a magic instant cure by the doctor – they expect a prescription to solve everything for them. Doctors are overworked and have to deal with each patient in a few minutes. Writing a prescription is almost always quicker than any other form of treatment, especially when the details of inhaler technique and follow-up can be handed over to the asthma nurse. (It is interesting to note that the training of asthma nurses is partially funded by some of the drug companies.)

To make matters worse, there is a shortage of resources for other treatment options. In Britain, particularly, there is a lack of trained consultant allergists. It is scandalous that 90 per cent of children with asthma are known to have allergies, yet only a tiny minority are ever referred to an allergist for specialist treatment. Skin-prick testing, a cheap and easy procedure that any GP or trained asthma nurse could carry out (see p. 301), is often unavailable.

Treatments that are known to help asthmatics – even orthodox and uncontroversial treatments such as physiotherapy, exercises to strengthen the breathing muscles, training in better patterns of breathing, or relaxation and stress-management techniques – are very rarely offered within Britain's National Health Service. These treatments won't cure asthma, but they may well stabilize it and help the sufferer to avoid severe attacks. Patients tend to need fewer drugs if they have these kinds of additional treatment, and many have a better overall quality of life. The heavy emphasis on drugs within conventional asthma treatment does tend to squeeze out these other options.

Fortunately, asthmatics can explore many of these other treatment options for themselves. One objective of this book is to help you in this exploration of other treatments (see pp. 2–6) which may reduce your need for drugs.

How safe are asthma drugs?

Asthma drugs, like all drugs, have some side-effects. What doctors try to decide is whether these side-effects outweigh the possible benefits of the drugs. Doctors make these decisions on the basis of the 'average patient'. For example, the average patient who is allergic to house dust mites would rather use drugs than go to the trouble of reducing house dust mite levels in their home.

You are not average: the fact that you are bothering to read a book about asthma shows this. Clearly, you are interested in taking an active part in your own treatment. You may decide that you would rather reduce house dust mite levels and (if that does the trick and your asthma improves) cut down on drugs, or even stop them altogether if you can. In the long term, your overall health would probably benefit from this.

To make such decisions, you need to know just how safe or dangerous asthma drugs are.

We will discuss this for each different type of drug in turn because there are huge differences between the various groups of drugs. It is vital to realize that the safety issues surrounding inhaled steroids are totally different from those surrounding B-2 relievers, for example. (If you are not familiar with names such as these, turn to p. 370, where you can find the brand-names of your drugs and discover which drug groups they belong to. For more detail on what each type of drug does, see pp. 334–49.)

How safe are short-acting B-2 relievers?

In general, asthmatics worry too much about steroids and not enough about B-2 relievers. Most people are less anxious about B-2 relievers than they should be because these drugs are familiar (almost all asthmatics have had a Ventolin or Bricanyl inhaler at some time), they've been around a long time, and they work straight away with few obvious side-effects: all very reassuring.

It took an epidemic of asthma deaths in New Zealand, between 1976 and 1988, to make doctors aware of how dangerous these drugs could be. For several years, the death rate was two to four times its previous level. Over 1000 New Zealanders died who might otherwise still be alive.

Most researchers now believe that the main cause of the epidemic was a new brand of inhaler which delivered a double dose of the drug fenoterol, a short-acting B-2 reliever. Subsequent research suggested that the same brand of inhaler was linked to increased death rates in Canada and Germany. The problem was probably worst in New Zealand because sales of the new inhaler were highest there, and because patients tended to get their inhalers through repeat prescriptions, without seeing the doctor: in New Zealand, doctors' appointments are expensive whereas these drugs were heavily subsidized.

As a result, many patients whose asthma was deteriorating badly were not seen by a doctor. They went on using fenoterol or other B-2 relievers, and inhaling them more and more frequently, without taking a preventer drug as well.

This is now known to be a major cause of asthma deaths. Firstly, the reliever covers up the effects of the severe inflammation of the airways. This inflammation can eventually lead to a very serious, and potentially fatal, asthma attack. Secondly, the airways become less and less responsive to the B-2 reliever itself (see below), so that when a serious attack occurs, and the asthmatic is rushed to hospital, huge doses of B-2 reliever are needed to open up the airways. These huge doses carry a risk of serious, and potentially life-threatening, side-effects involving the heart.

There is still heated debate over the details of the New Zealand epidemic. What was the exact cause of the deaths? Was it fenoterol itself, which is stronger than other B-2 relievers? Or was it just the fact that the inhaler delivered a double dose with each puff? In other words, would any short-acting B-2 reliever be dangerous at twice the normal dose? Or was it over-use of all B-2 relievers and lack of preventer drugs?

In practical terms, until this is resolved, it seems wise to assume that any of these possibilities could be correct. Our recommendations, following the New Zealand epidemic, would be:

- Avoid fenoterol (still available in lower-dose inhalers).
- Avoid double-dose inhalers of any short-acting B-2 reliever (those that deliver 200 µg/micrograms per puff). And don't routinely take two puffs of your single-dose inhaler if you only need one: but check with your doctor first if you have been told to always take two puffs.
- Use all short-acting B-2 relievers only 'as needed', not regularly. If needed more than once a day (British guidelines) or three times a week (international guidelines), take a regular preventer drug as well. (The US guidelines are different again – see p. 343.)
- Remember, however, that during a full-blown asthma attack, you really do need a B-2 reliever, and you should take as many puffs as necessary – up to a total of 30 (see p. 51) – to get your airways open. *There is a risk of death if you don't use the reliever fully in this situation.*

'Is the cure the cause?'

The New Zealand epidemic raised a lot of questions about the safety of short-acting B-2 relievers in general. Researchers discovered that patients given salbutamol (Ventolin, Aerolin, etc.) four times a day had more irritable airways (when tested in a particular way) after just two weeks, and that their airways were also less responsive to the drug.

Alarm bells began to ring. There had been a small but steady increase in asthma deaths throughout much of the Western world since the mid-1970s, and some doctors suggested that the increasing use of short-acting B-2 relievers could be behind this.

This question was raised by an article published in 1992 in the respected British medical journal *The Lancet*. The article, entitled 'Worldwide worsening wheezing – is the cure the cause?', went further. It suggested that the rise in the number of cases of asthma could be *due to* these drugs: perhaps children with mild wheezing, which would have gone away in time if left untreated, were becoming long-term asthmatics because they were now being given inhalers such as Ventolin.

Many doctors and researchers became very concerned about these questions. But since 1992 much more has been discovered about short-acting B-2 relievers, and while there are still unanswered questions, most of the serious concern about these drugs has died down. The anti-drug books and pamphlets we described at the beginning have not caught up with these developments: they are still reporting the situation as it was in 1992. They have taken up that question posed in *The Lancet* – 'Is the cure the cause?' – as a war-cry, without realizing that research has, quite clearly, shown the answer to be 'no'.

The new findings are:

1. Since about 1990, the death rate seems to have been falling, particularly in countries with a policy of reducing use of B-2 relievers and increasing inhaled steroids. The death rate in New Zealand is now the lowest it has been for 50 years, and at the same level as other Western countries. If this world-wide fall in the death rate continues, doctors will know that they are now using the drugs correctly, but only time will tell.

2. In the light of the now-falling death rates, it seems likely that the small, steady worldwide rise in asthma deaths which began in the mid-1970s was due to increasing severity of asthma, combined with over-use of short-acting B-2 relievers and under-use of inhaled steroids. (The high-dose fenoterol inhaler may have boosted the death rate a little in several countries, and a lot in New Zealand.)

3. New research has shown that short-acting B-2 relievers, used regularly, make the airways more sensitive to allergens, and to exercise. This means that the asthmatic who is allergic to dust, or cats, for example, reacts to them at much lower levels in the air. The B-2 drugs are powerful enough to open up the airways in spite of this increased sensitivity, so you may not notice any change. But there could well be an increase in the underlying inflammation of the airways, which could be damaging in the long-term. This is an additional reason for avoiding regular use of B-2 relievers, if at all possible.

4. The idea that short-acting B-2 relievers could increase the number of cases of asthma (as opposed to the number of deaths) no longer seems plausible. But it is still important that wheezy children (those with mild or moderate asthma) use them only when needed, and not more than once a day.

Making decisions about B-2 relievers

Most patients with mild or moderate asthma, who are willing to inhale a preventer drug, will be able to use their short-acting B-2 reliever infrequently, in accordance with the new guidelines. In this case, there is absolutely no risk of making the asthma worse: it is only regular use that is damaging and dangerous.

A few patients will still face a dilemma, however, because they need more frequent doses of B-2 relievers to control their symptoms. These are patients with moderate to severe asthma who are still breathless and wheezy, even though they are inhaling moderate doses of a steroid preventer every day. Doubling the dose of inhaled steroids is often no use, and it increases the risk of side-effects, whereas taking a long-acting B-2 reliever may have great benefits.

These long-acting drugs are very similar to the short-acting B-2 relievers, but their effects last for about 12 hours (see p. 344). Research has shown that the long-acting forms make the airways slightly more irritable, just as the short-acting drugs do, and that the response to the drug (and to short-acting B-2 relievers) declines in the same way. It is possible that they also increase the response to allergen and to exercise, but this has not yet been investigated.

Such effects are obviously worrying, but the overall conclusion at present is that the long-acting drugs taken twice a day are considerably safer than short-acting drugs taken regularly four times a day. Because long-acting B-2 relievers often work wonders for patients with moderate or severe asthma who have not responded fully to other drugs, doctors generally believe that they should be used. But most doctors would probably waste no time in switching these patients on to a new drug (such as zafirlukast – see p. 340) if it looked as though it could do the same job with fewer risks. Older drugs such as theophylline (see p. 346) may also be worth a try.

A few patients need to take regular doses of short-acting B-2 relievers as well as taking long-acting B-2 relievers. If this applies to you, you obviously have severe asthma *so you should follow the advice of your asthma specialist closely*, and not change your drug programme without his or her approval. However, it might be worth discussing other options, such as the newer anti-inflammatory drugs.

If the previous four paragraphs apply to you, read on. Anyone taking long-acting B-2 relievers (especially those who also need regular doses of short-acting B-2 relievers) should take every opportunity to reduce their asthma symptoms in other ways. For example, if there is anything you can do to avoid cigarette smoke and other asthma triggers (see pp. 2–3) or reduce allergen exposure (see pp. 127–78), you really should do this, as it may lessen your need for drugs. There are also many other ways to tackle asthma that may allow you to cut down on drugs (see pp. 3–6).

How safe are inhaled steroids?

Most asthmatics worry about steroids. It is such a problem that doctors have coined a name for it: 'steroid phobia'.

Some people are worried because they confuse the steroids used for asthma (corticosteroids) with the anabolic steroids taken illegally by athletes: in fact they are different substances with completely different effects (see p. 296).

Others are worried because they (rightly) see corticosteroids as powerful drugs with dangerous side-effects, and do not realize that *the dose makes all the difference* with these drugs. Serious side-effects do occur when steroids are taken *in tablet form* for long periods or at high doses. But when steroids are inhaled, much lower doses are used, and the severe side-effects are generally avoided.

Full details of side-effects from inhaled steroids (mostly minor ones), and the sort of dosages that will produce more serious effects, are given on pp. 351–60. There is also information on ways of preventing these side-effects, and on recognizing the early warning signs. We hope that this section will help to put your mind at rest about these drugs, because they are extremely useful in treating asthma.

The main advantage of taking inhaled steroids is that they control the inflammation of the airways, which is the underlying problem in asthma. So the benefits you get from inhaling steroids are real benefits, whereas the benefits from using B-2 relievers can be illusory: your airways open up, but underneath they are still inflamed and sore.

Bear in mind that the inflammation of the airways does long-term damage. The walls of the airways change, becoming thicker and tougher. This extra thickness makes for even more troublesome symptoms, and increased narrowing whenever the airway muscles contract. Such changes cannot be reversed, so the damaged airways are permanently narrowed. This is why, in people with lifelong asthma, the relievers and other drugs come to have less and less effect. New evidence shows that corticosteroids, used early on in the disease process, can prevent this kind of long-term damage. This alone is a powerful reason for using inhaled steroids.

In many countries, doctors are now using inhaled steroids at quite an early stage, even for mild asthma among young children. Parents may be worried about children inhaling steroids, but the evidence shows that a few years later, such children have healthier lungs than children who have gone without steroids.

These children are not necessarily going to be inhaling steroids for ever. A typical pattern is for a wheezy child to be given a steroid inhaler during the winter, when infections bring on wheezing, but to stop using it during the summer. The steroids calm the inflammation down, and as long as the child does not develop allergies, and is not breathing cigarette smoke at home, it is often possible to stop the steroid treatment after two to three years. You can help to prevent allergies from developing (see pp. 89–93).

For over ten years Swedish doctors have been using steroids for most wheezy children, and there has been a striking drop in the number of Swedish children dying from asthma or needing emergency hospital treatment, even though asthma itself has become more common in that time. Fewer hospital admissions is just the tip of the iceberg: it means that more Swedish asthmatics and their families are living a normal life, not staggering along from one crisis to another, their lives dominated by asthma attacks.

Making decisions about inhaled steroids

If you are still worried about inhaled steroids, there are various other treatment options that you can explore:

- Ask the doctor to try out cromoglycate (see p. 338) for six to eight weeks. This is another preventer drug, with no serious side-effects. It does not work for all adults, but it often works for children.
- Try to identify any allergies (see p. 113) and see whether there are changes you can make to reduce exposure to the allergen (see pp. 127–78).
- If the allergen is difficult to avoid, consider a desensitization treatment (see pp. 197–202) to reduce your reaction.
- Reduce your exposure to irritants such as tobacco smoke, traffic fumes, airborne chemicals at work (see p. 268), and other pollutants, whether indoor (see pp. 221–6) or outdoor (see pp. 204–15).
- Ask your doctor to let you try one of the new leukotriene-antagonist drugs (see p. 340).

You could give these alternative measures a year to take effect. If there is no benefit, and the asthma is still bad, you should not hesitate to take inhaled steroids, because uncontrolled asthma begins to inflict permanent damage on the airways after a year or two.

Taking a long-term view, going without inhaled steroids now may mean taking more drugs in the long run. If the inflammation is not controlled, it may well become worse and eventually need higher doses of drugs, or a wider range of drugs, to keep it under control.

How safe are other asthma drugs?

If you want to reduce your risk of side-effects to an absolute minimum, the two safest drugs are cromoglycate (a preventer) and ipratropium or any other anti-cholinergic reliever. Unfortunately, these do not work for everyone, but they are worth trying. Even anti-cholinergics should not be taken continuously, however, as they make the airways more sensitive and likely to contract if they are taken regularly several times a day.

Theophylline has its own problems, quite different from those of the other asthma drugs (see p. 367). There is no risk of it making the asthma any worse, but it is very toxic if you take too much. However, it can be a useful drug, and the risks are fairly small when taken at low doses.

Of the other anti-inflammatory drugs (see p. 363), several have previously been used for other diseases, but not for asthma, such as cyclosporin and methotrexate. The advantage of these is that the side-effects are very well known from their use (usually at higher doses) in diseases such as rheumatoid arthritis. Monitoring techniques, such as blood tests which look for the first signs of kidney damage, are well developed. The fact remains, however, that these are powerful drugs which can have serious side-effects.

The newer anti-inflammatories known as leukotriene antagonists (see p. 340), developed in the past few years specifically for asthma, seem to have far fewer side-effects. This is the conclusion from the trials carried out before the drugs were released on to the market, but (as with all new drugs) these are trials with limited numbers of people for a couple of years at most. Only time will tell if this good reputation holds up once they are used by large numbers of people for long periods of time: side-effects that only occur in a tiny minority of people, or after many years, will not show up until drugs have been widely used for a while. We would not want to discourage you from trying these new drugs, because they may well be the answer for many asthmatics, but it is also sensible to keep an eye out for unusual side-effects while taking them.

Steroid tablets, taken every day, are the most worrying of the asthma drugs. One study showed that 10 per cent of people over 40, taking steroids in this way, had suffered broken ribs or crushed vertebrae, as a result of osteoporosis. This is only one of the distressing side-effects that can come from long-term use of steroid tablets. *If you need these drugs, you need them, and you must follow your doctor's instructions to the letter*. But if there is anything you can do to reduce the dose of steroid tablets, such as avoiding cigarette smoke or reducing your allergen exposure, you really should take these steps. Check all the suggestions on pp. 2–6.

Occasional short courses of steroid tablets are much less problematic, but it is wise to keep these to a minimum by taking other precautions, including your inhaled steroids.

> ### *'. . . one of my patients did refuse and she died unnecessarily . . .'*
>
> Dr Joe Collier is a pharmacologist at a major London teaching hospital and author of a book that is highly critical of the drugs industry, entitled *The Health Conspiracy: how doctors, the drug industry and the government undermine our health.* He is a fierce and informed critic of the excessive or inappropriate use of drugs. But this is his view of asthma drugs: 'Patients must ask whether the pharmaceutical industry's success in business is matched by similar achievements in improving health. Unquestionably it has successfully produced many important medicines which provide enormous benefit. The prospects for patients with peptic ulcers, heart disease, asthma and diabetes have been improved out of all recognition by the introduction of new medicines. For example, corticosteroids will, with few exceptions, relieve even the most severe forms of asthma . . .
>
> 'In fact, a doctor who declines to give corticosteroids to severe asthma sufferers might be considered negligent, and in my experience, asthmatics rarely refuse this treatment.
>
> 'Tragically, one of my patients did refuse and she died unnecessarily at the age of 31, leaving behind a devoted husband and a four-year-old son.'

Other questions often asked about asthma drugs

'Are asthma drugs addictive?'

None of the asthma drugs is addictive in the sense that heroin, cocaine or nicotine are addictive: that is, they are not the type of drug that is both physically addictive and causes a substantial change in the state of mind of most people who use it.

What worries most people about asthma drugs, especially when they are taken by children, is that taking any drug every day, or several times a day, is equivalent to 'drug addiction'. This fear is completely unfounded: there is no similarity at all between inhaling cromoglycate four times a day, for example, and being addicted to a drug such as heroin or cocaine.

A few people taking steroid tablets will experience a mood of euphoria (or, in some cases, depression), but this is unusual. The B-2 relievers do make some people feel jittery and wide awake, and very rarely this is experienced as a positive feeling, especially by those who are normally lacking in energy. In extremely rare cases these drugs have been misused by people who find this feeling enjoyable – but most people find it thoroughly unpleasant and ask the doctor for a different brand of inhaler with fewer of these side-effects.

There have been a few cases of teenagers (both asthmatic and non-asthmatic) misusing aerosol inhalers of B-2 relievers, but they are generally addicted to the propellants in the aerosol, not to the drug itself. These are often the same types of propellant as found in other aerosol cans, so this behaviour is a form of 'glue sniffing'.

Needless to say, overusing B-2 inhalers – whether for the drug itself or the propellant – is extremely dangerous, and could lead to a severe asthma attack, or to fatal effects on the heart. One teenage boy suffered a major epileptic fit as a result of abusing his inhaler in this way.

No parent should ever prevent their child from having an inhaler for fear of this risk of misuse – it is an extremely small risk, far outweighed by the dangers of asthma itself. But any parent noticing that their child is using very large numbers of inhalers, or needing a prescription more and more frequently, should take action. Teachers should also be aware of this possibility, and watch for non-asthmatic children and teenagers using inhalers, or asthmatics using them excessively.

For those asthmatics who are addicted to the propellants, dry-powder systems (see p. 379) are a useful alternative.

'Why does asthma treatment vary from one country to another?'

If you move from one country to another, you will probably be surprised at the differences in the asthma treatment you receive. For medical researchers, these differences can be useful in discovering more about the best use of asthma drugs: some of the differences in New Zealand 25 years ago, and Sweden today, have already been considered.

There are still widespread differences in guidelines on B-2 relievers, and how often they should be used (see p. 343).

In addition, two countries continue to have radically different drug strategies from most other countries: Japan and the USA. What might be learned from these differences in approach?

The two most popular asthma drugs in Japan are ketotifen (see p. 340) and terfenadine. This is curious because ketotifen is regarded as 'disappointing' in its effects on asthma by British doctors and pharmacists, and little used. Terfenadine, an anti-histamine mainly used for hayfever in Britain, is not used at all for asthma, as anti-histamines are believed to have no effect on asthma.

It is possible that many Japanese do benefit from these drugs. About 40 per cent of Japanese and other Asiatic people have an unusual reaction to alcohol (see pp. 265–6) and develop an asthma attack whenever they drink. This reaction is blocked by anti-histamines, and by ketotifen. (Some non-Asiatics have this reaction too, and they could benefit from the same drugs.)

But the unusual reaction to alcohol amongst 40 per cent of the population cannot fully explain the very high use of these two drugs in Japan. It seems that there is some strangely unscientific behaviour going on, in which doctors prescribe the drugs which are believed to work by their elders in the local medical community. What they have been told works does work, to a degree – the patients get some benefit from pure placebo effect, and the doctors' expectations are confirmed. They pass on their wisdom to the next generation of medical men and women, and so it continues.

In the USA, one unusual aspect of asthma treatment concerns the drug theophylline (see p. 346). In most other countries, this is regarded as a rather risky drug that may sometimes be added to the drug regime of people with severe asthma who are not responding well. The drug is used as a type of reliever, for which high doses are needed. There is a substantial risk of toxicity and patients have to be monitored very carefully.

In the USA, the same drug is given to people with mild asthma at lower doses: too little to act as a reliever, but carrying much less risk of toxicity. At one time it seemed – to doctors outside the USA – that the use of this drug at low doses was a matter of faith rather than one of science, with American doctors loyal to a time-honoured practice that did not actually work.

Recent evidence, however, suggests that theophylline *does* have a useful anti-inflammatory effect at low doses: in other words, it acts as a preventer, not a reliever. The American doctors were right all along.

Because they have had low-dose theophylline in their armoury for so long, American doctors have been slower than others to prescribe inhaled steroids. Many more American asthmatics could benefit from these drugs, but are not yet receiving them. Consequently, B-2 relievers are used more frequently in the USA than in other countries (see p. 343), a policy which may increase the risk of severe asthma attacks (see pp. 322–3).

'. . . I remember my uncle living the life of an invalid . . .'

Sally is in her forties. 'I've got asthma and both my children have it badly. Henry is the worst – he's had it since he was six months old. Most of my cousins and second cousins have severe asthma, and so did my uncle.

'One of the reasons I'm quite happy to use the modern asthma drugs is that I remember my uncle living the life of an invalid. Physically he was hunched over, his rib-cage and back very deformed from struggling to breathe. He died in 1978, when he was in his fifties, and by that time the asthma had taken such a massive toll on his heart and lungs that he had serious heart problems and was in hospital for months. There were some good asthma drugs by then, but for him it was too late, the damage had been done.

'He actually stopped taking the asthma medication in the end. He just said he'd had enough. Although it said "Asthma" on his death certificate, really it was just that he'd had enough, that he'd got no sort of life.

'So when I think of him, and then I think of my childhood, struggling to breathe and missing school for months, I don't feel any qualms about the modern asthma drugs. I think, "At least my children have got the choice of having really sickly lives dominated by asthma or of taking these drugs and running around."

'I sometimes stand by the school playground and see Henry running like the wind along with the rest of them, and I think "That's absolutely wonderful". I went through the whole of secondary school never doing school games because I was never well enough.'

WHAT ARE THE DIFFERENT DRUGS SUPPOSED TO DO?

This section describes asthma drugs in terms of the different types or categories they belong to. These category names will probably be unfamiliar, and to make sense of the information given here you need to know, for example, that Ventolin is a short-acting B-2 reliever. To relate the brand-names of the drugs you are taking to the category names used here, turn to pp. 370–5. You can fill in the relevant information below (use pencil in case your drugs change in future):

Brand-name of drug	Generic name of drug	Colour of inhaler	Preventer or reliever?	Category of drug
———	———	———	———	———
———	———	———	———	———
———	———	———	———	———
———	———	———	———	———
———	———	———	———	———
———	———	———	———	———
———	———	———	———	———
———	———	———	———	———

The different kinds of asthma drug

There are basically two kinds of drug used for asthma: relievers and preventers.

Relievers (or bronchodilators) simply make the muscles around the airways relax, so that the airways widen temporarily.

Preventers treat the underlying problem, the inflammation of the airways which causes swelling of the airway lining and over-production of mucus (see p. 22). They therefore have long-term benefits in reducing asthma severity. Once the inflammation is reduced, the muscles around the airways tend to relax of their own accord.

To put it simply, relievers give short-term relief, and no more, while preventers tackle the root cause of the asthma.

Relievers, especially the short-acting B-2 relievers (see p. 342), have a very rapid and noticeable effect, which is often a great relief to the asthmatic. They can easily seem more powerful and effective than any other drug. Preventers, on the other hand, make no difference at first. They take days or weeks to reduce the inflammation, and have a much more subtle (*but eventually more valuable*) effect on the symptoms.

Asthmatics sometimes say of their preventer: 'Oh, I don't bother with that one because it doesn't do the trick for me.' They are mistakenly comparing the preventer with the immediate and noticeable impact of the reliever. If this leads someone to use too much of the reliever and too little of the preventer, their mistake may have serious consequences, and could even put their life at risk (see p. 322). This is why it is so important to understand the differences between these drugs.

Alternative names for drug groups
You may need to understand these terms if you come across them in other books or pamphlets, or hear them from your doctor or asthma nurse.

Steroids	Corticosteroids
Cromoglycate-type drugs	Mast-cell blockers
	Anti-allergic drugs
B-2 relievers	B-2 agonists
	Beta-2 agonists or β-2 agonists
	B-2 bronchodilators
	Selective B-2 adrenoceptor stimulants
Anti-cholinergics	Anti-muscarinic bronchodilators
	Atropine-type drugs
Theophylline-type drugs	Xanthines
	Methylxanthines

Preventers
There are several basic types of preventer, but the two most widely used are corticosteroids and cromoglycate-type drugs. Both reduce the inflammation in the airways but they work in different ways.

Steroids (corticosteroids)
These are nothing whatever to do with the steroids that are used illicitly by some athletes (see p. 296). Corticosteroid drugs are designed to mimic a hormone called cortisol which is produced

naturally by the body. They are useful in asthma because they are very effective in damping down inflammation, the reaction of the body's immune system which plays a major role in asthma (see p. 22).

Inhaled steroids
Brand-name of your inhaled steroid:
Corticosteroids are powerful drugs, and doctors use them with caution. But when they are taken by inhaler, only very small doses are needed, because the drug goes directly to the airways. At low or moderate doses, inhaled steroids can be used quite safely. There are relatively few side-effects at such doses, and no serious risks as long as they are used correctly. Indeed, they can prevent permanent damage to the lungs, which may occur with severe uncontrolled asthma. The widespread fears about taking inhaled steroids are largely unfounded (see p. 326).

Far more worrying is the recent evidence about some of the short-acting reliever drugs, showing the ill-effects of relying heavily on these. Using short-acting B-2 relievers more than once a day can make asthma worse and in those with severe asthma it can increase the risk of a fatal attack (see pp. 322–3). By taking inhaled steroids regularly asthmatics can reduce their need for reliever drugs. This is now seen as the best possible option for all asthmatics, even those with mild asthma. Patients who might only have been given a reliever in the past are now being given a steroid inhaler as well, because this is in their best long-term interests.

Inhaled steroids must be taken twice a day for about a week before they begin to have any noticeable effect on asthma symptoms. Within a few weeks, if you are feeling better, it should be possible to use your short-acting B-2 reliever less often.

At present, inhaled steroids are not given to asthmatics unless they have persistent symptoms. Some doctors believe that the earlier use of inhaled steroids, even for patients with intermittent symptoms, could be valuable in reducing the long-term severity of asthma. This idea is currently being tested in a scientific trial.

Practical points:
- Always take inhaled steroids at regular intervals: get into a routine and they will be much more effective.
- Wash your mouth out well afterwards – and spit the water out. This reduces side-effects (see p. 352).

- If you do forget a dose, take it as soon as you remember, or double the next dose, but avoid doing this regularly.
- Don't stop taking steroids because you have infrequent symptoms, or are symptom-free. If you have been symptom-free for three months, it is then worth discussing the possibility of reducing the dose with your doctor. *This must be done slowly and with medical supervision.*
- If you are using an aerosol inhaler (an MDI or 'puffer'), you get less of the drug into your lungs. Ask your doctor about the possibility of having a spacer or a more modern inhaler device (see p. 379).
- Special care is needed when inhaling steroids from a nebulizer (see p. 387).

Steroid tablets
Brand-name of your steroid tablet:
When asthma is very severe, steroids are used in tablet form ('oral steroids'), to suppress the inflammation as effectively as possible. The tablets are usually taken for a short period of time only, because of the risk of side-effects. Short courses generally last about five days, and no more than three weeks.

Some patients with very severe asthma have to take steroid tablets continuously. They are carefully monitored for possible side-effects.

Practical points:
- It is important to start taking the steroid tablets at an early stage: they are much more effective if used at the beginning of an attack. There should be some noticeable response after about three hours, but the maximum effect takes nine or more hours to develop.
- Generally speaking, steroid tablets should always be withdrawn gradually, by changing to a lower dose before stopping completely, otherwise the inflammation may flare up again. Ask for specific instructions from your doctor.
- If you are taking steroid tablets continuously, the consequences of stopping abruptly are particularly dangerous. Never stop taking the tablets without first talking to a doctor. Make sure you always have enough tablets with you if travelling.

- If taking steroid tablets for more than three weeks carry a Steroid Card (see p. 359) and wear a Medic-Alert bracelet (see p. 459). Continue with this for two years after taking long-term steroids.
- Taking all the day's tablets at once, after breakfast, seems to produce the best effect and reduces the risk of major side-effects. The risk is reduced even further by taking steroids on alternate days, but you must have your doctor's permission to try this (see p. 359).
- Taking the tablets with food, not on an empty stomach, reduces the risk of stomach upsets.
- Women on the contraceptive Pill require a lower dose of steroid, because the two drugs interact. If you decide to stop taking the Pill, your dose of steroid may need to be increased.

Cromoglycate-type drugs
Brand-name of your cromoglycate-type drug:
There are just two drugs in this group, sodium cromoglycate and nedocromil sodium. Both are believed to work at an early stage of the inflammation process, stopping it before it even starts. If, for example, you are allergic to pollen, cromoglycate will prevent immune cells known as mast cells from responding to the pollen grains in the air, so that the allergic reaction doesn't happen. (In this way, cromoglycate-type drugs differ from steroids which damp down inflammation that has already occurred.) For cromoglycate or nedocromil to work, they must get to the mast cells in advance of a reaction – they are useless if taken later.

These drugs are extremely safe, with few or no side-effects in most people, and they can be useful in reducing the dose of steroid needed to control asthma. Unfortunately, they do not work for everyone. Children are more likely to benefit from them than adults.

Like steroids, cromoglycate-type drugs build up to their full effect slowly. They need to be taken regularly for at least four weeks before their impact on symptoms can be assessed realistically.

Practical points:
- When they are being taken continuously, these drugs need to be inhaled three or four times a day, at regular intervals: get into a routine and they will be much more effective. (Occa-

sionally, a more frequent inhalation may be recommended: six or even eight times a day.)

- If you do forget a dose, take it as soon as you remember. There is nothing to be gained by doubling the next dose, if you have completely missed one.
- Once asthma is well controlled, it may be possible to reduce the dosing regime to three times a day, or just twice, but ask your doctor first.
- If taken on an 'as-needed' basis, cromoglycate-type drugs must be taken in advance: 30 minutes before an allergen is encountered, for example, or 30 minutes before a bout of exercise if they are being used to control exercise-induced asthma. This can be an extra dose, on top of your regular four-times-daily inhalation.
- Children may respond differently, getting protection from exercise-induced asthma immediately. However, the effect may only last for two to three hours.
- Make sure you know how to use your inhaler device properly (see p. 376).
- Do not stop taking these drugs without first talking to your doctor. It is best to reduce the dose slowly over a period of a week. You may need to introduce (or reintroduce) steroids at the same time, to maintain control of your asthma.

Theophylline-type drugs
Brand-name of your theophylline-type drugs:
Theophylline is now known to have an anti-inflammatory action and is increasingly being seen as a type of preventer (see pp. 332–3). But these drugs are traditionally regarded as relievers (bronchodilators) and are therefore dealt with on p. 346.

Anti-histamines
Anti-histamines are drugs used to treat hayfever and other allergic reactions. They are not normally used to treat asthma, except in Japan (see p. 332). However, one anti-histamine can be useful for exercise-induced asthma (see p. 72) and there may also be a place for these drugs where asthma is made worse by alcohol (see p. 332).

Ketotifen
Brand-name of your ketotifen:
Ketotifen is more than just an anti-histamine: it can also prevent inflammation occurring, by acting in a similar way to cromoglycate. For this reason it may help some asthmatics.

On the whole, ketotifen has not proved quite as useful for asthma as was widely hoped, but some people do find it effective. If it works for you, it may allow you to reduce the dose of steroids taken. One advantage of ketotifen is that you take it by mouth (in capsules, tablets or syrup) not by inhaler.

Practical points:
- Ketotifen requires several weeks to take effect, so continue taking your previous drugs (e.g. steroids) for at least two weeks, or you will risk losing control of your asthma.

Leukotriene antagonists
These drugs work in a completely different way from either steroids or cromoglycate. They reduce levels of inflammation, by interfering with inflammatory messages carried by natural chemicals which the body produces, called leukotrienes.

Zafirlukast
Brand-name of your zafirlukast:
This is the first example of a new type of drug, called a leukotriene receptor antagonist.

Practical points:
- Zafirlukast can be inhaled or taken as tablets. For those who dislike inhalers, the fact that this drug can be taken as tablets makes it an attractive option.
- If you are taking it for the first time, it takes about three days for any noticeable effects to occur.
- Once you are taking it regularly, each dose requires two to four hours to have its full effect, but goes on working for 12–24 hours in total.

Montelukast
This is taken in tablet form, once a day but not with food. Like other leukotriene antagonists it is a preventer drug, and is of no value for

immediate relief during an asthma attack. So you must still have a reliever inhaler.

Zileuton
Brand-name of your zileuton:
This tackles inflammation in a similar way to zafirlukast (see above), but it works by stopping the production of the leukotrienes altogether. It belongs to a group of drugs called 5-lipoxygenase-inhibitors.

Zileuton is not used for children under 12. If theophylline is also being taken, the dose of theophylline should be halved. This is a preventer drug, and of no use during an asthma attack.

Zileuton is taken in tablet form once a day. It should begin to produce an improvement in symptoms within the first week, with maximum effects reached after four months. There is usually a reduction in the need for B-2 relievers and courses of steroid tablets.

Other anti-inflammatory (preventer) drugs
Methotrexate and gold salts
These are powerful drugs that suppress the immune system, and are used to treat rheumatoid arthritis. They are being tried as experimental treatments for severe asthma, for those on high doses of steroid tablets, and for the very small minority of patients who do not respond to steroids. Careful monitoring for side-effects is essential.

Cyclosporin
This is another immune-suppressing drug, used to treat leukaemia. It may be useful for some patients with very severe asthma who do not respond to steroids or other drugs.

Intravenous immunoglobulin
This is an effective but extremely expensive form of treatment, used only for those with very severe asthma.

Relievers
There are four kinds of reliever:
1. Short-acting B-2 relievers
2. Long-acting B-2 relievers
3. Anti-cholinergics
4. Theophylline-type drugs

Short-acting B-2 relievers
Brand-name of your short-acting B-2 reliever:

Both types of B-2 reliever (short-acting and long-acting) work by stimulating targets in the airways called B- (pronounced *beta*)-2 receptors. These targets are normally stimulated by adrenaline (epinephrine), the chemical which we naturally produce when alarmed, angry, excited or preparing for strenuous physical activity. By opening up the airways it enables us to run faster or punch harder.

Adrenaline and similar chemicals were among the earliest treatments for asthma. However, adrenaline also stimulates the heart to beat faster, raises the blood pressure and has other effects on the body which are unwanted in asthma treatment. The B-2 relievers overcome these problems by selectively working on the airways. At normal doses they have little effect on the heart and other organs.

Inhaled forms

These take effect within moments of being inhaled, and give full relief after about 15 minutes. The effect should last three to six hours, usually for about four hours, although rimiterol tends to last for a shorter time.

Generally speaking, they should only be used when needed, that is, when the airways have already narrowed, resulting in wheezing, breathlessness, a tight chest or coughing.

There are exceptions to this rule, however: occasionally you can take the drug in advance of symptoms. For example, if you know that you get asthma during or after exercise (see p. 68), the doctor or asthma nurse may recommend that you use your reliever inhaler before exercising. Similarly, if you are about to be exposed to an allergen which you know will affect you (for example visiting a house with a cat, if you are allergic to cats), and cannot avoid the exposure, you could use your reliever inhaler in advance. However, it would be much better to use inhaled cromoglycate which blocks the allergic reaction (see p. 338): ask your doctor about prescribing this.

All that short-acting B-2 relievers do is to make the airway muscles relax: they do not tackle the underlying problems. In fact, if overused, they can make the problem worse (see pp. 322-3).

Medical attitudes to short-acting B-2 relievers have changed in the last few years, as the potential dangers of these drugs have been realized. At one time, most people with mild asthma had an inhaler of

this kind, and nothing else. Now, anyone who has night-time symptoms, or who needs to use a short-acting B-2 reliever more than once a
day, should be given a preventer as well. (This is the British guideline:
the international guideline is more stringent, and says that if a short-
acting B-2 reliever is needed more than three times a week, a
preventer should also be prescribed. US guidelines are less stringent,
and allow three or four doses a day before a preventer is added: British
and European doctors consider this to be much too frequent.)

Practical points:
- Make sure you have an inhaler device that suits you and that
  you know how to use it properly (see p. 376). It is important
  to inhale slowly, and then to hold your breath for ten seconds.
- If you are using your short-acting B-2 reliever more than once
  a day (or more than three times a week: see above), ask your
  doctor about adding a preventer, or increasing the dose of your
  preventer if you are already taking one. Over-using a short-
  acting B-2 reliever, or relying on it too heavily, is the most
  dangerous thing an asthmatic can do: it is a major cause of
  death among asthmatics.
- Unfortunately, some people with severe asthma still need to
  use a short-acting B-2 reliever more than once a day, despite
  being treated as thoroughly as possible with preventers. Even
  these patients should not use this inhaler more than three or
  four times a day.
- If you have symptoms at night, tell your doctor. You should be
  taking a preventer as well as your short-acting B-2 reliever. If
  you still have troublesome symptoms, you may also need a
  reliever that lasts longer (see p. 344).
- Always keep your short-acting B-2 reliever inhaler with you,
  even if you have not needed it for ages: asthma is unpredictable, a severe attack can happen out of the blue, and in an
  emergency this reliever could save your life.
- If you ever find that you need to use a short-acting B-2 reliever
  more than once every four hours, this indicates a serious asthma
  attack and you need urgent medical help (see pp. 51–2).
- If you ever find that your short-acting B-2 reliever no longer
  seems to be working (if it has no effect within 15 minutes),
  you need urgent medical help.

- During a severe asthma attack, while getting to hospital or waiting for a doctor to arrive, 15–30 puffs of a short-acting B-2 reliever can be taken as an emergency treatment. A spacer (see p. 380) may be helpful if it is difficult to use the inhaler. An improvised spacer can be made from a plastic drinks cup (see p. 384).

Tablets or syrup

Tablets or syrup may be prescribed for those who have difficulty using an inhaler, but they have serious disadvantages. When taken in tablet or syrup form, the drug has to be absorbed into the bloodstream and only reaches the airways via the blood, so a much larger dose of B-2 reliever is needed to produce an effect on the airways. Consequently, side-effects, such as a pounding heart, trembling hands or insomnia, are more likely.

Given the concern about B-2 relievers, taking large doses regularly in tablet or syrup form is undesirable. Ask your doctor if there are any other drugs that could help you.

Other forms in which these drugs are taken

Patients with very severe asthma may need to have these drugs delivered directly into the body, by a continuous infusion into the bloodstream or under the skin (parenteral bronchodilators). This requires wearing a small device, strapped around the waist, containing a pump which delivers the drug at regular intervals.

Long-acting B-2 relievers

Brand-name of your long-acting B-2 reliever:

These drugs are very similar chemically to the short-acting B-2 relievers, and they can produce an initial effect almost as quickly, within five to ten minutes. Where they differ is that the effect goes on building up, reaches a maximum after an hour or so, and then lasts for another nine to eleven hours. When taken regularly (twice a day) for several days, there is a gradually increasing benefit.

These drugs are especially useful for nocturnal asthma (see p. 76) and for marathon runners (see p. 294).

Unfortunately, like the short-acting B-2 relievers, a drug of this type can make asthmatic airways less responsive to the benefits of the drug itself and to other B-2 relievers (see p. 325). However, it seems to be safer to take a long-acting B-2 reliever twice a day, rather than a short-acting one four times a day.

Practical points:
- Take regularly, once every 12 hours.
- Do not take additional doses in between: these are not 'as required' drugs. They should not be used if you have a sudden and more serious asthma attack.
- Do not stop taking your preventer drug, even if you feel considerably improved: these drugs are not a substitute for preventers.
- Make sure you know how to use your inhaler device properly (see p. 376).

Anti-cholinergics
Brand-name of your anti-cholinergic:
These drugs work in an entirely different way from the B-2 relievers, by blocking the effects of a set of nerves called the parasympathetic nervous system. These nerves have many effects on the body, including sustaining muscle tone in the airways (see p. 418).

Anti-cholinergics take 30–90 minutes to achieve their full effects, and should continue working for three to six hours.

Anti-cholinergics are generally less effective than B-2 relievers for most asthmatics, especially those with a strong allergic component. But for those with chronic bronchitis as well as asthma, the anti-cholinergics can be as effective or even more effective than B-2 relievers. For those with severe asthma, they may be combined with B-2 relievers. They are particularly useful for asthma with a lot of mucus production.

Anti-cholinergics are also useful in children under one year, who may not react to B-2 relievers.

Practical points:
- Make sure you know how to use your inhaler device properly (see p. 376).
- If taking these drugs with a nebulizer, be very careful that the mask fits well (see p. 387).

Theophylline-type drugs

Brand-name of your theophylline-type drug:

These drugs are chemically similar to caffeine, the stimulant found in tea and coffee. They cannot be inhaled, unlike the other three types of reliever, so they are taken in tablet form, or as a syrup. They take 30 minutes to start working and their effects last for about six to eight hours. The slow-release forms are slower to start working (90 minutes) but last for 12–24 hours.

Side-effects are common with these drugs (see pp. 366–8), and there is a very narrow margin between the dose that opens up the airways and the overdose that causes unpleasant, or even dangerous, reactions. Such side-effects usually occur in the early stages, when the doctor is still trying to work out the correct dose (which varies from one person to another).

However, once asthmatics are established on a safe dose (and provided their general health and their intake of alcohol, tobacco and other drugs are stable – see below) they can usually go on taking theophylline on a long-term basis without serious side-effects.

Because of the difficulty of establishing a safe dose for each individual, theophylline-type drugs are not much used in Britain, except for those with severe asthma, and for brittle asthma (see p. 32), where theophylline can be useful as an additional treatment for 'smoothing out' the unpredictable variations in symptoms.

Theophylline remains popular in the USA, however, and is even part of the first line of treatment for mild asthmatics (see p. 332). Recent research has shown that by taking low doses of theophylline, asthmatics can reduce their use of B-2 relievers. Given the concern now felt about B-2 relievers, low-dose theophylline could be an attractive option.

New forms of theophylline-type drugs are under development, which may have fewer side-effects.

Practical points:
- When first taking theophylline, blood samples must be taken regularly to check the levels of the drug in the blood. Don't miss your appointments.
- If you give up smoking, or cut down, or (are you crazy?) take it up, tell your doctor. Your dose of theophylline will need to change immediately as smoking affects the breakdown of the

drug. (So will any other source of nicotine, such as chewing tobacco or nicotine chewing-gum.)

- Heavy drinking also changes the effects of the drug, and the dose will need adjustment if your alcohol intake changes.
- Avoid sudden, major changes to your diet, and high-fat foods.
- Taking contraceptive Pills, and a variety of other drugs, alters the dose needed. Check with your doctor or pharmacist before starting any new drugs, or coming off the Pill.
- Viral infections, flu vaccinations, heart disease and liver disease also change the effects of theophylline. Watch for side-effects and consult your doctor immediately if you are concerned.
- Simply getting older changes your reaction to this drug: your dose may need to change as you age.
- Be very careful never to take a double dose by mistake: if you are at all forgetful about tablets, keep a careful record of taking your theophylline.
- Always report any side-effects to your doctor immediately. If concerned, stop taking the drug.

Older types of reliever drug

There are several old-fashioned asthma drugs (see pp. 372–3) which are quite similar, chemically, to the natural adrenaline molecule. They therefore work in much the same way as the B-2 relievers, but are far less selective for the airways: they also affect the heart and this can produce unpleasant side-effects (see p. 368).

Older patients, who have had asthma for many years, may still be using these drugs. For anyone taking such drugs, it would be wise to talk to a doctor about switching to a newer form of asthma drug which will be more effective as well as having fewer side-effects.

Adrenaline (epinephrine) inhalers and injection kits

Patients with severe asthma triggered by serious allergic reactions (see p. 111) can be given an inhaler containing adrenaline (epinephrine). *These are for emergency use only, not daily use.*

Introduction of a new standard for inhaler design has meant that the adrenaline inhaler formerly available in Britain, the Medihaler-Epi, has recently been withdrawn. Some doctors are so concerned about this that they are now bringing in small supplies of an American adrenaline inhaler called AsthmaHaler Mist for their patients. Pharmacies can also order this inhaler for you (see p. 469). For more information, speak to your doctor or specialist, or contact the Anaphylaxis Campaign (address on p. 453). In the USA, the AsthmaHaler Mist and another brand, Primatene Mist, can be bought without prescription.

Those who have suffered from anaphylaxis in the past should also be carrying injectable adrenaline, known as an Epi-pen, Anapen, Anakit, Anaguard or Anahelp (see p. 375). (In Britain these are only issued for those known to suffer from anaphylactic shock – see p. 48 – but in some countries, asthmatics who do not suffer anaphylaxis but are prone to rapid asthma attacks and who live some distance from the nearest hospital or ambulance station, may be given an adrenaline (epinephrine) injector kit for use in an emergency.)

Both injectable and inhaled adrenaline can be used during a severe attack (see p. 55).

Mixtures of drugs

Various drug mixtures have been tried in the past, including mixtures of a preventer and a short-acting B-2 reliever (e.g. Ventide). This is no longer recommended for asthma treatment in Britain because doctors feel these drugs should be inhaled separately, so that the preventer can be taken regularly, while the reliever is used only when needed (see p. 323).

One of the older drug mixtures, Combivent, which combines two different forms of reliever, may be useful for those with COPD (see p. 32). Generally speaking, however, the use of the older drug mixtures is being phased out.

Two new mixtures of drugs have been introduced recently, both for people with quite severe asthma. One (Seretide) combines a steroid preventer with a long-acting B-2 reliever. This makes sense as both drugs need to be taken regularly, twice a day (see p. 336 and p. 344). The other new mixture (Aerocrom Syncroner) contains the preventer cromoglycate and the short-acting B-2 reliever salbutamol. The cromoglycate needs to be taken regularly four times a day to be effective, so the salbutamol is also taken four times a day. We would question the wisdom of this kind of regular dosing with a B-2 reliever. It is only acceptable for those with very severe asthma which has not been controlled by other drugs (see p. 343).

Cough medicines and other over-the-counter drugs
Cough medicines
If your main asthma symptom is coughing, it may be tempting to use cough medicines. Parents of asthmatic children often want to use these to help the child during an attack, or even to replace asthma drugs.

Don't be tempted. Cough mixture will not help with the asthma, and it could even make matters worse by making the mucus in the airways more sticky. If it does succeed in reducing the coughing, it could also conceal the severity of the asthma, so that you are not aware when emergency treatment is needed.

Expectorants
These drugs help to clear mucus from the lungs, and may be helpful if you produce a lot of mucus and it tends to accumulate. Ask your doctor for advice. (Although many cough medicines contain expectorants, they also contain other drugs that are not at all beneficial for asthma – see above.)

Inhalations
These can be very useful for loosening thick sticky mucus in the airways. Chemists' shops sell traditional inhalation capsules, which you add to hot water. Put a towel over your head and inhale the steam. Simply inhaling steam from plain hot water will also be useful. Note that many inhalation capsules contain menthol: some asthmatics are sensitive to this and should therefore avoid it (see p. 234).

See also:

Certain other drugs, including common ones such as aspirin, may make asthma *worse* (or, more rarely, better). For details see pp. 257–66. Herbal remedies and homeopathic medicines are discussed on pp. 407–9.

SIDE EFFECTS:
WHICH ONES ARE WORTH WORRYING ABOUT?

Everyone's body chemistry is different, so side-effects are very variable. You may well have no side-effects at all. Most of the commonly used asthma drugs have no inevitable side-effects.

The exceptions to this are:
- Steroid tablets, which if taken continuously and at high doses, have inevitable (and potentially dangerous) side-effects for anyone.
- Theophylline-type drugs, which will poison anyone if the dose is too high – even if only slightly too high.
- Short-acting B-2 relievers (Ventolin, Bricanyl, etc.) which are probably dangerous to all asthmatics if over-used (see p. 322). If you have been asthmatic for a long time, note that what counts as 'over-use' now is an inhalation of a short-acting B-2 reliever (e.g. Ventolin) more than once a day or more than three times a week (depending on which guidelines are used – see p. 343). This would have been considered perfectly normal and safe 20 years ago, when many doctors were happy for their patients to use short-acting B-2 relievers four or more times a day. More is now known about the effects of these drugs.

If you are taking any of these three drugs, you should be aware of the dangers listed above, and alert for signs of trouble. But in general, if you are just starting on a new drug, it may be best not to read this section yet: many people only have to know about a side-effect to start suffering from it. (This is why doctors generally don't tell patients about side-effects.) It may be better to wait and see how the drug is for you.

Please read this before you go any further!
Reading long lists of side-effects can be very frightening or depressing, especially if you are dependent on drugs to keep your asthma under control. It is very much like reading about muggings or car accidents: you have to try to keep things in perspective, and remember that it is probably *not* going to happen to you, especially if you are sensible and careful. Bear the following points in mind:

- All the most common side-effects are minor ones. A minor side-effect may be unpleasant or inconvenient, but it does not mean that the drug is doing you any serious damage.
- If the drugs are used in the correct way, most people taking them will not suffer any major side-effects.
- You can avert major side-effects by being vigilant about early warning signs: this section is designed to help you in this (not to make you feel alarmed or anxious about your drugs).
- Uncontrolled severe asthma is more dangerous than the drugs.
- You should always talk to your doctor before stopping any drug or changing the dose.

Steroids (corticosteroids)

These drugs are associated with fairly high levels of side-effects when taken in tablet form, but are much less troublesome when inhaled. For general information on steroids see pp. 326–8 and pp. 335–8.

Inhaled steroids

In general, inhaled steroids are far, far safer than steroid tablets. For anyone with moderate to severe asthma, who sometimes needs courses of steroid tablets, there are huge advantages to taking your inhaled steroids regularly: this will keep your asthma under control and reduce the number of courses of steroid tablets that you need.

The dose is the crucial factor as regards side-effects from inhaled steroids. Before reading any further, check what dose of inhaled steroid you are taking.

	Adults, children over five years:	*Children under five:*
A *low* dose	100–400 mcg per day	less than 200 mcg per day
A *moderate* dose	500–800 mcg per day	250–400 mcg per day
A *high* dose	more than 800 mcg per day	more than 500 mcg per day

These figures are for budesonide or beclomethasone (this is the generic name, not the familiar brand-name – see p. 370). For fluticasone (Flixotide), halve these figures (i.e. 400 mcg is a high dose). If you are taking any other type of steroid, check with your pharmacist.

(Note that mcg stands for microgram. It may also be written 'µg'.)

To work out your total daily dose:
- You need to know how many mcg (micrograms) you are getting per inhalation. Look on the leaflet in the inhaler package for this information. Note that some brands come in several different strengths: Becotide, for example, comes as Becotide 50 (50 mcg per puff), Becotide 100 (100 mcg per puff) and Becotide 200 (200 mcg per puff).
- If you are not sure how much is in each inhalation, ask your pharmacist.
- Write down how many inhalations you take each day.
- Multiply this by the number of mcg per inhalation, to get the total daily dose.

If you are on a low or a moderate dose, you have very little to worry about as regards more serious side-effects. Only those inhaling high-dose steroids for many years need feel concerned about these.

Minor side-effects
Hoarseness and short-lived coughing due to direct irritation of the throat.

Throat infections: Steroids reduce the body's ability to fight infection and a common side-effect of inhaling them is an infection of the throat by *Candida*, which is a yeast (a type of fungus). It is the same microbe that causes vaginal thrush. As well as soreness, there are often white spots on the throat, hence the name thrush.

Oesophageal infections: These are rare but can happen – again, it is *Candida*. The symptoms are heartburn and indigestion.
Prevention:
- Washing your mouth out and gargling with warm water after each inhalation should prevent this. (Spit the water out afterwards: don't swallow it as this will increase the amount of steroid absorbed into the bloodstream.) Inhaling your steroids morning and evening, just before brushing your teeth, is a good idea, as you will automatically rinse your mouth out afterwards.
- If you still suffer from this problem, there are anti-fungal lozenges that can help.

Note that the risk of chest infections is not increased by using inhaled steroids (see pp. 238–9). (But steroid tablets may increase this risk.)

Cold sores: Herpes infections around the mouth (cold sores) can also be made worse by contact with steroids.

Prevention:

- Keep your inhaled steroids away from your lips if you suffer from cold sores.

More serious side-effects

There are more likely to be serious side-effects if a large amount of the steroid is swallowed, because this gets absorbed into the bloodstream. Studies have shown that most people using an aerosol inhaler, even those with good technique (see p. 376), inhale as little as 10 per cent of the drug. The other 90 per cent is deposited in the mouth and swallowed.

Prevention:

- After using your inhaler, always rinse your mouth, gargle, and spit the water out.
- Using a large-volume spacer (see p. 380) or changing to a newer type of inhaler (see p. 379) will increase the amount of steroid inhaled. Ask your doctor about prescribing one of these.

Growth suppression: Children's growth can be stunted by long-term use of inhaled steroids, but only if relatively high doses are taken for many years. On low to moderate doses, most children will be fine: although they may have a short-term slow-down in growth, their eventual height will be normal.

There are a few children, however, who react differently, and whose growth is stunted even by relatively low doses of inhaled steroids. There is no way of predicting which children will be affected in this way. However, if it is noticed in good time, and if the steroids can be withdrawn safely, the child's growth rate will almost certainly recover.

You may notice that your child does not need new clothes as often as expected, or takes sizes smaller than expected for his age. Point this out to the doctor or asthma nurse. Measuring the child regularly is also a good idea.

Remember that uncontrolled severe asthma stunts children's growth.

Osteoporosis: The risks are much less with inhaled steroids than with tablets, but there may be significant and damaging bone-mineral loss if high doses are taken for long periods of time. See below, under steroid tablets, for ways in which you can protect yourself.

Potentially dangerous side-effects

Adrenal suppression: There is some possibility of adrenal suppression (explained below, under steroid tablets) but *only* with high doses of inhaled steroid. Periodic check-ups and blood tests should be carried out.

Recurrence of tuberculosis: See below, under steroid tablets.

Effects on the eyes and the skin of the face: Special care is needed when inhaling steroids from a nebulizer (see p. 387).

Taking steroid nose or eye drops as well as a steroid inhaler

Many people feel concerned about their total dose of steroid when they are given an inhaler as well as steroid drops. There is no need to worry about this unless you are taking very high doses of inhaled steroid, in which case talk to your doctor. The amount in nose or eye drops is quite small, because, as with inhalers, it is going straight to the place where it is needed. Relatively little gets into the bloodstream.

Using steroid nose drops can be very helpful for asthma (see p. 253).

Steroid tablets (oral steroids)

Of all the anti-asthma drugs, these carry the highest risk of side-effects. However, doctors are thoroughly aware of the dangers, and you should be given extremely careful supervision if taking steroid tablets continuously.

Occasional short courses (usually about five days, and no more than three weeks) at high dose have far fewer serious side-effects than prolonged courses at lower doses. Indeed, short courses can be taken several times a year, with no ill-effects.

Prevention:

- Always follow your doctor's instructions to the letter when it comes to steroid tablets: you cannot afford to be careless about these drugs.
- Anything you can do to reduce your need for steroid tablets (see pp. 2–6) will be extremely beneficial.

Minor side-effects

Hunger, nervousness and insomnia: Increased appetite for food. Feeling 'hyped up' and edgy during the day, and not sleeping at night.
Prevention:
- You don't actually need more food, unfortunately. It is very important not to increase your calorie intake, as you will put on weight quite quickly and obesity makes asthma worse (see p. 255). To cope with the hunger pangs, eat more fruit, vegetables and starchy foods such as bread, rice and potatoes, while cutting down on fat and oil. This will satisfy your appetite with extra bulk while not piling on the calories.

Periods: With prolonged use, some women may suffer irregular periods.

Diabetics may need more insulin.

Wounds may be slow to heal, and they are also more likely to become infected because of reduced immunity.
Prevention:
- Keep all cuts and grazes as clean as possible.

More serious side-effects

Raised blood pressure: This can occur even with short-term use of steroids, so your blood pressure should be checked regularly by the doctor.
Prevention:
- Eating less salt will reduce this risk, and is good for asthma too (see p. 100).

Growth suppression: Children may stop growing, or grow more slowly, if taking steroid tablets. Sometimes they make up for this later, but sometimes the effect is irreversible. Your child's growth should be watched carefully by a doctor or asthma nurse, and you should also be vigilant.
Prevention:
- Taking steroids every other day (see below) can prevent growth problems. Ask your doctor about this.

Cushing's syndrome: Long-term use at high doses can result in Cushing's syndrome, characterized by deposits of fat on the shoulders and abdomen, and around the face ('moon face'), easy bruising, acne, muscle wasting, water retention producing puffiness, and weakening of the bones leading to easy breakage. All these changes are due to effects of corticosteroids on other body processes apart from inflammation. Some of the effects are reversible, if corticosteroids are withdrawn, but there can also be permanent damage.

The steroids must be withdrawn slowly, under close medical supervision.

Prevention:

- Weigh yourself daily. If your weight suddenly starts to increase, despite normal food intake, consult your doctor: this may be a sign of water retention, which is a feature of Cushing's syndrome.
- If you develop swollen ankles, acne, or muscle weakness, tell your doctor.

Mental disorders: Psychological side-effects may occur, particularly in those with a history of psychological problems. In the worst cases, there may be paranoia or severe depression, with a risk of suicide. Some people experience an exaggerated sense of well-being (euphoria).

Prevention:

- Do tell the doctor if you have had psychological problems such as depression, psychosis or schizophrenia in the past.
- If you notice mood changes when taking steroid tablets, tell your doctor.

Stomach ulcers: A few patients may be more likely to develop stomach ulcers, or inflammation in the oesophagus (the tube leading down to the stomach) or serious problems in the intestine. The risk is quite small.

Prevention:

- There are coated forms of the tablets that may reduce the risk. Ask your doctor if it would be a good idea to prescribe these.
- Taking the tablets after food helps.
- Contact your doctor if you have persistent indigestion while taking these drugs.

- If you notice that you are producing black, tarry stools, contact the doctor immediately. This is a sign of bleeding from the digestive tract.

Eye problems: Steroids can increase the risk of glaucoma and, with prolonged use, cataracts.
Prevention:
- Get your eyes checked regularly by an optician, who will be able to detect these problems before there is irreversible damage.

Thinning skin: With prolonged use of steroid tablets, the skin may become thin, and the small blood vessels beneath it more fragile, leading to easy bruising and stretch marks (striae). Elderly patients are much more susceptible to this problem.

Diabetes: Patients who have the potential to develop diabetes may be more likely to do so if taking steroid tablets long-term. When the steroids are stopped, it should disappear.
Prevention:
- You should be given regular tests for diabetes.
- Consult your doctor if you are excessively tired, unusually thirsty, or need to urinate much more often than usual.

Impotence: With long-term use, a minority of men may suffer impotence. Hormonal treatment may help in some cases, so don't hesitate to talk to your doctor about the problem.

Osteoporosis: With prolonged use, there can be loss of calcium and phosphorous from the bones, leading to thinning and fragility (osteoporosis). Nothing is noticeably wrong for many years. Eventually, a decade or more later, there may be fractures of the wrist and/or hip, collapse of the vertebrae producing a 'dowager's hump', or broken ribs. Osteoporosis (which is common even among elderly people not taking steroids) is painful and disabling.

Men, on the whole, are less affected by osteoporosis than women, but long-term use of steroids increases the risk for them as well.
Prevention:
- Keep as active as possible, with plenty of exercise such as

running or tennis. This is the best possible defence against osteoporosis. (Uncontrolled asthma often stops people taking exercise, and this in itself greatly increases the risk of osteoporosis. If taking steroids allows you to take active, vigorous exercise, the benefits in terms of avoiding osteoporosis probably outweigh the risks.)

- Don't get too thin, as this is a risk factor.
- Smoking is also a risk factor (but you are surely not smoking if you have severe asthma?)
- If you go through the menopause before age 55, you should seriously consider taking hormone replacement therapy (HRT) as this protects against osteoporosis (but see p. 263 for precautions). Any woman whose ovaries have been removed surgically should take HRT.
- Make sure you get plenty of calcium, magnesium, Vitamin D and green leafy vegetables in your diet. Reduce your salt intake. Don't drink too much alcohol as this increases the risk.
- Your doctor should order a bone-density measurement periodically. There are also drugs that may help prevent osteoporosis, and your doctor may be able to prescribe these.
- Report any unusual back pain to your doctor: this can be an early sign of osteoporosis.
- If you fracture your wrist in a fall (a Colles' fracture) make sure your GP knows about this. You should be given urgent treatment for osteoporosis if this happens.

Contraception failure: High-dose steroids can reduce the effectiveness of IUDs (which work by inducing a mild inflammation in the womb) and lead to pregnancy.
Prevention:
- If you have an IUD, ask your doctor about switching to another form of contraception.

Potentially dangerous side-effects
Adrenal suppression: If corticosteroids are taken for more than three weeks, the body's natural ability to produce its own steroids is suppressed. The longer the steroids have been taken, the greater the effect will be. This is called adrenal suppression. As long as you go on taking the steroids, everything will probably seem to be fine. But

stopping the drug abruptly leaves the body without corticosteroids, which can lead to collapse in the worst cases, or greater vulnerability to physical stress (including such things as surgery, an accident, serious illness or childbirth). Adrenal suppression can last for 6–12 months after the treatment with steroids has ended. It can take up to two years before a major stress such as surgery can be dealt with by the body unaided: your doctor will need to start you on low doses of steroids again to get you through stress of this kind.

Prevention:

- Taking all your daily steroids as a single dose in the morning reduces the risk of adrenal suppression.

- Even better protection comes from taking steroids every other day (as a single dose in the morning). The 'day off' between doses encourages the body to maintain its own steroid-making abilities. Not all asthmatics can keep their asthma under control with this regime, but for those who can there are enormous advantages in terms of avoiding side-effects. Some experts believe that everyone on long-term steroids should at least try taking them in this way. If you want to do this, you must consult your doctor. The dose may need adjusting.

- It is important that your dentist, or anyone treating you in a medical emergency, should know that you have been taking steroid tablets (even if you stopped up to two years earlier). In case you are unconscious, or unable to speak following an accident, *you should always carry a Steroid Card*, available from your doctor. Make sure you have such a card, even for short courses of steroids. It is also a very good idea to wear a Medic-Alert bracelet (see p. 459).

- Because of the risks of adrenal suppression, steroid tablets should never be stopped abruptly if they have been taken for more than two to three weeks. The body must be given time to recover its natural level of activity, by gradually reducing the dosage. Your doctor will tell you how quickly or slowly you can reduce the dose.

- If, while reducing the dose of steroids, you suffer any of the symptoms of adrenal suppression, do not delay contacting your doctor. The symptoms can include: muscle weakness, muscle and joint pain, feeling 'under the weather', mental changes, scaly or flaking skin, breathlessness, lack of appetite, nausea and vomiting. Other symptoms that might be experienced are fever, a runny or congested nose, red eyes, weight loss and painful itchy lumps on the skin.

Increased risk of infections: Because steroids suppress inflammation, which is a valuable part of the body's fight against disease, these drugs tend to make infections more likely. Viruses and fungi (e.g. *Candida*), in particular, are likely to flourish. Wounds may become septic more readily.

Additionally, infections may be masked by the drugs because they tend to suppress fever. So a disease may not become evident until it has already reached an advanced stage.

Common childhood diseases such as chickenpox or measles can be more serious, or even fatal, if steroid tablets are being taken, or have been taken within the last three months.

Vaccination with live vaccines can produce problems for those taking steroid tablets. Other vaccines are safe.

Elderly people who suffered from tuberculosis (TB) as children, may suffer a recurrence of the disease if treated with high-dose steroids.

Prevention:

- You should get detailed instructions from your doctor about what to do if you develop any kind of infection or suffer an accident. It is often necessary to increase the dose: follow these instructions carefully.
- Asthmatics who have never had measles or chickenpox should take particular care not to catch these diseases. Avoid contact with anyone suffering from chickenpox or from shingles (*Herpes zoster*) which is caused by the same virus. *Seek urgent medical attention if there is any contact with someone infected.* Emergency treatment to combat the virus can be given, but it should be started within three days of contact with the infected person, and no later than ten days after contact. The same advice applies to measles: avoid contact with anyone infected, and seek urgent medical attention if contact occurs.
- If you are being vaccinated, make sure the doctor or nurse knows that you are taking steroid tablets.
- Tell your doctor if you have ever had TB.

Cromoglycate-type drugs

These preventer drugs have far fewer side-effects than steroids, and make a good alternative if they work well for you (see p. 338). For asthma, they are taken by inhalation only.

Minor side-effects

Coughing: The powder often irritates the throat and produces coughing. Occasionally this may lead to wheezing, because the irritation of the powder has caused a temporary tightening of the airways. The standard advice is to use a short-acting B-2 reliever (such as Ventolin or Bricanyl) beforehand, to overcome this problem. However, this would involve using the bronchodilator four times a day, which is no longer considered advisable, except for some people with severe asthma (see p. 343). Talk to your doctor about this.

Prevention:
- These problems mainly occur with dry-powder inhalers (see p. 379). Switching from a dry-powder inhaler to an aerosol inhaler (with a spacer if necessary) often solves the problem of throat irritation.

Headache, nausea and vomiting are occasionally reported.

More serious side-effects

None for nedocromil sodium. Cromoglycate can cause joint pain and swelling, or a severe allergic reaction in certain patients, but both these reactions are extremely rare.

Potentially dangerous side-effects

None.

Anti-histamines

For more on these drugs see pp. 339–40.

Ketotifen

Minor side-effects

Nausea and headache.

Increased appetite and weight gain.

Prevention:
- Try not to eat more, as putting on weight is bad for asthmatics.

Drowsiness, dry mouth, slight dizziness.

Prevention:

- Do not drive until you are certain that the drug does not make
  you drowsy. Alcohol may have a more powerful effect than
  usual, so drink cautiously at first. If drowsiness is a problem,
  take the drug at bedtime. It is worth persisting, as the sleepy
  feeling may wear off after a few weeks of taking the drug.

More serious side-effects

None, except if taken with drugs for diabetes.

Leukotriene antagonists

For more on these drugs see p. 340. As with any new drug, you should
report any unusual symptoms just in case they are rare or delayed
side-effects (see p. 329).

Zafirlukast

Minor side-effects

The side-effects reported from pre-release trials of this drug are all
minor ones: headache, upset stomach, sore throat, and a blocked or
runny nose.

Montelukast

Minor side-effects

Headache, in children taking this drug. Other side-effects reported
from pre-release trials included headache, abdominal pain, cough and
flu-like symptoms, but they were no more frequent than in patients
taking the placebo (dummy drug).

More serious side-effects

A few asthmatics suffer anaphylaxis (see p. 111) from this drug, or
other reactions of an allergic nature, such as itchiness, nettle rash
(urticaria) or swelling and water-retention (angioedema).

Very rarely, some people taking this drug in addition to several
other asthma drugs have suffered a condition called systemic eosi-
nophilia, in which there is inflammation of the blood vessels, similar
to a disorder called Churg-Strauss syndrome. The symptoms may

include a rash, a flu-like illness, worsening asthma, and numbness or tingling in the limbs. This reaction may not be due to montelukast itself.

Zileuton

Minor side-effects
Indigestion

More serious side-effects
Liver damage can occur in a minority of patients.
Prevention:
- Asthmatics with active liver disease should not take this drug.
- All patients should be monitored regularly: once a month at the outset, then every two to three months. Don't miss these appointments.

Because this is a new drug, you should report any side-effects promptly – see above.

Other anti-inflammatory drugs
For more on these drugs see p. 341.

Methotrexate, gold salts and cyclosporin
These can have quite serious side-effects (which your consultant will probably describe to you before prescribing these drugs) but fairly small doses are all that are needed to control asthma. The small-scale trials carried out so far suggest that they do not cause any very severe reactions in asthmatics, and if they allow the dose of steroid tablets to be reduced, the overall effect should be beneficial.

Short-acting and long-acting B-2 relievers
There is some controversy surrounding the long-term effects of these drugs, which is discussed on pp. 322–6. For general information on these drugs see p. 342. New and chemically purer forms of these drugs (e.g. levalbuterol, brand-name Xopenex) are now being introduced, which have fewer side-effects. At present, these are only available for nebulizer treatment.

Inhaled B-2 relievers

Minor side-effects
Headache, nervousness, shakiness, trembling hands, flushing, dry
mouth, anxiety or restlessness, muscle cramps. These usually wear
off within a short time. Trembling hands may be a problem for those
doing manual work that demands great precision. Children may
become more excitable and restless.
  Prevention:
  • If tremor of the hands is a problem, an anti-cholinergic drug
    (see p. 345) may be a better option.

Nausea: Some long-acting B-2 relievers may cause nausea and vomiting.

More serious side-effects
Heart rhythm: A pounding heart is usually a relatively minor side-
effect, but it can be more serious and should be discussed with your
doctor.

Wheezing: A minority of people find that their airways tighten up
when these drugs are inhaled, rather than dilating (this is called
'paradoxical bronchoconstriction'). Some people have allergic reactions to the drugs.
  Prevention:
  • If your airways tighten up after inhaling these drugs, stop using
    them immediately and see your doctor as soon as you can.

Mental effects: Very, very rarely, these drugs cause hallucinations,
usually in children or the elderly. Seizures (fits) have also been
reported occasionally.

Rashes, including nettle-rash (urticaria), are another extremely rare
side-effect.

Special note on eformeterol (Foradil):
Rashes and itchiness are slightly more common with eformeterol
(Foradil) than with the other drugs in this group. It can also irritate the
mouth and eyes, cause swelling of the eyelids, nausea, insomnia and

taste disturbances. This drug should not be used during pregnancy or breast-feeding.

Potentially dangerous side-effects
An irregular heartbeat may be a sign of a dangerous side-effect (loss of potassium from the blood), although it can also be a harmless minor side-effect. Low potassium is only likely to occur in those taking large doses of these drugs, or taking other drugs, mainly steroids, theophylline-type drugs, digoxin (for heart problems) and/or diuretics (for water retention). Consult your doctor promptly if irregular heartbeat ('palpitations') occur.

Prevention:
- If you buy over-the-counter diuretics, tell the pharmacist that you are also taking a B-2 reliever, and ask which types of diuretic are safe.
- If you have a thyroid condition, high blood pressure or a heart problem, make sure the doctor remembers this when prescribing these drugs.
- Finally, over-use of short-acting B-2 relievers increases the risk of a serious, and possibly fatal, asthma attack (see pp. 322–3). This is not a 'side-effect' in the conventional sense of the word, but it is a cause for serious concern, and something that every asthma sufferer should be aware of.

B-2 relievers in tablet or syrup form
All the side-effects listed above may occur when these drugs are taken as tablets or syrup. *They are more likely to occur, and to be severe, because a larger dose is needed (see p. 344).*

Parenteral B-2 relievers
When B-2 relievers are infused directly into the bloodstream, or under the skin (both are described as 'parenteral bronchodilators'), for the treatment of severe asthma, high doses are used. The side-effects will be similar to those listed above, but are likely to be more severe than with inhaled relievers.

Anti-cholinergics
These are another type of reliever drug, with fewer side-effects than B-2 relievers. There is general information on these drugs on p. 345.

Minor side-effects

Dry mouth, blurred vision, constipation, irritation of the mouth and throat. More rarely, nausea or difficulty in passing urine.

Potentially dangerous side-effects

These are rare. An increase in the stickiness of the sputum coughed up by children is a cause for concern. If there is an increase in wheezing or coughing, stop taking the drug.

If you already have glaucoma or prostate problems you should be monitored carefully by your doctor.

Like short-acting B-2 relievers, these drugs should be taken when needed, not regularly several times a day. If used regularly, they can make the airways more sensitive, just as short-acting B-2 relievers can (see pp. 322–3).

When these drugs are used in a nebulizer, it is vital that the mask fits well (see p. 387). Contact with the eyes can cause glaucoma.

Theophylline-type drugs

For more on these drugs see p. 346. They can have quite serious side-effects at higher doses, and should be treated with respect.

Minor side-effects

None are minor – any side-effect of these drugs should be taken seriously and reported to your doctor.

More serious side-effects

Nausea, anxiety and heart problems: Nausea, stomach pains, vomiting, diarrhoea (often bloody), headache, insomnia, anxiety, restlessness, dizziness, pounding heart or irregular heartbeat.
   Prevention:
   • See your doctor as soon as possible. If you cannot get an appointment within the next few days, it may be advisable to stop taking the drug before seeing the doctor, as long as you have other asthma drugs to control your symptoms. Telephone the doctor for advice on this.

Pregnancy: Although the drug does not affect the vast majority of unborn or newborn babies, there are occasional reports of toxicity.
   Prevention:
   • While pregnant or breast-feeding, it may be advisable to stop

taking theophylline: this is something to discuss with your doctor.

Behaviour and learning problems: The theophylline-type drugs may produce behavioural problems and learning difficulties in young children but seem to be safe for children over six.

Potentially dangerous side-effects
Shaking, vomiting, thirst, irregular heartbeat, etc.: Unfortunately, it is all too easy to overdose with these drugs (see p. 346) and such overdoses can be fatal. The warning signs are: shaking, repeated vomiting, excessive urination, severe thirst, feeling unusually hot, maniacal behaviour and irregular heartbeat (palpitations). Delirium and convulsions may follow. Hospital treatment is needed *urgently* in these circumstances.

A serious overdose can sometimes occur as a result of long-term therapy, without the prior appearance of milder side-effects to warn that anything is wrong. Regular blood tests protect against this possibility.

Prevention:
- There are now slow-release forms of theophylline, which last up to 12 hours and are useful for nocturnal asthma. There are fewer side-effects than with the ordinary forms of the drug.
- Avoid fatty or oily meals. Eating a lot of fatty food has a bad effect on these slow-release drugs, causing too much of the drug to be released at once. This increases the risk of side-effects.
- Check if your dose of theophylline needs changing:
  o whenever you start taking a new drug of any kind
  o if you change your consumption of nicotine or alcohol
  o if you stop taking the contraceptive Pill
  o if you develop certain illnesses (see p. 347 for details). See the doctor *promptly* if you have a viral infection as this can increase the level of theophylline in the blood
- Many drugs interact with theophylline, and you should always check, but there is a particular problem with the antibiotics ciprofloxacin (Ciproxin) and erythromycin, and with cimetidine, used to treat stomach ulcers and heartburn. (The last two drugs are sold under various brand-names – check with a pharmacist.)

- Wear a Medic-Alert bracelet (see p. 459) saying that you are taking theophylline. If you have a severe asthma attack and are taken to hospital, it is important that medical staff know this, so that they do not give you more drugs of this type.

Older types of reliever drug

These drugs are listed on pp. 372–3. They no longer have any place in asthma treatment: much better and safer drugs are now available. Ask your doctor to prescribe something different.

Minor side-effects
Headache, anxiety, restlessness, insomnia and dizziness.

Major side-effects
Urination: Difficulty in passing urine.

Potentially dangerous side-effects
Heart problems: Pain in the chest, irregular heartbeat ('palpitations').

Side-effects from other substances used in inhalers
Aerosol inhalers
Some aerosol inhalers contain as many as five other ingredients besides the drug itself: they are known as propellants and surfactants and they are there to keep the drug thoroughly dispersed in the liquid, and to make sure it shoots out of the canister in an even spray. Some asthmatics are sensitive to one of these added substances, and they either cough or get tight airways when they inhale them. Estimates of the numbers of asthmatics affected range from 1–2 per cent to a staggering 33 per cent.

In addition, aerosol inhalers once contained CFCs, which are very inert gases (at ground level) and perfectly safe to inhale. However they cause serious damage in the ozone layer high above the earth. They are being phased out in asthma inhalers, as in all aerosols. New propellants, such as hydrofluoroalkanes (HFAs) are being introduced instead. They are thought to be very safe, but may cause reactions in a tiny minority of people: this is one of those problems that will only show up when very large numbers of people are using them. Tell your doctor if your reaction to your usual inhaler seems to change suddenly.

Dry-powder inhalers

Dry-powder inhalers do not contain propellants or surfactants, so they are suitable for anyone sensitive to these. But they may contain lactose, a sugar, in addition to the drug. Enough lactose is deposited in the mouth and swallowed to provoke symptoms in some patients who are lactose intolerant. They usually suffer from diarrhoea, bloating and wind as a result.

You would probably know already if you were lactose intolerant: the main sign is suffering from violent diarrhoea and wind if you drink milk or, in severe cases, if you eat any milk product.

Note that many people who cannot tolerate milk are not lactose intolerant – they are sensitive to something else in the milk, usually milk proteins. A few ultra-sensitive individuals might react to traces of milk protein that are found in lactose, but such a reaction would be extremely rare.

'Each time he has made me go on taking it for a month'

Sarah Morrison is in her late fifties, and has had severe asthma since her childhood. She suffers from a rare reaction to inhaled steroids called paradoxical bronchoconstriction. 'Each of the three inhaled steroids that I've tried have pushed my peak flow reading down to about 60 overnight. And each time the GP has said "Well, I can't send you back to the specialist straight away" and he has made me go on taking it for a month, just to see that it really was having this effect. After a month of that I'm really bad.

'The last time I was given a steroid inhaler and this happened, the specialist then wanted me to go on to steroid tablets as well, because my asthma had deteriorated so much. I said to him "Look – just take me off the inhaled steroids. This is what happened the last time I took them." So he took me off them, and it did improve as soon as I stopped taking them.'

As Sarah's case shows, it pays to be well-informed about your drugs and to take careful notice of what happens when you take them. Don't be intimidated by doctors – be prepared to calmly tell them what you think. You have a right to discuss your treatment with them and to take an active role in decisions.

IDENTIFY YOUR DRUGS

This section will help you to identify your own inhaler, tablets or syrup, and discover what *type* of drug it is so that you can relate the information about different types of asthma drugs (see pp. 334–69) to the brands you actually take. You may want to fill in the blank sections on p. 334 with the names of your own drugs.

New brands are introduced all the time, and if your brand came on the market after this book was published, the **brand-name** (names shown with a capital letter, such as Aerobec or Becotide) won't appear here. Brand names can also vary in different countries, and American readers might not recognize some brand names. The chances are, however, that the drug itself is not new or different – just the brand name. So look for the **generic name** of your drug: this should be given in small letters somewhere on the package or the leaflet that comes with the drug. These names are shown without a capital letter here (e.g. salbutamol, beclomethasone) but they may appear differently on the drug package. Then look for the generic name in the lists below. This will tell you what type of drug it is.

Entirely new drugs with new generic names are also introduced from time to time, so you still may not be able to identify a drug from these lists. In that case, ask your pharmacist, doctor or asthma nurse which group your drug belongs to. Note that they may use different names for the drug categories – see p. 335 for what these mean.

In Britain, most reliever drugs are packaged in blue inhalers, to avoid confusion with other kinds of inhaled drugs. Steroids, the most widely used type of preventer, are usually packaged in a brown inhaler.

Inhaled drugs
Preventers
Steroids (see p. 336)

BRAND-NAME	GENERIC NAME OF DRUG
AeroBec	beclomethasone
Aerobid	flunisolide
Asmabec	beclomethasone
Azmacort	triamcinolone
Beclazone Easi-Breathe	beclomethasone
Becloforte	beclomethasone
Beclovent	beclomethasone

Becodisks	beclomethasone
Becotide	beclomethasone
Dalalone	dexamethasone
Decadron	dexamethasone
Filair	beclomethasone
Flixotide	fluticasone
Flovent	fluticasone
Hexadrol	dexamethasone
Decadron	dexamethasone
Pulmicort	budesonide
Qvar	beclomethasone
Vanceril	beclomethasone

Cromoglycate-type drugs (see p. 338)

Cromogen	sodium cromoglycate
Intal	sodium cromoglycate
Tilade	nedocromil sodium

Relievers (bronchodilators)

Short-acting B-2 relievers (see p. 342)

One of these drugs has two different generic names: it is called either salbutamol or albuterol.

Aerolin-Auto	salbutamol
Airomir	salbutamol
Asmasal	salbutamol in Britain, albuterol in the USA
Asmaven	salbutamol
Berotec	fenoterol
Brelomax	tulobuterol
Brethaire	terbutaline
Brethine	terbutaline
Bricanyl	terbutaline
Bronchodil	reproterol
Exirel	pirbuterol
Maxair	pirbuterol
Maxivent	salbutamol
Monovent	terbutaline
Proventil	albuterol

Pulmadil	rimiterol
Respacal	tulobuterol
Rimasal	salbutamol
Salamol Easi-Breathe	salbutamol
Salbulin	salbutamol
Salbuvent	salbutamol
Steri-Neb Salamol	salbutamol
Tornalate	bitolerol
Ventodisks	salbutamol
Ventolin	salbutamol in Britain, albuterol in the USA
Xopenex	levalbuterol

Long-acting B-2 relievers (see p. 344)

Bambec	bambuterol
Foradil	eformeterol
Oxis	eformeterol
Serevent	salmeterol

Anti-cholinergics (see p. 345)

Atrovent	ipratropium
Ipratropium	ipratropium
Oxivent	oxitropium
Respontin	ipratropium
Steri-Neb	ipratropium
–	butethamate
–	atropine

Note that in some countries, but not in Britain, Atrovent also contains a short-acting B-2 reliever.

Older types of reliever drug (see p. 347)

Alupent	orciprenaline
CAM	ephedrine
Ephedrine	ephedrine
Fedrine	ephedrine
Isoproterenol	isoprenaline
Isuprel	isoprenaline
Medihaler-Iso	isoprenaline

Metaprel	orciprenaline
Metaproterenol	orciprenaline
Neo-respin	ephedrine
Numotac	isoetharine
Promeva	orciprenaline
–	phenylephrine

Adrenaline/Epinephrine Inhalers (see p. 347)

This drug has two different generic names: It is commonly called adrenaline in Britain, but epinephrine in the USA.

AsthmaHaler Mist	adrenaline/epinephrine
Bronkaid	adrenaline
Epiphrine	adrenaline
Medihaler-Epi	adrenaline (withdrawn from market, see p. 347)
Primatene Mist	adrenaline

Drugs in tablet or syrup form
Preventers
Steroid tablets: 'oral steroids' (see p. 337)

Azmacort	triamcinolone
Deltacortril Enteric	prednisolone
Deltasone	prednisolone
Deltastab	prednisolone
Hydeltrasole	prednisolone
Kenacort	triamcinolone
Kenalog	triamcinolone
Ledercort	triamcinolone
Precortisyl	prednisolone
Prednalone	prednisolone
Prednesol	prednisolone (soluble form)
Prednisolone	prednisolone
Sintisone	prednisolone

These are the most commonly prescribed steroid tablets. However, there are many other steroid drugs, and many brand-names: far too many to list them all here. If you have been given tablets that are not listed here, and you are not sure what they are, ask your pharmacist, doctor or asthma nurse.

Anti-histamines (see p. 339)
Zaditen   ketotifen

Leukotriene antagonists (see p. 340)
Accolate   zafirlukast
Leutrol   zileuton
Singulair   montelukast
Zyflo   zileuton

Relievers (bronchodilators)
B-2 relievers in tablets or syrup (see p. 344)
Asmaven   salbutamol
Bricanyl   terbutaline
Bronchodil   reproterol
Exirel   pirbuterol
Monovent   terbutaline
Salbulin   salbutamol
Salbutamol   salbutamol
Salbuvent   salbutamol
Ventmax   salbutamol
Ventolin   salbutamol in Britain,
                                 albuterol in the USA
Volmax   salbutamol in Britain,
                                 albuterol in the USA

Theophylline-type drugs (see p. 346)
Biophyline   theophylline
Bronchodyl   theophylline
Brondekon   choline theophyllinate
Choledyl   choline theophyllinate
Elixophyllin   theophylline
Labophylline   theophylline
Lasma   theophylline
Nuelin   theophylline
Pecram   aminophylline
Phyllocontin Continus   aminophylline
Pro-Vent   theophylline
Sabidal   choline theophyllinate
Slo-Bid   theophylline

Slo-Phyllin	theophylline
Theo-Dur	theophylline
Uni-dur	theophylline
Uni-phy	theophylline
Uniphyllin Continus	theophylline

Adrenaline/Epinephrine injections (see p. 348)

This drug has two different generic names: it is commonly called adrenaline in Britain, but epinephrine in the USA.

Anapen	adrenaline/epinephrine
Ana Guard	adrenaline/epinephrine
Anahelp	adrenaline/epinephrine
Epi-pen and Epipen Junior	adrenaline/epinephrine
Epi E-Z Pen	adrenaline/epinephrine
Mini-I-Jet	adrenaline/epinephrine

Mixtures of drugs
Older mixtures (see p. 348)

Bronchilator	isoetharine + phenylephrine
CAM	butethamate + ephedrine
Combivent	ipratropium + salbutamol
Duovent	ipratropium + fenoterol
Franol	theophylline + ephedrine
Medihaler-Duo	isoprenaline + phenylephrine
Tedral	theophylline + ephedrine
Ventide	salbutamol + beclomethasone

Generally speaking, these older mixtures are no longer recommended for asthma treatment, though there are exceptions (see p. 348).

Newer mixtures (see p. 348)

| Aerocrom Syncroner | cromoglycate + salbutamol |
| Seretide | fluticasone + salmeterol |

HOW TO USE INHALERS, SPACERS AND NEBULIZERS

'Inhaler' is a general name for any small, portable device that delivers anti-asthma drugs directly to the lungs. It includes the old-fashioned 'puffers' or aerosol inhalers (correctly called pressurized metered-dose inhalers or MDIs), as well as the many new devices that deliver drugs in dry-powder form.

A spacer is a large empty chamber that can be fitted to an aerosol inhaler, to make it more effective and easier to use.

A nebulizer is a much larger piece of equipment that delivers high doses of inhaled drugs in an easily inhaled form. It is generally used for severe asthma only, or in an emergency to relieve asthma attacks.

Inhalers
Why use an inhaler instead of taking tablets or syrup?
An inhaler is to the lungs what ointment is to the skin: it gets the drug to the place where it's needed quickly and efficiently. The major advantage is that a far smaller dose is required, because the drug is not travelling all the way around the body in the blood, before reaching the lungs. The smaller dose means far fewer side-effects.

Inhaler technique: doing it well
Everyone given an inhaler should be shown how to use it by a doctor or asthma nurse. There is no substitute for this.

Many studies have shown that a high proportion of asthma patients are using their inhalers incorrectly. This usually results in them getting too little of the drug. Unfortunately, this can lead to their asthma getting out of control.

In many cases of unsuccessful treatment, only the inhaler is a problem, not the choice of drugs.

It may be possible to improve your inhaler technique with help from a doctor or asthma nurse, or you could switch to a different kind of inhaler. A great many people find one type of inhaler difficult (particularly the aerosol inhalers or 'puffers'), but do well with another type. If you are not succeeding with your inhaler, ask the doctor if a different one can be prescribed. There should be several different inhalers available for you to try out, to see which one suits you best.

Arthritis and inhalers

Patients who have arthritis in their hands often find inhalers difficult to use. There are several aids now available to help with this problem, including the Haleraid (for Becotide and Ventolin inhalers – available on prescription from a pharmacy), and the Turbohaler arthritis aid (available free from Astra Pharmaceuticals if requested by your doctor).

The different types of inhaler

The advice for using inhalers given here is intended only as a guide, and there is no substitute for having your doctor or asthma nurse check your technique.

Whatever type of inhaler you have, be sure to read the instruction leaflet that comes with the inhaler: it is an excellent source of information.

Aerosol inhaler

The oldest type of inhaler, often called a 'puffer'. It is a miniature aerosol canister which produces the drug in a fine liquid spray. (Also called a pressurized metered-dose inhaler, a metered-dose inhaler or an MDI)

Practical tips:

- It is vital to shake the inhaler well or you will not get the right dose.
- You must get the in-breath coordinated precisely with pressing the canister down: this is the part that many people find difficult.
- You must breathe in slowly and deeply, otherwise you do not get much of the drug into your airways.
- When your lungs are full, hold your breath for at least ten seconds.
- Try to wait at least another 30 seconds before breathing in again.
- Get the asthma nurse to check your technique every time you visit the asthma clinic, to make sure you have not got into bad habits.

Problems with this type of inhaler:
- Many people automatically stop inhaling when the cloud of cold droplets hits the back of the throat. (As well as the drug, these droplets contain the liquid propellant, which is what makes them so cold.) This is a reflex response to cold liquid that may be impossible to control. If so, you need a dry-powder inhaler (see below), or a spacer (see p. 380) to use with your aerosol inhaler.
- With steroids, other types of inhaler may be better for getting more of the drug into the lungs and for avoiding side-effects (see p. 353).
- It is difficult to tell when these inhalers are running empty. The answer is to place them in a bowl of water: if they sink they're full, if they float horizontally they're nearly empty. If they float vertically, nozzle downwards, they're half full. You could, alternatively, use a dose-counter that attaches to the inhaler (see p. 469). Always order a new inhaler in good time, well before the old one runs out. Some asthmatic keep a spare inhaler to ensure they are never without their asthma drugs.
- When almost empty, aerosol inhalers produce propellant only – no drug – so they are not effective *even though they still 'puff' as usual.*

Breath-operated aerosol inhalers
These are an improved form of the traditional aerosol inhaler. The best-known device is called an Autohaler.

With these devices, you do not have to push the canister down because your in-breath automatically triggers the release of the drug. They can be useful for those who find ordinary aerosol inhalers too tricky.

Practical tips:
- Be careful not to block the air-intake holes with your hands.
- Don't stop breathing when you hear the inhaler click.
- If there is no click, you have not breathed in with enough force to activate the device, and no drug has been inhaled.
- When your lungs are full, hold your breath for at least ten seconds.

Problems with this type of inhaler:
- As with ordinary aerosol inhalers, it is difficult to tell when these are running out (see above).

Dry-powder inhalers
These include the Spinhaler, Rotohaler, Diskhaler, Accuhaler, Click-haler and Turbohaler. They release a measured dose of the drug, in powder form, for you to inhale.

Because there is no aerosol device in these, nothing pushes the drug into your mouth and lungs: you have to do the work yourself. This means you have to breathe in quite hard and fast to get the powder into your lungs.

Each type of dry-powder inhaler is different in design and the way you use it. If one does not suit you, another may be better, so ask to try different brands. The Diskhaler is generally thought to be the most successful device.

If you are the parent of an asthmatic, and would like to keep an eye on how much of each drug your child is using, most of the dry-powder inhalers (except the Turbohaler) allow you to do so. Ask your asthma nurse or doctor to show you the different inhalers available.

Practical tips:
- Breathe in as hard and fast as you can to get the powder into your airways.
- When your lungs are full, hold your breath for at least ten seconds.
- Never let the inhaler get damp. With the exception of the Diskhaler, they are all damaged by moisture.

Problems with this type of inhaler:
- During a severe asthma attack you may not be able to breathe in hard enough to get a good dose of the drug. If you have experienced this problem, or are concerned about it, talk to your doctor or asthma nurse. It may be possible to have an aerosol inhaler, perhaps combined with a spacer, for use during severe attacks.

Special points about the Turbohaler:
- The advantage of this inhaler is that it already contains the

drug (200 doses) so you do not have to put in capsules or blister packs of the drug.

- It is impossible to tell how many doses have been taken or how full the inhaler is. And with each individual dose, there is no way to tell if the full dose has been taken. This is not the case with the other dry-powder inhalers.
- The Turbohaler is particularly sensitive to moisture: never breathe out with the mouthpiece still in your mouth.
- Children under six may not be able to breathe in hard enough to make the Turbohaler work.
- Always hold the Turbohaler vertically when twisting the device before inhaling: it will not load properly if clicked when not vertical.

Questions that are often asked about inhalers

'Are there other ingredients in the inhalers, and what effect do they have?'

Yes, there are other ingredients, particularly in the aerosol inhalers. Some of these can cause side-effects (see pp. 368–9).

'What happens to all this powder I'm inhaling – does it just accumulate in my lungs?'

No. The particles other than the drug itself are relatively large in size, so they do not travel right down into the lungs. They are deposited in the upper part of the airway and coughed up soon afterwards. The drug does go down into the lungs, but it dissolves in the film of liquid that covers the inside of the airways. The lungs are well equipped to clear out any deposits in the airways, bringing them up by means of mucus, which also traps natural particles such as dust and pollen.

Spacers

A spacer is just a large empty chamber with a hole at either end. It can be used with any aerosol inhaler ('puffer'). The aerosol sprays the drug into one end of the spacer, and you breathe in from the other end. There is a valve at the end where you breathe in.

Spacers are useful because they allow the aerosol propellant (see p. 378) to evaporate, leaving tiny droplets of the drug to be inhaled. It is the cold droplets of propellant that cause most difficulties for people using aerosol inhalers.

Note that spacers are for aerosol inhalers only. Neither a real spacer device, nor an improvised emergency spacer, will be of any use with a dry-powder inhaler.

Spacers are particularly useful:
- for babies and small children, who cannot yet coordinate the in-breath with pushing the aerosol canister down.
- in an asthma attack, because you can still get some of the drug into your airways even if you are unable to take a deep breath.
- for taking steroids, since they get more of the drug into your lungs and leave less in your mouth. This increases the benefits of the drug, and decreases side-effects.

There are several brands of spacer, including the Volumatic, the Nebuhaler, the Fisonair, and the Aerochamber, which is smaller than the others. Most of the spacers only fit on to particular brands of inhaler: check with your pharmacist before buying one.

For babies and toddlers, there is the Babyhaler or special forms of the Aerochamber, Nebuhaler or Volumatic. All these have masks that fit over the nose and mouth, as it is too difficult for children under two years to use a mouthpiece.

Some inhalers now have a small built-in spacer, such as the Becloforte Integra and the Beclazone Easi-Breathe, a breath-activated inhaler.

There is also a collapsible spacer, made in the USA, called the E-Z Spacer (see p. 469). It folds up into a plastic case small enough to be slipped into a pocket. In a severe asthma attack, having such a spacer with you could be a life-saver.

Practical tips:
- Remember to shake the inhaler before spraying into the spacer.
- Puff the inhaler into the spacer once only. Breathe in within five seconds of spraying the inhaler. During an asthma attack, you can keep adding another dose from the inhaler every ten seconds, until the attack begins to subside (see p. 51).
- With a spacer, if you are short of breath, you can just breathe normally: you don't have to take all the drug in at once, or hold your breath after you've inhaled, if this is too difficult. (But you should still try to breathe in fairly deeply to get the

drug deep into your airways, and should try to hold your breath for up to ten seconds.)

- Use a large-volume spacer for taking steroid inhalers, to get the maximum benefit.

Practical tips for babies and children:
- For young children, the following routine is recommended:
  - Take the cap off the inhaler, shake it well, and fit it to the spacer.
  - Put the mouthpiece into the child's mouth, or put the mask on.
  - Get the child to breathe in and out steadily and listen for the valve clicking as it opens and shuts.
  - When the breathing is regular, squirt a single dose of medicine from the inhaler into the spacer.
  - Make sure the child breathes in and out five to eight times before taking the spacer away.
- If using the Nebuhaler or Volumatic with a mask for a baby or toddler, hold it tilted upwards, with the inhaler higher than the mouthpiece. This ensures that the valve stays open.
- A spacer can be used on a baby while it is asleep, which may be easier if the baby gets distressed by the spacer.
- If you need to use the spacer while the baby or toddler is awake, stroke its cheek with the mask first to get it used to the feel. Make sure that the child feels secure – keep smiling and talking so that the situation doesn't seem so frightening. If the baby does start to cry, keep the mask in place. Both during and after crying it will breathe in sharply and so get a good dose of the drug.
- For an older child, coloured stickers can be added to the spacer, making it more like a toy. It may help to let the child pretend it is a trumpet (blowing into the mouthpiece will not harm it). Let the child play with it so that it becomes a familiar object, not something frightening that only appears during asthma attacks.

Problems with spacers

Some types of plastic spacer (those made of polycarbonate) have an electrostatic charge: the same sort of force that makes some clothes crackle when you take them off, or makes a scrap of paper stick to a TV screen. Unfortunately, this electrostatic charge causes the drug to stick to the inside of the spacer. You won't be able to see the drug as it forms a very thin coating.

This is generally not a problem for anyone aged over four years. The drug does not stick to the plastic immediately, and it takes nine seconds for the dose of drug in the chamber to be halved, which is plenty of time for most adults and older children to inhale the drug. In any case, once you have used the spacer 10–20 times, there will probably be enough drug stuck to the spacer walls to prevent any more sticking.

For children under four, who take more time to inhale the drug from the spacer, steps must be taken to overcome the electrostatic problem. Fire the inhaler into the new spacer about five times in succession and just allow the drug to settle on the spacer walls. This should coat the plastic thoroughly with the drug so that when you come to use it, there is no problem. If you wash the spacer, the drug is removed, and you are back to square one, so repeat this treatment on a newly washed spacer. Making spacers from metal would be another answer, but these are not available at present.

Making a spacer in an emergency

During a severe asthma attack, when it is difficult to inhale deeply, it often helps to use a spacer to inhale reliever drugs, rather than inhaling them directly from an aerosol inhaler. More of the drug can get to the airways this way.

A plastic cup can be converted into a spacer, for use with an aerosol inhaler, as shown on p. 384.

Use a thin-walled smooth plastic cup. Do not use a polystyrene cup (the kind with thick sides and a rough surface) as this carries an electrostatic charge (see above).

A paper bag can also be used in an emergency. Cut a small hole in the bottom, and fit it tightly around the inhaler mouthpiece. Bunch up the open end of the paper bag around your mouth, fire the inhaler, and breathe in.

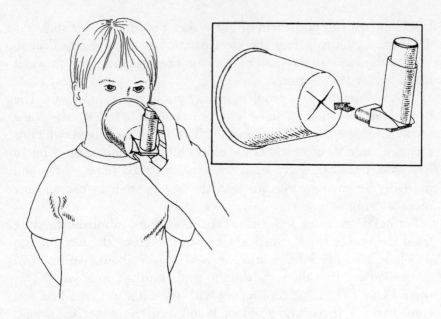

Nebulizers

A nebulizer is a machine that turns a liquid drug into a very fine mist that can be breathed in through a mask or mouthpiece. It delivers a much larger dose of the drug than an inhaler does.

Nebulizers can be attached to an oxygen cylinder, which enriches the air/drug mixture with oxygen. This is useful in severe asthma, when oxygen levels in the blood can get very low.

Nebulizers are useful:

- in an emergency involving a severe asthma attack, when large doses of B-2 reliever drugs are needed. If you go to a hospital or GP's clinic with such an attack, you will be given drugs from a nebulizer. Only those people whose asthma can deteriorate very suddenly and sharply need to keep a nebulizer at home for emergencies.
- on a daily basis, for a very small minority of asthmatics with brittle asthma, who need large doses of their drugs.
- on a daily basis, for some very small children with severe asthma, because it is the easiest way for them to take their drugs.
- on a daily basis, for some elderly people with severe asthma who have difficulty in using inhalers.

Getting your own nebulizer

Because nebulizers are so effective in an emergency, some people see them as 'magic machines' which can cure asthma, and think that owning a nebulizer would be the answer to all their problems. This is a mistake: the nebulizer only works so well because it delivers a much higher dose of the reliever drug. This higher dose also carries a higher risk of side-effects, and you would not want to use such high doses on a regular basis – they are for emergencies only. No one should buy a nebulizer unless the doctor has advised them to do so.

In most countries, if you are advised by the doctor to keep a nebulizer at home you will have to buy one. In Britain, if you need a nebulizer you should not have to pay for it yourself: ideally the National Health Service should be able to provide one, but the process is not necessarily straightforward, and it depends where you live.

These are the options:
- If you need a nebulizer occasionally for emergencies, your GP practice may be able to lend you one. For those who need a nebulizer constantly, it may be possible to borrow one from your hospital clinic or local health authority on a long-term basis.
- Nebulizers can be prescribed on the NHS by hospital consultants, but not by GPs.
- Some people, unfortunately, do have to pay for a nebulizer themselves but they may be able to get some financial help: ask the Citizens' Advice Bureau what help is available locally.
- Whatever you do, don't pay VAT on your nebulizer: ask your doctor for a letter to send with your order form, claiming exemption from VAT.

Choosing a nebulizer

Obviously you should ask the advice of your doctor or consultant about choosing a nebulizer. But it may be helpful to have some information in advance about the different kinds available:
- Ultrasonic nebulizers make the liquid drug into a mist by bombarding it with ultrasound. They are quieter than others, and the battery-operated ones are small enough to be carried around. The mist they produce is not quite as good as that from a jet nebulizer.

- Jet nebulizers produce a mist by pumping air or oxygen through the liquid drug. They are noisier but may be cheaper.

When it comes to buying a nebulizer, these are the choices you will have to make:

- Ultrasonic or jet nebulizer? The ultrasonic neubulizers are particularly good for elderly people because they are quieter and because the production of the mist is only triggered with breathing in. This allows the asthmatic to have a rest without switching off the machine and without wasting any of the drug. However, these machines are not particularly good for small children taking regular doses of asthma drugs. A battery-operated ultrasonic nebulizer gives you more mobility because you can use it anywhere.
- If you have decided on a jet nebulizer: should you choose an electric pump or foot pump? Most jet nebulizers have an electric pump but some are available with a foot pump, or even a hand pump. These are much cheaper, but it is essential for somebody fairly energetic to be present whenever the nebulizer is needed, to operate the pump.
- Do you ever need a nebulizer when travelling in the car? If you do, there are some which can run off a car battery, by plugging into the cigarette lighter on the dashboard.
- Do you travel abroad often? If buying a plug-in nebulizer, check that it can adapt to a different voltage easily.

Using a nebulizer wisely
If you have a nebulizer you should also have detailed written in-structions from your doctor about when and how to use it. In particular, make sure that you know:

- how to set up the nebulizer and pump.
- how to keep it clean.
- how to add the drug and how much to use.
- if the nebulizer is for emergency use: what should prompt you to use it.
- if you have begun using the nebulizer for an emergency, the signs which suggest you are losing the battle, and should call the doctor or go to the hospital now. (Generally speaking, if the reliever drug given by nebulizer is not working quickly, or

if another dose is needed in less than three hours, this is a sign
that you should seek medical help.)

- after you have used the nebulizer for an emergency, and the
  crisis has passed, what your next steps should be.

Practical tips:
- Nebulizers need servicing regularly, usually every three
  months. This can create enormous difficulties since the servicing usually takes about ten days, and few people can afford to
  have a second nebulizer to cover this period. Help is now at
  hand. One of the drug companies offers while-you-wait
  servicing at asthma clinics. There is no catch and no cost,
  and you don't even have to be using one of the drugs that this
  company makes. Your asthma nurse or doctor should know all
  about this scheme. (If you are wondering why the drug
  company should do this for nothing, they are hoping to create
  'goodwill', and it also gives their representative an extra
  chance to call in and mention his latest products to the asthma
  nurse!)

Problems with nebulizers:
- Owning a nebulizer may give you a false sense of security
  during emergencies, and delay you from getting expert medical help when you need it. Never put off ringing the doctor or
  going to the hospital if an asthma attack is getting worse.
- Be careful, when using a nebulizer, not to allow the mist to
  escape around the face, and especially the eyes. Repeated
  exposure to steroid mist can cause cataracts in the eyes, and
  thinning of the skin. Anti-cholinergics (Atrovent, etc.) can
  cause glaucoma if they go directly into the eye. Placing a soft
  scarf around the upper edge of the mask to block any gaps will
  help reduce this problem. Washing the face after using the
  nebulizer is also a good idea.

DECISIONS ABOUT DRUGS:
WHAT TO TAKE, HOW MUCH AND WHEN

This section deals with two different topics:
- the decisions that your doctor makes in the surgery or clinic
- the decisions you make at home, on a day-to-day basis – decisions about which drugs to take and when to take them

Both sets of decisions should involve you fully. For the best possible outcome, you should participate in the decisions the doctor makes in the surgery, as well as making thoughtful, considered choices about your drugs on a day-to-day basis.

Many asthma patients don't do this. Instead, they accept what the doctor prescribes without any discussion, but then don't take the drugs as often as they should, or stop taking them altogether, or halve the dose, or chop and change in a haphazard way because they are not really sure what they feel about taking the drugs. For some, this leads to worsening asthma, with potentially dangerous consequences. For many it produces a very poor quality of life, with unmanageable symptoms and constant interference with everyday activities.

It would be much better for everyone concerned if patients were more outspoken in the surgery, voiced their misgivings about drugs, discussed the pros and cons with the doctor or asthma nurse, and then agreed to a treatment regime that they were prepared to stick to. (This might be a totally drug-based treatment, or one that combines drugs with other treatments, or one that is drug-free.) You should find that your doctor is happy to discuss the issues with you and to treat you as an intelligent partner in your own treatment: with asthma this is *essential*, and most doctors now recognize this fact. If you are unlucky enough to have the old-fashioned type of doctor who wishes to be obeyed without question, consider changing to one of the younger GPs in the practice, or going to another practice altogether.

To be able to agree on a treatment plan, you may first need to sort out your conflicting feelings about drugs (and, possibly, about what it means to have asthma in the first place). Often people are unwilling to accept that they have asthma, and this makes them 'forget' to carry their inhaler, or to use it regularly. Reading pp. 319–32 may help in sorting out your feelings about the drugs, and pp. 306–14 could be useful if you are not totally convinced you have asthma.

Stepping up and stepping down

For the past 25 years or so, the standard approach to asthma treatment has been to start patients on a simple reliever treatment (usually a short-acting B-2 reliever) and then add other drugs if there are still troublesome symptoms ('stepping up'). The standard steps are as follows (if the terms for drugs used here are unfamiliar, turn to p. 370 to relate them to the names of your drugs, and p. 334 for a description of what they do):

1. For mild symptoms: a short-acting B-2 reliever only.
2. For more troublesome symptoms: add cromoglycate or low-dose inhaled steroids.
3. If symptoms are not well controlled, try a higher dose of inhaled steroid or a long-acting B-2 reliever.
4. If symptoms are still interfering with daily life, try out each of the following in turn: theophylline, anti-cholinergic drugs, cromoglycate and higher doses of B-2 relievers (either inhaled or as tablets/syrup).
5. If there is no success in controlling symptoms, add regular steroid tablets.

Short courses of steroid tablets may be used at any stage, for the control of sudden, severe attacks.

(Note that doctors in some countries, particularly the USA and Japan, have a different strategy – see pp. 331–3).

A major change has occurred in the last ten years, as a result of the New Zealand asthma epidemic (see p. 322). The regular use of short-acting B-2 relievers is discouraged, and inhaled steroids are now given to most asthmatics, even those with mild asthma. Few people are now kept on Stage 1, unless they have symptoms only very occasionally. Experience in Sweden, where inhaled steroids are used more extensively than anywhere else, suggests that this policy works well and is much better for asthmatics in the long run (see p. 327).

Once a person's symptoms are well controlled, and have been so for three to six months, a cautious process of 'stepping down' begins. The drug doses are reduced, or certain drugs cut, to see what happens. If the symptoms remain stable, that's fine. If not, the dose goes up again.

A different basic approach is now being tried out in some countries: starting *immediately* with moderate to high doses of inhaled steroids (equivalent to Stage 3) to get the inflammation under control, and then 'stepping down'. For some patients, this may be the best strategy.

Adding a steroid inhaler to your treatment programme

Most asthmatics will now be asked to try out an inhaled steroid. It will probably be a low-dose inhaler, and the risks of side-effects from this are very small (see pp. 351–2).

If you are still worried, in spite of all our reassurances, there are various suggestions for other options listed on p. 328. But please don't delay using an inhaled steroid for too long, as this could damage your airways permanently.

Are you being over-treated or under-treated?

Some patients with asthma are being over-treated: taking drugs that they don't need. If your asthma has been stable and causing you little or no trouble for three to six months, ask your doctor about experimenting with lower doses of some of the drugs, to see if you can manage on less. You must have medical supervision for this – don't try reducing the dose without your doctor's agreement.

Many more asthmatics are being under-treated: not getting the drugs that would help them lead a more normal life. This is true of both children and adults. They may not be aware of how much they have unconsciously limited their activities to fit in with their asthma, or how much better they could feel with good treatment.

Under-treatment also means the airways are permanently inflamed, and therefore at risk of sudden severe asthma attacks which need emergency treatment in hospital, and could even be fatal.

You are being under-treated if any of the following are true:
- You cannot keep up with most other people your age when engaged in any strenuous physical activity, such as playing sport, running or walking fast.
- You are frequently breathless due to asthma, when climbing stairs or walking uphill.
- You often wake up in the night because of asthma.
- Your asthma varies a lot from one day to the next, from morning to evening, or from one week to the next.
- You have a persistent cough that is not due to a chest infection (one that does not produce green or yellow phlegm).

- You regularly need to use your reliever inhaler more than once a day (see p. 343).
- You frequently have asthma attacks that require steroid tablets to get them under control: it is much, *much* safer (in terms of fewer side-effects) to use inhaled steroids regularly (see p. 326).
- You frequently have asthma attacks that require hospital treatment.

Make sure your doctor knows about symptoms such as these to ensure that you are given the treatment you need. If you are given preventer drugs, do take them regularly and at the correct dose, and check that your inhaler technique is good (see p. 376).

Day-to-day management
You should have been given a written asthma management plan by your doctor or asthma nurse. If you have not received one of these, ask for one now. Make a photocopy, in case you lose it, and keep that in a safe place. Keep the written management plan with you at all times.

Dealing with severe attacks
Your management plan should tell you how to recognize a severe attack coming on, and what to do about it. Look also at pp. 45–7 for more details on recognizing severe asthma attacks in their early stages.

Following a management plan
Your management plan should tell you how often to take your drugs under normal circumstances, and what to do when your asthma gets worse. Make sure that the actual brand-names of your drugs (and/or the colour of the inhaler) are written on the management plan, and that everything about the plan is crystal-clear to you. Don't leave the surgery or clinic until you are absolutely sure you know how the guidelines relate to the sort of real-life situations that you actually experience – would it have helped during your last asthma attack, for example?

If you have a peak-flow meter, there should be peak-flow values filled in on your management plan, showing you the values that indicate a need to take more preventer, or call the doctor.

However good your management plan, real life is usually much

more complicated and confusing, so you may sometimes find it hard
to know what to do. Any time you find the management plan difficult
to follow, or just inappropriate to what is happening with your
asthma, write down your exact circumstances, and the reason for
your uncertainty about what should be done. Contact your doctor
immediately if your asthma is getting worse, and explain what is
happening. If things get better without needing to contact the doctor,
save your notes for the next time you attend the surgery or clinic
(don't rely on your memory) and ask what you should have done in
those circumstances. In this way you will gradually build up a valuable
detailed knowledge of how to manage your own asthma in all the
different circumstances that you come up against.

Whatever you do, never ignore asthma symptoms. Learn to recognize them before they get troublesome (see p. 49), and to take
action immediately.

'It's very much better to keep it under control.'

Susan has severe asthma, and so do two of her children. 'Generally, with all three of us, we aim to use as little Ventolin as
possible. One of the problems with asthma is that if you let it
build up, it can be quite difficult to get it under control. What
we've learnt by trial and error is that it's very much better to
keep it under control, rather than let it go out of control.
Generally speaking, once we are in the realm of using Ventolin,
it has gone out of control. That means asthma attacks in the
middle of the night, rushing to hospital sick with worry, and all
that awful business.'

12

Alternative medicine

> '. . . it is important to remember
> to treat the individual and not the label.'

Andrew Ferguson is an osteopath in London, and he sums up his
approach to treating conditions such as asthma: 'Labelling a
condition has some uses, but it is important to remember to treat
the individual and not the label.' This attitude is typical of
osteopaths and many other alternative practitioners in their
approach to ill-health.

Most conventional doctors would agree with Andrew Ferguson wholeheartedly. They share the belief that it is often very
useful to look at the whole person, and not just one disease in
isolation. Unfortunately, the amount of time required to put this
holistic approach into practice is simply out of the question for
most busy general practitioners. One of the benefits of seeing an
alternative practitioner is that they have the time to apply this
holistic approach to your asthma.

WHAT CAN ALTERNATIVE MEDICINE OFFER?

Many people with asthma try out one or more forms of alternative medicine, usually because they are anxious about drug therapy. There can be enormous benefits from trying these different approaches, but it is important to recognize that none of them is truly an 'alternative' to conventional treatment of asthma. You may, in time, be able to reduce your use of drugs by using some of these methods, especially if you combine them with other approaches, such as avoiding allergens, but it is risky to start cutting down on your drugs before you are ready.

Useful therapies

These are the four most useful forms of therapy for asthma. They will probably benefit all or most asthmatics, and will be even more powerful if you combine all four.

Correcting hyperventilation

Hyperventilation often plays a large part in asthma, and the success of the Buteyko Method (see p. 423) suggests that more asthmatics hyperventilate than doctors previously realized. Sorting out hyperventilation – which can be done with a variety of different practitioners (see pp. 422–3) – may be a useful first step to gaining control over asthma.

Osteopathy

It may well be useful to see a good osteopath, to loosen up any parts of your rib-cage or shoulders that are seriously 'stuck' in an unnatural position as a result of having over-inflated lungs during asthma attacks. This can be valuable to loosen you up before you begin working with some other kind of alternative approach (such as Feldenkrais, breathing exercises, yoga or a martial art). Go again, a month or two later, if you can afford it. The osteopathic treatment should produce further benefits at this stage.

Learning to stay calm under stress

The benefits to asthmatics of being more calm and relaxed are accepted as much by conventional doctors as by alternative therapists. For some asthmatics, this can make a huge difference in terms of reducing the number of asthma attacks or improving the way attacks are handled. There are many different approaches to relaxation (see pp. 446–51), and you may have to try several before you find one that works for you. It is useful to see this as a journey of self-exploration rather than something that quickly 'fixes' a problem. There could be many benefits in other areas of your life.

Yoga (see p. 397) is excellent for producing a calm, relaxed attitude to life, and it will loosen up your chest area and help improve your breathing as well. Martial arts, if studied properly (we are not talking kung-fu movies here), also encourage a state of inner calm and have a similar all-round benefit to breathing and physique (see p. 429).

Strengthening the breathing muscles
Special exercises to strengthen the breathing muscles (see pp. 430–45) have been shown to improve the health of asthmatics and reduce their need for asthma drugs.

Things to avoid
Some alternative practitioners, especially those specializing in allergy, may offer you diagnostic tests for allergies. Unless these are skin-prick tests (see p. 304) you should refuse. There are several other tests, which may analyse samples of blood or hair, or test muscle strength or electrical conductance of your skin. Some of these are complete nonsense. Others are partially accurate, but cannot be relied on.

Choosing a therapist or teacher
Personal recommendation is usually the best way to choose someone, because it is often the personal qualities of a therapist or teacher that make all the difference in alternative medicine. But do check on qualifications as well. Don't take strings of letters after the name at face value – ask what they stand for, and for the addresses of the professional organizations that award the qualifications. You can also contact these bodies to check that the person concerned really is a member if you are in doubt. Alternatively, contact the professional organization at the outset (see p. 460) and ask for names of practitioners in your area.

Steer clear of anyone who tells you to stop taking your asthma drugs. This is extremely irresponsible, and suggests that they do not understand much about asthma, or the serious dangers it can pose. A good therapist will advise you to talk to your doctor before reducing preventer medication, and will encourage you not to decrease any drugs until there is very clear improvement in your asthma.

'It's much more empowering to do techniques for yourself . . .'

Peter Blackaby is both an osteopath and a yoga teacher, with much experience of treating and teaching asthmatics. 'It's much more empowering to do techniques for yourself, to know ways of helping yourself. That's why I would prefer asthmatics to learn yoga rather than coming for endless osteopathy treatments, or other kinds of treatment – if you do this you are asking the therapist to solve your problems and handing over responsibility to someone else.

'But if you are just starting out on yoga therapy, or some other training, then it's good to get checked out by an osteopath who can improve the movement of the chest region and pick up any underlying problems. A good osteopath will also try to teach you how to get yourself out of trouble, and how to avoid getting into the habits of asthmatic breathing.'

'I'm not aware of any restrictions on my singing . . .'

'I saw the doctor recently, because I had an asthma attack, and he did various measurements of my breathing. He was really surprised – because he could hear the degree of asthma that I had at the time – at how much lung strength I had. I said, "Perhaps that's because I sing in a choir" and he said "Oh yes, that'll be it . . ."

'I'm not aware of any restrictions on my singing from the asthma. Singing is really less to do with pure lung capacity, than to do with controlling what you have. I feel sure the training that we have for singing has helped with my asthma.' See p. 429.

YOGA AND YOGA THERAPY

Yoga originates in India, and was traditionally a spiritual discipline, part of Hinduism. In its most complete form it works on the physical, mental, emotional and spiritual levels, as well as providing a complete philosophy for living. Accomplished yogis (people who have practised yoga seriously for many years) achieve great calmness and concentration, and a remarkable level of control over bodily functions. For example, many can control their blood pressure, heartbeat or other 'autonomic' functions (ones that are not normally under voluntary control) purely by power of thought. These fundamental changes are achieved through a combination of yoga postures (asanas), breathing exercises (pranayama), meditation, cleansing practices and careful attention to diet and way of life.

The different forms of yoga

Yoga has now been practised in the West for over a century, and during that time it has been gradually 'Westernized' – more so in some traditions than others. It is possible now to be taught forms of yoga that are little more than stretching exercises plus relaxation. Such classes are widely available, and if this is what appeals to you most, then that's what you should try. It may well help by giving you a more relaxed outlook which helps you cope better with your asthma, and by loosening up areas of your neck, chest and back that have become stiff and contracted as a result of repeated asthma attacks.

However, for the greatest benefits from yoga, look for classes with a broader approach, especially those that include yoga breathing exercises. Meditation can also be very valuable in dealing with the panicky feelings that accompany asthma attacks.

As a general guide, teachers of Iyengar Yoga concentrate on postures, as do some of those teaching Hatha Yoga, although others include breathing exercises and meditation as well. Teachers of Kundalini Yoga are likely to place greater emphasis on breathing. You will probably have to talk to the teacher personally to find out what is on offer.

If you are going to a class that includes breathing exercises, make sure the teacher is really experienced in yoga teaching, and has some knowledge of working with asthmatics. It is possible to do yoga breathing badly, making the breaths too deep, and for this to turn into hyperventilation. Being tense and 'trying too hard' is another major obstacle to doing yoga breathing correctly. Relaxing as you breathe is vitally important. Apart from anything else, make sure that the teacher seems like a relaxed person (no one can teach relaxation if they themselves are tense), as well as being someone who is perceptive, adaptable and concerned about your asthma.

Whatever kind of yoga you take up, do be sensible about things and don't overdo any of the very vigorous breathing exercises.

What evidence is there that yoga helps with asthma?

Many asthmatics will tell you that they have been helped greatly by practising yoga. There have also been several studies of yoga and its effects on asthma. Unfortunately, most of these are not good scientific trials with a control group, so the apparent benefit could just be placebo effect (see p. 36). There is, of course, no harm at all in placebo effect if it reduces the number of attacks, improves your peak flow and helps you manage with fewer drugs – in some of these studies, asthmatics practising yoga did reap all these benefits.

There have also been a few rigorous scientific trials. One showed that yoga breathing exercises which extend the out-breath so that it takes twice the time of the in-breath made asthmatic airways less likely to tighten up when challenged. In another study, doctors in Belgium compared advanced practitioners of Hatha Yoga with people of the same age and sex, and found that they breathed more slowly and had higher levels of carbon dioxide in their blood. This suggests that yoga would be useful for anyone with hyperventilation (see p. 419) as well as asthma.

Yoga therapy

A fairly new development, yoga therapy aims to use yoga techniques and apply them to the treatment of specific medical problems. This approach is an interesting marriage of traditional yoga methods and a modern understanding of health problems based on conventional Western medicine.

Yoga therapy begins with a one-to-one consultation in which the teacher asks about your asthma and other medical problems. The classes then consist of eight weekly sessions of teaching, during which you will be taught standard basic yoga, plus special postures and breathing exercises that are particularly useful for asthma or for any other medical condition you may have.

Teachers of yoga therapy are well trained, and will know how to teach yoga breathing exercises correctly.

'. . . asthmatics are often very tense around the chest and diaphragm . . .'

Robin Monro trained as a research scientist and is now director of the Yoga Biomedical Trust. He is particularly concerned that yoga should be taught well. As he points out, 'The most essential part of pranayama is relaxation – if you try to do these breathing exercises without relaxing you will not get any benefit. This is one of the least developed sides of yoga teaching in the West, because the main emphasis is on asanas, or poses, and a lot of teachers do very little pranayama.

'But if yoga is taught well, by good and intuitive teachers, it can be very valuable to asthmatics. One reason is that it teaches breathing with movement, and asthmatics are often very tense around the chest and diaphragm, very "locked" in their breathing. Yoga can teach asthmatics to relax and open up the diaphragm, so that they learn to use it properly.

'Before people start, though, they should ask whether it's appropriate for them – they should have the motivation, and the time to practise every day. They also need to have the right home situation and family members allowing them the space. Unless they can do at least 30 minutes a day there won't be any effect – and 60 minutes a day will be more helpful.'

OSTEOPATHS AND CHIROPRACTORS

Osteopaths and chiropractors work with the bones, joints, muscles, tendons and ligaments, but they see their work as affecting health as a whole, allowing improvements to occur in *general* health, not just in the musculo-skeletal system. Their fundamental belief is that the body heals itself if given a chance – that it has its own methods of getting back to the equilibrium called 'health', but that misalignments in the skeleton can block the body's efforts to achieve that equilibrium. By putting the skeleton back into its correct alignment (or at least an improved alignment) the osteopath or chiropractor can encourage healing.

Chiropractors tend to focus more on the spine than osteopaths, and are more inclined to use X-rays in diagnosis.

In addition to the ideas already described, there is a traditional belief in osteopathy that the manipulations of the skeleton can be used to influence the autonomic nervous system – which controls the body's automatic functions (including control over the narrowing and widening of the airways – see pp. 417–8). There is no strong evidence for this and it is a controversial belief even among osteopaths.

Most of the ideas and methods of osteopathy and chiropractic are perfectly compatible with orthodox medicine, and osteopathy, in particular, has an excellent track record with problems such as back pain that doctors find difficult to treat. It is a great mystery why these approaches are still rejected as 'alternative' by the medical establishment, especially when they have so much to offer.

An osteopath approaches an asthmatic client with several objectives in mind:

1. To look for misalignment of the rib-cage, shoulders, neck and upper spine that have occurred as a result of the lungs being over-inflated during asthma attacks, and for muscles that are over-contracted or over-stretched as a result of abnormal breathing patterns (see p. 415).

2. To correct these problems, to loosen up stiff areas and to give greater freedom of movement. This allows healthy breathing patterns to occur more easily, because the muscles and bones are in the best possible position mechanically, rather than working at a disadvantage.

3. To suggest ways in which the posture could be improved, so that healthy breathing comes more naturally.

4. To teach exercises that will maintain the mobility and correct alignment of the chest region, plus exercises that will strengthen the diaphragm.
5. If the asthmatic does not normally breathe with the diaphragm, to teach this, and to discourage breathing with the upper chest (see p. 421). To try to correct mouth-breathing if this is also part of the picture.
6. To address any obvious psychological problems related to breathing, or to asthma attacks. Some practitioners will be better at this than others.
7. To try to influence the autonomic nervous system, by manipulating the neck and spine, so that the branch which makes the airways get narrower becomes less powerful. Not every practitioner will include this approach.

Chiropractors vary, but in general they do not take such a broad approach to asthma as osteopaths.

The evidence for benefits in asthma

There has been no scientific research into the effects of osteopathy on asthma. It would be difficult to carry out such research, because osteopaths are not claiming that they can actually reduce symptoms of airway narrowing, or reduce drug use – although some clients do report that this happens. What they do claim to do is to minimize the impact of asthma on the skeleton, avoid deformities of the chest region and improve breathing dynamics. The treatment will have different kinds of benefits for different asthmatics, which makes any kind of trial difficult to devise.

There are very good common-sense reasons for believing many of the claims made by osteopaths in relation to asthma. Such treatment may well help you, particularly if you have severe asthma, if you have a typical asthmatic posture (see p. 415) or if you hyperventilate (see p. 419). Children are likely to be helped by osteopathy, and if their asthma attacks are severe, it may prevent them from developing deformities of the chest region.

One study of chiropractic has been carried out with asthmatics in Denmark. The researchers found no difference in asthma symptoms or use of asthma drugs after the patients had chiropractic sessions twice weekly for four weeks. As with osteopathy, however, it is unrealistic to look for substantial changes in asthma symptoms as a result of chiropractic: that is not the point of the treatment.

'Osteopaths are neither magicians nor miracle workers . . .'

Robin Shepherd has been an osteopath for over ten years. This is his outlook on asthma:

'Osteopaths are neither magicians nor miracle workers. The osteopathic treatment of asthma is directed at improving breathing mechanics, undoing posturally related problems and removing as many stresses, mechanical, and if possible psychological, from the scene. If the treatment and exercises are carried out with integrity and common sense they cannot be anything but beneficial for the patient.

'Physiotherapists will say they can perhaps do all of these techniques, and that they share similar considerations. I do not claim that osteopathy has patents on any. In fact I would encourage practice nurses, physiotherapists and even family members of asthmatics to learn some of the simple techniques . . . They may well save the NHS something from its drug bill and will certainly let asthmatics feel they can do something to improve their quality of life.'

ALEXANDER TECHNIQUE AND FELDENKRAIS METHOD

Neither of these techniques has been tested scientifically in relation to asthma, but successes have been reported by many asthmatics. If you feel your breathing may need 're-education' (see p. 422), either of them could be useful. Experienced teachers who have worked with other asthmatics should be able to check whether you are breathing well, using your diaphragm. They will also be able to help you correct some of the unhealthy changes in posture that are a result of asthma (see p. 415). It might be a good idea to have a treatment from an osteopath as well (see p. 400).

Of the two, Alexander Technique is much more widely taught and better known, but Feldenkrais, which was introduced more recently and is still not widely known, is probably more appropriate for asthmatics. Alexander Technique can be rather static, whereas Feldenkrais is more movement-oriented and should bring benefits to asthmatics more quickly. To find a local teacher see Useful Addresses.

Alexander Technique

The aim of this method is to correct bad posture, and particularly to get your head in its correct position in relation to your spine. Alexander Technique teachers believe that this will automatically improve your breathing and re-educate your body to move in its correct and natural way. The teaching of Alexander Technique can sometimes be quite rigid, but the teachers do vary considerably in their approach.

The technique is not aimed at specific problems and you won't be working exclusively on your asthma. Alexander Technique does not regard itself as a therapy. It is concerned with a more efficient (that is, less effortful) use of the self, by teaching greater awareness of the body and alternatives to damaging habitual use. Benefiting from the Alexander Technique may be a question of finding the right teacher, preferably someone who has worked with other asthmatics and is willing to focus on your breathing as well as your posture.

Because our habitual posture is so deeply ingrained, it can take a very long time to achieve lasting change. A course of ten lessons is usually the minimum required.

Feldenkrais Method

The Feldenkrais Method has some things in common with the Alexander Technique, but it focuses more on how people move and use their bodies than on static posture. It encourages you to find out for yourself what are the best ways to do things, rather than laying down a 'right way' that applies to everyone. The Feldenkrais Method also emphasizes that movement in one part of the body is linked to movement in almost every other part, so that the whole body is a complex connected structure. This can be very valuable for asthmatics.

The principle of Feldenkrais is that you experiment for yourself, trying out different ways of moving or breathing, doing everything slowly, gently and quietly so that you notice the effects of different approaches.

There are two ways in which Feldenkrais is taught:
- one-to-one sessions called 'Functional Integration'
- general classes known as 'Awareness Through Movement'

For anyone with asthma, Functional Integration is recommended. You may need only one or two sessions.

The Feldenkrais teacher will first get you to observe your own breathing, and then encourage you to play around with your breathing patterns – for example, first to exaggerate what you normally do, and then to do the exact opposite. The idea is that somewhere in this process the part of your brain which controls the muscles involved in breathing will work out a better way of doing things, a way that is more efficient and less effortful. For this process to occur, it is important that you relax during the session, and don't 'try too hard' – the process is largely an unconscious one, so just let it happen. One of the interesting things about a Feldenkrais session is when, at the end of the hour, you try again to do things in your 'old way' and discover what incredibly hard work it is.

You will also be given some simple explorations to try out, which again are intended to open up new possibilities for your breathing patterns. There is no 'right way' to do these either – they are just another method of exploring your own breathing. Typically, once you have done these explorations you find that there has been a subtle loosening-up of your breathing, and something which felt difficult before now feels easier. Again it is your subconscious mind which has adjusted your breathing movements to a better pattern.

The changes brought about by the Feldenkrais Method are small and subtle at first, and you may find you slip back into your bad old habits, but if you keep experimenting with the explorations regularly, and go back for another session now and again, it should produce long-term changes in your breathing which are highly beneficial.

Two simple Feldenkrais Explorations

Remember that the whole point of these explorations is to *notice* how your body feels, and *experiment* with different ways of doing things. Don't try too hard, and don't force anything. Bear in mind that you would get a great deal more out of working with a qualified Feldenkrais teacher.

1. Lie on your back and get comfortable, with your legs bent, feet slightly apart.
   - *Observation stage*: Place one hand on your belly, and one on your upper chest, with your elbows supported by cushions. As you breathe in try to raise the hand on your belly a little, using your in-breath (keep the hand and wrist floppy). Do it again and try to raise the hand on your chest a little. Which of these feels more difficult?
   - *Exploration stage*: Now take in a fairly deep breath and hold it. While holding your breath, use the muscles in your chest and abdomen to push the air down into your belly as far as you can, and then push it up into the top of your chest as far as you can. Keep pushing it backwards and forwards and notice how your hands move as you do so. (Don't go on too long and make yourself feel ill.) Stop and breathe normally for a while, until you feel ready to do the exploration again. When you have done it three times, go back to the observation stage.
   - *Observation stage*: Observe again, as described above. Does anything feel different now?
2. Do this exploration lying down, then do it sitting up for comparison.
   - *Observation stage*: Breathe normally and observe which feels more difficult – is it the in-breath or the out-breath? (For most asthmatics the out-breath feels more difficult.)

- *Exploration stage:* Work with whichever breath felt easier – for example, if you found the out-breath more difficult, work with your in-breath. Take your in-breath in several very small stages, with tiny pauses in between, rather than a steady flow. Once the lungs are comfortably full, let the out-breath occur naturally. Do this several times.
- *Observation stage:* Now return to the observation stage. Does your out-breath feel any easier?

'You can work it out, and I can help you . . .'

Ilana Nevill has been a Feldenkrais teacher for ten years. 'The important thing about Feldenkrais is that it doesn't tell you what to do. We believe that trying to "get it right" is often part of a person's problem. Our rationale is that the human nervous system is highly intelligent and that this intelligence can be relied on to find a way that is right for yourself.

'So when I work with the breathing of a person who has asthma I am not saying to them: "I will show you how to do it". I am saying "You can work it out, and I can help you to discover things you never would have thought of before." I get them to try anything – the crazier the better, even doing it very badly – that's good too, that's how you learn.

'Moshe Feldenkrais, who devised the Method, was adamant that teaching people about "correct" breathing is stupid because breathing changes all the time, with what you do and how you feel. Any ideas about how one "should" breathe interfere with that spontaneous process.'

HERBAL REMEDIES, HOMEOPATHY AND AROMATHERAPY

Herbal remedies

Many plants contain chemical substances which have a drug-like action on the human body. Indeed, many modern drugs were originally derived from plants – cromoglycate for example, was first extracted from the roots of ammivisnaga, a plant found in Egypt.

There are many different herbal remedies that are said to help with asthma – some can be bought in health food shops, while others are only available from registered herbalists. People often feel safer taking a herbal remedy than a drug, because they assume that something 'natural' is automatically safe. But if something affects the body sufficiently to treat an illness it is quite likely to affect the body in other, less welcome, ways as well. Herbs can be just as toxic as drugs (how many wayside plants could you eat without ill-effects?) and they have been tested much less rigorously for side-effects. You should bear this in mind if you decide to take a herbal remedy. Keep an eye out for side-effects and stop taking the herb promptly if any develop.

Most herbal remedies have never been tested scientifically, but in the following cases there is research to show that they may have some effect:

- *Coleus forskholii*, a herb used in Ayurvedic medicine, has a powerful effect on the airway muscles, making the airways open up in a similar way to B-2 reliever drugs.
- *Cannabis sativa* has a similar effect. The well-known side-effects include a decline in short-term memory, a slowing-down of mental function and, in most countries, getting arrested.
- *Tylophora asthmatica* is used in Ayurvedic medicine, and some studies show benefits in asthma. However, side-effects are also common, including nausea and soreness in the mouth. This herb is not readily available in Western Europe.
- *Ginkgo biloba* seems to reduce the sensitivity of the airways, and may improve lung function, reduce the reaction to allergens, and protect against exercise-induced asthma.
- Saiboku-to comes from a Japanese plant and has been investigated more carefully than most herbal remedies. Several

studies suggest that it has good long-term effects and can allow asthmatics to reduce their dose of steroids.

- *Lobelia inflata* and *Ephedra sinica* are also known to have some benefits in asthma.

A herbal treatment called Ma-huang, included in some dietary supplements, is a source of ephedrine (see p. 372) and over-use can cause a vascular spasm of the blood vessels in the brain or heart, resulting in injury or death.

If you are allergic to pollen, you should avoid any preparation containing royal jelly, as this has caused near-fatal anaphylaxis (see p. 111) in some asthmatics. Propolis should also be treated with great caution.

Homeopathy

All homeopathy is based on the principle that diluting an active substance in a particular way (with a special shaking-and-tapping technique known as 'percussing') can make the active substance *more* powerful, despite the dilution. In fact, homeopathic remedies are all diluted to such an extent that there is unlikely to be even one molecule of the active substance in the remedy that the patient finally takes. It is rather like pouring a cup of coffee into the Atlantic Ocean, letting it all swirl around for a while, then drinking a cupful of seawater. You might just get a molecule of caffeine, but the chances are you won't – and you certainly wouldn't expect the seawater to keep you awake at night. According to homeopathic lore, if you had mixed it into the sea in the right way, with percussing, the seawater would acquire all the potency of the original coffee and actually be more powerful – though it might produce the *opposite* effect to caffeine and send you into a deep sleep.

This is a theory that we personally find difficult to swallow, but there are many people (including some doctors) who believe, on the basis of their own experience, that homeopathy can work.

Some of these doctors have tested out homeopathic treatments for allergic asthma. They have apparently been successful in reducing asthma symptoms by taking the allergen to which the asthmatic reacts – pollen or dust mites, for example – diluting it according to homeopathic practice, and using this as a remedy. This form of homeopathy is known as homeopathic immunotherapy or HIT.

This is unlikely to be the treatment you will get if you go to see a homeopath. Most homeopaths use a technique called classical homeopathy, in which a person's symptoms (not just asthma, but any other symptoms as well) are compared to the known effects of a range of toxic plant and animal extracts. The extract that matches your symptoms best is given as a remedy in homeopathic dilution, with the aim of *curing* the same symptoms that it would *cause* if taken at full strength.

There is a third approach called complex homeopathy, which uses a mixture of herbal remedies and homeopathic treatments, and you may be given this type of treatment. There is no evidence that either this or classical homeopathy can help with asthma – the evidence about HIT is not really relevant to these forms of homeopathy.

Many people with asthma are helped by seeing a homeopath, however, because homeopaths take a broad view of most illnesses, and they often give some advice on diet, lifestyle and allergen avoidance as well. Many will recommend avoiding certain foods, on the basis of assumed food intolerance, although they rarely use an elimination diet to achieve accurate diagnosis (see p. 181). Additionally, homeopaths have time to talk in detail about any emotional problems that are contributing to the asthma, and offer advice and support. This can be very helpful for many asthmatics. Seeing a good counsellor (see p. 451) would give you the same sort of help with the emotional aspects of asthma, and this book provides you with more comprehensive and up-to-date advice on diet and allergen avoidance than most homeopaths could give.

Homeopathic remedies bought from a shop will follow either classical or complex homeopathy.

Aromatherapy

Many people use aromatherapy oils, often combined with massage, as an aid to relaxation and general well-being. It can be useful, but be aware that strong smells can trigger asthma attacks (see p. 232) and there are reports of some aromatherapy oils having this effect. Stop using the oil promptly if your chest feels tight, and ventilate the room thoroughly.

ACUPUNCTURE AND SHIATSU

Acupuncture originates in China and is part of traditional Chinese medicine. It is based on the concept that there is life-energy, called *chi* or *qi* or *ki*, flowing through the body along channels known as meridians. The acupuncturist takes the pulse at several different places on the body, and uses this to identify imbalances and blockages in the flow of *chi*. The treatment is then tailored to the individual, with the aim of controlling, strengthening or redirecting the flow of *chi*, as appropriate, to promote health and combat illness.

The best-known technique involves pricking the skin with needles at particular points along the meridians, known as acupuncture points. However, there are also other methods of stimulating the acupuncture points, ranging from a traditional technique called moxibustion (in which herbs are burned in an inverted glass vessel, creating a vacuum and suction over the point) to the use of simple pressure with the fingers (acupressure) or high-tech stimulation with lasers.

Acupuncture has some quite stunning effects, which Western medicine is still at a loss to explain, such as the suppression of pain. It is possible to carry out certain surgical operations using only acupuncture as the anaesthetic. However, acupuncture is not always so successful in other areas, and the claim that it is a complete medical system with a cure for everything is exaggerated. It is worth remembering that in China the majority of people use Western medicine, despite the widespread availability of acupuncture.

Does acupuncture work for asthma?
There have been quite a number of studies, and the overall impression is that acupuncture can indeed help the airway muscles to relax during an asthma attack, although it has a less dramatic effect than a puff of Ventolin. When it comes to long-term benefits such as reducing inflammation in the airways, acupuncture does not seem to be effective. The short-term benefits in opening up the airways are probably achieved by affecting the autonomic nervous system, which controls the muscles around the airways.

However the sort of acupuncture used in a scientific study is nothing like an individual acupuncture treatment. For a rigorous scientific study it is important to standardize treatment and to needle exactly the same points in everyone. This is fundamentally different from a proper acupuncture treatment, where the points are chosen as much for the person as for the disease. Perhaps an individualized acupuncture treatment has benefits for some asthmatics that are not seen in scientific trials. It is interesting that a survey in the Netherlands found that almost 25 per cent of family doctors believe acupuncture to be helpful for asthma. There may also be general health benefits, such as an increase in well-being and relaxation, which many people report after an acupuncture treatment.

Choosing an acupuncturist

Acupuncturists vary enormously in their skill, and you should ask around locally for recommendations, rather than just choosing someone at random. Ask how long they have trained for, and what qualifications they have. Check that the sterilization procedure used for the needles is adequate, or that disposable needles are used, because there is a potential risk of infection with HIV or hepatitis C. Most acupuncturists are extremely careful to avoid this.

Acupuncture can produce emotional responses in some people, and a good practitioner should be able to deal with these constructively and help the client to find ways of coping with their problems. This can sometimes be the most beneficial part of an acupuncture treatment. It is important that you find the acupuncturist congenial and sympathetic – someone you can talk to – for this kind of work to be successful.

Shiatsu

This technique originated in Japan in the 1920s, but is based on traditional Chinese acupressure (see above). Shiatsu practitioners require a much shorter period of training than acupuncturists, which is one reason for its popularity in the West. It aims to prevent illness by helping the body achieve its own equilibrium and by strengthening self-curative powers. One benefit often reported is a reduction in fatigue and tension. This may be useful in a general way for asthmatics, but there are no studies to show any particular effects of shiatsu on asthma symptoms.

> *'. . . my asthma started clearing up from the very first treat-*
> *ment.'*

Vanessa is a healthy 28-year-old, who was once asthmatic. 'I
never have any attacks now. I don't even have an inhaler, and I
used to be the sort of person who, if I'd come out without it or
lost it, would immediately panic and that would bring an attack
on. I used to feel less strong if I didn't have the inhaler with me. If
it wasn't by my bed at night I couldn't sleep.

'I had asthma quite badly as a child and it got worse when I
was in my teens, so I had to have Ventolin three times a day. My
doctor wasn't really doing anything except prescribing more and
more Ventolin. Then, when I was at college, I developed Chronic
Fatigue Syndrome (CFS). The doctor was obviously fed up with
me, and she wanted me to go and see a counsellor but I said no. I
don't think that would have helped, because, although I think the
asthma and the CFS both had psychological roots, the problems
were just too deep to be sorted out by talking.

'A friend came to see me when I was absolutely at my lowest,
almost suicidal with the CFS, and she suggested I see an acupuncturist. So I did, and my asthma started clearing up from the
very first treatment. It was incredible. I was so elated after that
first treatment. The CFS took longer to clear up, but it did go in
time.'

To Vanessa, there is absolutely no doubt that acupuncture
cured her of asthma. It certainly helped her enormously, but was
she actually suffering from asthma at the time? Clearly Vanessa
was psychologically dependent (see p. 36) on her reliever
inhaler, and developed panicky feelings and asthma-like symptoms when it was not available. It is possible that by this stage she
had actually grown out of her asthma, as many young adults do,
but she was hyperventilating as a result of her underlying anxiety
(see p. 36) and the hyperventilation was bringing on attacks of
breathlessness which resembled asthma. Hyperventilation can
also produce a set of severe symptoms that are very much like
CFS. What the acupuncturist probably did was to correct the
hyperventilation, and build Vanessa's self-confidence so that her
dependence on the inhaler disappeared.

In a sense, it doesn't really matter *why* she got better. The important point is that she no longer needs asthma drugs, and now lives a much healthier and happier life. The acupuncturist achieved this when her doctor (who perhaps had no training in recognizing hyperventilation) could not help. Having plenty of time to spend with clients often allows alternative practitioners to help asthmatics more than doctors, especially in complicated cases where asthma is tied in with various emotional and family problems. The fact that asthmatics choose their alternative practitioners may also help – in this case Vanessa and her doctor were clearly disenchanted with each other, but Vanessa was able to strike up a good and trusting relationship with the acupuncturist, which aided her recovery.

'. . . I just see all these shoulders going up . . .'

Jill is a yoga teacher in California, and an asthmatic herself. She runs special yoga classes for people with asthma. 'The first thing I tell them is to breathe in through your nose. If you breathe through your mouth, you're breathing in particulates and harsh, dry air.

'Next I tell them to imagine they have a balloon in the abdomen. As you breathe in you're filling the balloon, as you breathe out you're emptying it, and you do that with a long, slow exhalation.

'I watch them try it, and at first I just see all these shoulders going up, because that's how they always breathe, with the upper part of the chest. They have to learn to breathe *past* that part of the chest and into the bottom of the lungs.

'Once you get the hang of this way of breathing with the diaphragm it's very relaxing, but it can feel strange at the start, if you're not accustomed to it. It's a question of learning it, the same way you'd learn to type or drive an automobile – so that when you do it, it's just automatic. You should practise twice a day, for about ten minutes. You can practise while you watch TV.'

For more on brathing with the diaphragm, see pp. 421–3.

BREATHING EXERCISES AND THE BUTEYKO METHOD

Knowing how to breathe well can help to improve control over the airways for people with asthma. Unfortunately, the conventional scientific understanding of breathing is still far from perfect because breathing is particularly difficult to study scientifically – as soon as you ask someone to breathe into a piece of scientific apparatus, their breathing is likely to change. But certain things *are* now understood and new ways of studying breathing are being devised. It seems likely that our knowledge of breathing will improve enormously over the next few decades.

The basic role of the lungs and airways in breathing is explained on p. 20. This section deals with the dynamics of breathing (how the muscles and bones of the chest make the lungs pump air), the control mechanisms involved, and the ways in which breathing exercises can improve asthma.

The dynamics of breathing

The rib-cage and the diaphragm are the main structures involved in the dynamics of breathing. The rib-cage can be felt through the skin, but you cannot touch your diaphragm and many people are not aware they have one. It is a thick, dome-shaped layer of muscle, that lies below the lungs and above the intestines. If you are breathing correctly, the diaphragm contracts and relaxes when you breathe.

The ribs have many small muscles running between them, called the intercostal muscles. By contracting or relaxing different combinations of intercostal muscles, we can make the rib-cage move and change shape in different ways.

Breathing in

When you breathe in, the diaphragm should power the in-breath by contracting. It is anchored around all its edges – to the spine and to the lower ribs. When it contracts, the diaphragm flattens out: so it becomes less dome-shaped and more like an upturned saucer. This exerts a downward pull on the chest cavity. The outer surface of the lungs is effectively 'stuck' to the chest cavity, so this downward pull enlarges the lungs and makes them suck in air. The action is similar to pulling on a bicycle pump so that air rushes into the pump.

As it moves downwards, the diaphragm presses on to everything that lies below: the stomach, intestines and bladder. They become increasingly squashed, and eventually stop the diaphragm moving any further. But the diaphragm goes on contracting, and this pulls the lower ribs upwards and, therefore, outwards. The action is like a bucket handle being pulled up from a resting position to a horizontal position: in coming up, it also swings outwards.

This action by the diaphragm on the ribs makes the bottom part of the rib-cage flare outward during the in-breath, expanding the lungs even further.

If you are at rest, the diaphragm should do most of the work, or even all the work, of breathing in. The intercostal muscles help to stabilize the rib-cage, but they should not be working to expand it. The upper part of the rib-cage should hardly expand at all during restful breathing.

When you are exerting yourself and need to breathe harder and faster, the upper chest expands as well as the lower chest. At this point the intercostal muscles become involved in breathing, and some other muscles, called the 'accessory muscles of breathing', may be used as well. Some of these run from the neck down to the topmost ribs and the collarbone, and can raise these bones by contracting. Others run from the shoulder across to the breastbone (the sternum) and can expand the rib-cage at the front by lifting the breastbone. When someone exercises so strenuously that they pant and gasp, these muscles all come into use.

During a severe attack, asthmatics may use the accessory muscles of breathing to try to take in more air. If attacks happen frequently, or if this way of breathing becomes a habit and persists between attacks, the chest may be distorted by the constant use of the accessory muscles, as well as by the over-inflation of the lungs. This is why severe asthmatics often have hunched shoulders and a 'barrel-chested' look.

Breathing out
When you breathe out, your diaphragm relaxes, which makes it become dome-shaped again, and allows the lungs to go back to their original size and shape. When the airways are healthy and open, there is no muscular force involved in breathing out during rest. The lungs are naturally elastic, like balloons, so they tend to force out the air once the external stretching pressure of the in-breath stops.

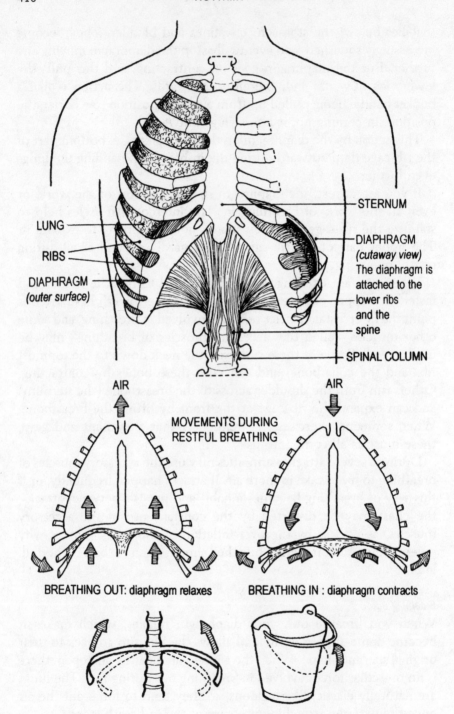

STERNUM

LUNG

RIBS

DIAPHRAGM
(outer surface)

DIAPHRAGM
(cutaway view)
The diaphragm is
attached to the
lower ribs
and the
spine

SPINAL COLUMN

AIR

AIR

MOVEMENTS DURING
RESTFUL BREATHING

BREATHING OUT: diaphragm relaxes

BREATHING IN : diaphragm contracts

During exercise, the out-breath requires more effort. To speed up breathing out, we contract the abdominal muscles (those across the belly) to exert pressure on the chest cavity from below, and pull the ribs down and in with the intercostal muscles. This pushes the stale air out and allows the next in-breath to start sooner.

The out-breath during an asthma attack

Breathing out is a different matter during an asthma attack. The narrowed airways make it hard for the air to escape quickly, and, even at rest, the natural elasticity of the lungs is not enough to overcome this obstruction. There are various breathing exercises that can help asthmatics improve their capacity to breathe out fully (see p. 429) but they should *not* be practised during an attack.

How breathing is controlled

Breathing is unusual among bodily actions because it is under both involuntary and voluntary control – most actions are either totally involuntary (e.g. the pumping of the heart) or totally voluntary (e.g. kicking the legs). Involuntary control of breathing can supply us with the right amount of oxygen for basic activities such as walking, running or swimming, but we need voluntary control as well to be able to talk, sing, whistle for the dog and cheer at football matches.

The involuntary control of breathing depends on the part of the brain called the respiratory centre. It receives information about the amount of carbon dioxide and oxygen in the blood, and uses this to adjust the breathing rate and depth of breathing. Normally, the level of carbon dioxide in the blood has a much more important effect on the breathing than the level of oxygen. During an asthma attack, however, if the level of carbon dioxide rises above a certain level, the respiratory centre switches to using oxygen as the main indicator of breathing need. This is what creates the feeling of extreme 'air hunger' that occurs during a severe asthma attack.

How the airway muscles are controlled

So much for the rate of breathing – what controls the widening and narrowing of the airways? There are two main mechanisms.

One involves the autonomic nervous system, which is responsible for controlling all involuntary muscles. There are two branches to the autonomic nervous system, the sympathetic and the parasympathetic.

The sympathetic nervous system is more active when you are frightened, angry, excited or stressed, and it makes the airways open up. Adrenaline is the messenger substance used by the sympathetic nervous system. This is why B-2 relievers such as Ventolin (see p. 342), which mimic the action of adrenaline on the airways, relieve asthma attacks.

The parasympathetic nervous system is more active when you are relaxed, and it makes the airways grow narrower, because less air is needed when you are less active. Anti-cholinergic relievers (see p. 345) act by blocking the action of the parasympathetic.

If you are someone whose asthma gets worse when you are stressed, this may all seem rather odd – surely, if stress stimulates the sympathetic nervous system, it should make asthma better not worse? For some people it does indeed make asthma better (see pp. 37–8). What is more, there are people whose asthma only gets worse once the stress is over. This too makes sense in terms of sympathetic/parasympathetic balance – as they relax after stress and the balance swings towards the parasympathetic, their airways tighten.

But what can explain the reaction of people whose asthma gets worse *during* stressful times? This is a puzzle that has not yet been resolved. One possible answer is that they are hyperventilating (see below) when under stress. They may be hyperventilating so slightly that it is unnoticeable, but it could be just enough to make their airways narrow. Breathing through the mouth more than the nose can also be part of the reaction to stress, and this irritates the airways because the air they receive is colder, drier and more dusty for not having been filtered through the nose. Anything that irritates the airway linings – which are already inflamed in asthma – can make the airway muscles tighten. There are local nerves running directly from the airway linings to the airway muscles which cause this reaction: this is the second major mechanism involved in airway narrowing.

For people whose asthma gets worse under stress, this local reaction seems to outweigh the effects of the sympathetic/parasympathetic balance.

There is one other interesting mechanism in the lungs of non-asthmatics which ensures that more air is inhaled easily when needed: if the airways are tight, taking a deeper breath than usual makes the airways muscles relax, so that the airways open up. The deep breath itself is stimulated by the brain, in response to rising levels of carbon dioxide in the blood, and the breath has a knock-on effect in opening up the airways.

Unfortunately, this mechanism does not work in about two-thirds of asthmatics: when they take a deep breath, the airways do not open up, and can even get tighter. These people tend to have more severe asthma than those asthmatics who respond normally to deep breaths.

Some researchers believe that this lack of response to deep breaths may occur because the lungs are so often over-inflated that the 'stretch receptors' (which sense a deep breath) have become over-stretched, exhausted and insensitive. Perhaps getting the asthma under control, so that the lungs are no longer over-inflated, would reverse the problem – as yet, this has not been investigated.

Hyperventilation – a common problem

Hyperventilation simply means 'over-breathing': taking in too much air. This makes the carbon dioxide (see p.21) level in your blood fall, or simply makes the level of carbon dioxide vary a lot, which upsets certain parts of the body, especially the nerve cells. The symptoms that can result from this changing level of carbon dioxide are many and varied. They include:

- dizziness
- tingling of the hands and feet, and often the tongue or lips
- numbness
- muscle cramps, aching muscles, twitches, tremors or sudden loss of strength
- migraine or headache
- spaced-out feelings, confusion, and even hallucinations
- panic attacks
- fear of sudden death (this can be overpowering)
- anxiety or depression, mood swings, phobias
- ringing in the ears
- blurred vision
- breathlessness or 'air hunger' (see p. 312)
- aching in the chest
- abnormal heart rhythm
- difficulty in swallowing

According to conventional medicine, there is more to hyperventilation than simply breathing too much air – in this respect, doctors differ from Buteyko practitioners (see p. 423) in their view of hyperventilation. Although there is no single accepted view of hyperventilation within the medical profession, most experts agree on the following points:

- Hyperventilation is linked with an abnormal pattern of breathing involving the use of the upper chest even when at rest, under-use of the diaphragm, and rapid, shallow breaths. The breathing is often quite irregular, and there may be deep sighing breaths at intervals, or frequent yawning.
- In order to treat hyperventilation, patients need to be taught to breathe slowly and deeply, using the diaphragm.
- There is usually anxiety or some other psychological problem underlying hyperventilation. (Some experts describe a typical profile for hyperventilators which includes perfectionism, very stressful recent events, and a sense of grievance or resentment.) Recognizing the link between emotions, breathing pattern and symptoms can be a key step in treatment.

How is hyperventilation linked to asthma?

Many asthmatics hyperventilate during attacks, and some breathe in this way most of the time. This will make asthma symptoms worse. Low levels of carbon dioxide in the blood can aggravate asthma in two different ways:

1. The involuntary muscles of the body – including those around the airways – tend to contract a little more when carbon dioxide levels in the blood fall.
2. Allergy-causing cells called mast cells become less stable when there is less carbon dioxide available. The mast cells then release histamine more easily, and it is histamine which brings on allergic symptoms and makes the airways become narrower.

Both these effects are relatively small, but they can make asthma and allergy symptoms worse.

Hyperventilation can begin quite easily for asthmatics. During an asthma attack, in an attempt to get more air, you are likely to start breathing with your upper chest, using the 'accessory muscles of respiration' (see p. 415) and breathing more rapidly. While the airways are narrow and breathing restricted, this may not reduce your levels of carbon dioxide much. But if this type of breathing pattern persists after the attack has ended – which it can easily do – the carbon dioxide levels will fall.

Rapid upper-chest breathing can also occur simply as a result of feeling anxious, in both asthmatics and non-asthmatics. If your airways are a bit tight, and you start to worry about this, you may begin taking deeper breaths just out of anxiety. This can develop into hyperventilation.

In addition to all this, hyperventilation can mimic asthma. A minority of 'asthmatics' do not have asthma at all, but are simply hyperventilating (see pp. 311–2).

Do you hyperventilate?

If may be difficult to tell if you hyperventilate or not, because your habitual pattern of breathing obviously seems 'normal' to you. You will not necessarily have many of the symptoms listed on p. 419.

If you do have some of the symptoms listed, and if you have them much of the time, not just during asthma attacks, you can try the 'paper bag test'. Hold a clean paper bag over your nose and mouth and breathe normally. By re-inhaling air that you have just breathed out, you will increase the level of carbon dioxide in the blood. If your symptoms promptly disappear, they are very likely due to hyperventilation. *Do not try this during an asthma attack.*

Another approach is to choose a time when you do not have symptoms, and deliberately breathe faster for a few minutes, to see if the symptoms appear.

Anyone who suspects hyperventilation should see their doctor, who should be able to make a diagnosis and refer them to a physiotherapist for breathing retraining.

Do you breathe with your diaphragm?

You can also check whether you are using your diaphragm or your upper chest in breathing, by lying on your back with your right hand on your upper chest, and the left one on your belly. Relax for a few minutes, then start to pay attention to your hands. When you breathe in, which hand rises? It should be the left hand that rises, with little or no movement in the right.

If that test feels difficult, or you are not sure, try the following experiment. Bend over and hold the back of a chair, with your back, head and arms forming a straight horizontal line at right angles to your legs (see below). In this position, breathing with the upper chest is very difficult, whereas breathing with the diaphragm is easy. If you find it reasonably easy to breathe while in this position, you are probably breathing well normally. If it is difficult to breathe in this position, you are not using your diaphragm, and would benefit from breathing retraining.

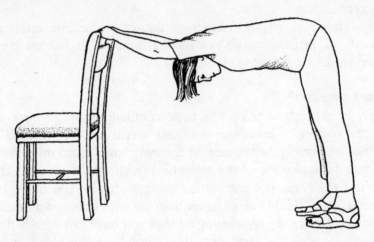

Overcoming hyperventilation

Conventional medicine treats hyperventilation by addressing any underlying psychological problems (see p. 420) and by retraining the breathing. This involves teaching the asthmatic to use their diaphragm rather than their upper chest, as well as slowing down the rate of breathing.

Breathing retraining can be taught by physiotherapists (ask your doctor to refer you), or by certain complementary therapists/teachers, such as osteopaths (see p. 400), Feldenkrais practitioners (see p. 404) and good yoga teachers (see p. 397). Learning to breathe with the diaphragm will tend to make you feel more relaxed – the in-breath disperses tensions in your abdomen.

In learning to breathe with the diaphragm it is important not to go too far and become a 'belly breather', whose abdomen bulges out with every in-breath. This is a mistake sometimes made by those who consciously set out to improve their breathing. The abdomen should resist the downward movement of the diaphragm to some extent, or else the lower ribs won't flare out and enlarge the chest as they should (see p. 415).

A physiotherapist can also teach you methods of clearing mucus from the airways which may be useful (see p. 59) while osteopaths will correct any structural problems in the chest area induced by asthma attacks and hyperventilation (see p. 400).

The Buteyko Method

There has been a great deal of publicity about the treatment programme for asthmatics devised by Professor Konstantin Buteyko. Initially most doctors were very sceptical about this treatment, but it seems clear that it does help many asthmatics.

The Buteyko treatment is really very simple, and has two main parts:

- unblocking the nose so that asthmatics stop breathing through the mouth
- training asthmatics not to hyperventilate

More details on how to practise the Buteyko Method are given below.

Professor Buteyko believes that *all* asthma is *caused* by hyperventilation. In fact he blames hyperventilation for causing no fewer than 150 different diseases, including allergies, insomnia, bronchitis, anxiety, eczema, headaches, emphysema, migraines, high blood pressure and haemorrhoids.

If you sign up for a course of Buteyko lessons (the most expensive of all the alternative therapies described in this chapter) you will be told that the treatment achieves astonishing things – for example, that it can get 97 per cent of asthmatics off most of their drugs and able to control attacks within a week of starting. Or that 'within a few weeks you will be able to live without medication and without asthma attacks'.

The reality is slightly less remarkable, though it is still impressive. In an 'open' study in Australia (this is a simple type of study, not made under rigorous scientific conditions) the Buteyko trainers reported that about 85 per cent of people going through the programme reduced their use of reliever inhalers, while 75 per cent had fewer asthma symptoms and 51 per cent found they could control all or most attacks.

In a more thorough scientific study of the Buteyko Method,

asthmatics were trained according to the normal Buteyko regime by an experienced Buteyko practitioner, and the results studied by Dr Simon Bowler and other doctors at Mater Hospital in Brisbane. They found that the overall use of reliever inhalers (e.g. Ventolin) by those trained in Buteyko, dropped substantially during the treatment programme and was still much lower three months later. On average, those who did the Buteyko training also felt a little better, but there was no change in their peak-flow or other tests that measure narrowing of the airways. This study averaged out the results for the whole group, so it is impossible to say what percentage of people benefited. However, there were clearly some asthmatics who did not benefit much, because 15 per cent were admitted to hospital with a severe asthma attack during the trial, and 30 per cent needed a course of steroid tablets during the eight months following the course.

In other words, Buteyko *does* work well for many asthmatics – but some of the amazing claims made by Buteyko practitioners are unjustified. The study also shows that, even though many of the asthmatics were using fewer reliever drugs after the course and feeling more in control of attacks, they still had narrow airways – just as narrow as before. This makes it clear that Professor Buteyko's claim to have discovered the *fundamental cause* of asthma is greatly exaggerated.

He has discovered something of great interest and usefulness, but it is neither the cause of asthma, nor a complete cure. The most likely explanation for the success of the Buteyko Method is that mouth-breathing is more of a problem for asthmatics than doctors thought, and there are many more hyperventilators among asthmatics (without any obvious symptoms of hyperventilation) than most doctors previously realized. In fact, some orthodox doctors had long been making this claim. Dr Claude Lum, a consultant chest physician, writing in 1987, stated that 'Most asthmatics breathe like hyperventilators . . .'

Dangerous advice
Some of the advice given by Professor Buteyko is positively dangerous – for example, according to one of Buteyko's followers, Alexander Stalmatski, the Professor advises you to refuse oxygen if you are taken to hospital with a severe asthma attack. He claims that the blood has plenty of oxygen even during an asthma attack, but that the oxygen cannot be off-loaded to the rest of the body because of a lack of carbon dioxide. This is simply wrong. Measurements show that the level of

oxygen in the blood is extremely low during a severe asthma attack. This lack of oxygen is the main cause of death from asthma during a fatal attack – refusing oxygen could kill you.

Another Buteyko suggestion is that you should not try to rid yourself of accumulated mucus on the chest because this 'protects you' against losing too much carbon dioxide. This is also mistaken. Mucus narrows the airways, and for some asthmatics it can even block an airway completely, causing the collapse of the part of the lung served by that airway. This is a serious and potentially damaging complication of asthma – don't risk it.

The claim, made by some Buteyko teachers, that inhaled steroids will make you more vulnerable to chest infections, is also wrong (see pp. 238–9).

Practising the Buteyko Method

You must get your doctor's permission before starting, and you should be careful to keep up your preventer drugs throughout. Keep your reliever inhaler handy while doing the exercises just in case they provoke an asthma attack. If after doing the exercises for a few weeks, you are feeling much better and want to reduce your dose of preventer, it is vital to talk to your doctor first.

The basic Buteyko exercises are:

1. First, unblock your nose. Sit or stand still and breathe normally. Wait until your breathing is steady before you begin. At the end of an ordinary out-breath, close your mouth and hold your nose. Stay like this for as long as you can without discomfort, while nodding your head, or walking around the room, or, if you are young and fit, while walking upstairs or squatting-then-standing several times. (Experiment with the different options to see which suits you best.) When you need to breathe in, stop all activity and release your nose while keeping your mouth firmly shut. Breathe in slowly through the nose. Repeat the exercise if your nose becomes blocked again.

2. Next check how long you can comfortably wait between your out-breath and your in-breath. Buteyko practitioners call this the 'control pause'. Sit in a relaxed posture in an

upright chair. Breathe out normally, then in and out again.
(Don't overdo it – you are not trying to empty your lungs.)
Hold your nose and count the number of seconds until you
feel uncomfortable and need to breathe in again. When you
do inhale, breathe slowly and calmly through your nose. If
you gasp for breath, or it takes more than a couple of breaths
to recover, you have waited too long. Buteyko practitioners
believe the control pause should be 40–60 seconds, and that
anything less than 30 seconds indicates a need for Buteyko
training. They suggest that you repeat this test before and
after you do the daily exercises, to check your progress.

All Buteyko teachers teach clearing of the nose and measuring the
control pause, but there are different versions of the other daily
Buteyko exercises:

- One version is known as 'shallow breathing' and tells you
  simply to sit still for three minutes and restrict the depth of
  your breathing a little, to the extent that you feel slightly
  hungry for air. Gradually build up to doing this for five
  minutes. Stop immediately if you feel unwell or have any
  visual disturbances. When you complete the exercise, it
  should take only 30 seconds to get back to feeling normal –
  if the recovery period is any longer, you have been overdoing
  it. This exercise should be done twice a day at first, building up
  to six times in each session, with the whole session repeated
  three times a day. Once there is a sustained improvement in
  the asthma, the number of repeats can be reduced. Note that
  this shallow breathing is just an exercise which, according to
  Buteyko teachers, will adjust the body's response to levels of
  carbon dioxide in the blood. Trying to practise shallow breathing all the time is *not* the objective and would be bad for you.
- A second version of the daily exercises consists of breathing
  normally, then stopping for as long as possible at the end of an
  out-breath. When you cannot continue with this any longer,
  begin breathing in (through the nose), but do so very gradually, with a series of small breaths. Return to breathing
  normally for five to ten minutes, concentrating on taking
  shallow breaths. When you feel fully recovered, repeat the
  exercise. This exercise is recommended several times a day.

- A third version of the daily exercises (recommended for children but also useful for some adults in place of the exercises above) instructs the asthmatic to place a finger along the top lip under the nose, breathe normally and to notice how the breath feels on the finger. Then try to make the breath so gentle that the finger can no longer feel anything. At the same time, try to make the breath very quiet, so that it cannot be heard at all. Children should try to sustain this for one or two minutes. Adults should start with three minutes, and build up to five minutes.
- A fourth exercise, designed solely for children, is very similar to the nose-clearing exercise (see above) in which the child holds the nose after an outbreath and walks around the room. After twenty steps, or when it becomes essential to breathe in, the child stops and inhales through the nose. The maximum number of steps allowed increases by ten each day, until it reaches fifty. After a couple of weeks at fifty, the number of steps increases further, to the maximum the child can manage.

With all these exercises, adult asthmatics should measure the control pause before and after each session. Children may not be able to measure the control pause easily.

Other Buteyko recommendations include:
- Breathe through the nose, not the mouth.
- Suppress the urge to gasp for air.
- Breathe less deeply whenever you think of it during the day.
- Sleep on your side, not your back, to encourage nose-breathing during the night.
- Cover the mouth with tape at night to prevent mouth-breathing. We think this could be dangerous but Buteyko teachers claim it is safe, providing you have not been drinking heavily and are not feeling nauseous. They say that, if you feel breathless, you will automatically pull the tape off in your sleep, and suggest using Magic Tape or the paper-based surgical tape sold by chemists, both of which come off easily. For children, they recommend using a long strip of tape running vertically from the top lip down onto the neck, to eliminate the chance of the child swallowing or inhaling the tape while asleep. We think it best not to use tape at all for sleeping children.

We have some concern about suppressing the urge to take a deep breath occasionally. This could, in some asthmatics, make the airways contract even more. As already described (see pp. 418–9) taking a deep in-breath helps the airways of non-asthmatics to open up, and while this response is absent in some asthmatics (an abnormality that contributes to their asthma) it does occur in others. For them, taking a deep but slow breath from time to time, when they feel the need, is probably a good idea, as long as the normal pattern of breathing is smooth, slow and regular, and they are breathing with the diaphragm. However, the large deep 'sighing breaths' typical of hyperventilators (see p. 420) are not healthy.

This difference of opinion reflects a fundamental disagreement between the Buteyko Method and the orthodox medical approach to hyperventilation. According to orthodox teaching, the important thing for those who are overbreathing is to slow the breathing down, not to make it more shallow. In fact, doctors would claim that many hyperventilators need to take slightly *deeper* breaths using the diaphragm, but to take them much more slowly.

One of the strange things about the Buteyko programme, in its original form, is that there is no training aimed at using the diaphragm rather than the upper chest to breathe. This is considered crucially important by conventional doctors treating hyperventilation. More recently, some Buteyko teachers have begun to include training in diaphragm breathing.

It would be enormously useful if doctors and medical experts on respiration could look more closely at the Buteyko Method, try to understand how it fits into the conventional picture of hyperventilation, and incorporate the useful aspects of the training into orthodox treatment.

Martial arts

Many asthmatics will tell you that learning a martial art, such as aikido or judo, helped them get control over their asthma. T'ai chi, which is basically a martial art, though a rather quiet and meditative one, has the same reputation. There have not been many scientific trials, but one carried out in Germany did show that children with asthma improved when they attended judo classes.

The benefits of these oriental martial arts probably comes from the emphasis on calm, steady, slow breathing – the common ingredient in all successful breathing exercises for asthma. Practising such breathing while in motion may also be helpful – one of the problems with asthma is that the chest and diaphragm can become locked and rigid, because there is tension and anxiety about breathing.

Singing lessons and learning a wind instrument

Many asthmatics report that learning to sing or play a wind instrument made a huge difference to them, and brought their asthma under control. Playing the flute has a particularly good reputation as an asthma treatment, and this has been studied by doctors in Slovakia.

Exercises to improve the out-breath

There are several simple exercises which are said to help asthmatics improve their ability to breathe out fully. Practising these exercises when you feel well pays dividends later, when you suffer an asthma attack. Some of these are adapted from yoga breathing techniques.

All the exercises should be done in a relaxed way without forcing or undue effort:

- Breathe out slowly and make a soft humming sound. Prolong the out-breath as much as possible without strain.
- Repeat this exercise, but make a buzzing sound. Listen to the sound you make. Notice when it changes and when you become breathless – stop then, pause for a moment, and breathe in gently.
- Pretend there's a candle in front of you and blow it out. Use your abdomen (belly) muscles to give a sharp out-breath – your abdomen should contract as you blow. Your upper chest should not be doing the work, and the out-breath should be a relatively quiet 'huff' (a loud 'whoosh' means you're using your upper chest). The in-breath should bounce back in naturally at the end of the out-breath. Repeat as many times as you can but stop as soon as you feel breathless. Build up to doing 30 or 40 in a row.
- Breathe in, then purse your lips and breathe out gradually in a succession of little puffs. Make the out-breath work against the pressure from your lips, using your abdomen to provide the force for the out-breath.

Some asthmatics find that they can abort an impending asthma attack by focusing on relaxed breathing out, emptying the lungs as much as possible, but very gently, and then trying to breathe in slowly and calmly, using the diaphragm.

Did you know?

Researchers in Germany tried out a device called a Nozovent on people with nocturnal asthma. This device keeps the nostrils open, so that people breathe through the nose rather than the mouth. Using the Nozovent halved the number of nights when these asthmatics were woken up by asthma attacks.

Exercises to strengthen the breathing muscles

Several different studies have shown benefits for asthmatics from increasing the strength of their breathing muscles.

If you are doing these or any other breathing exercises, make sure you do them in clean air, as free as possible from any allergens to which you are sensitive. Make sure you are as relaxed as possible while doing them, breathe slowly and calmly, and never force your breathing.

Before you start the programme, check that you do know how to breathe with your diaphragm (see pp. 421–2) and that you are not hyperventilating. You should also ensure that you are breathing through your nose, not your mouth.

The Powerbreathe device

This is a device which strengthens the breathing muscles (see pp. 414–5) by getting you to breathe in against resistance. The amount of resistance is gradually increased over the days and weeks, like slowly increasing the weights in a weightlifter's daily regime. Research in Israel has shown great benefit for asthmatics from strengthening the muscles that draw air into the lungs. They suffered fewer asthma symptoms, used fewer puffs of reliever drugs, and had fewer visits to hospital. Some were able to stop taking steroids.

The inventor of the Powerbreathe points out that you can achieve the same effect by inhaling through a small hole and progressively reducing the size of the hole, but suggests that the Powerbreathe is easier to use, and gives you more idea of your own progress.

If you buy a Powerbreathe (see pp. 469–70), make sure that you don't start hyperventilating. Breathe out thoroughly as well, pause slightly before your next in-breath, and always keep the breathing slow and steady – no gasping or straining.

A scientist in India, Dr Virendra Singh, has invented a device that does much the same thing as the Powerbreathe, but also imposes a pattern of breathing taught by yoga, where the out-breath lasts twice as long as the in-breath. He has shown that this produces excellent results for asthmatics, especially if the air inhaled through the device is also warm and moist. Unfortunately, this device (called, mysteriously, the Pink City Lung Exerciser) is not available commercially, but you could apply the findings by learning yoga breathing (see p. 397) as well as using the Powerbreathe. Steam inhalations to loosen mucus (see p. 349) could be used as a separate treatment.

Operatic exercises for the diaphragm
These exercises were originally devised for opera singers. When several asthmatics who had undergone operatic training reported a great improvement in their asthma, Dr Michel Girodo and other researchers at the University of Ottawa in Canada carried out a full scientific trial with asthmatics.

They found that, after doing these exercises for four months, the asthmatics were, on average, using 50 per cent fewer drugs. Their asthma attacks were much less severe than before, allowing them to engage in three times as much physical activity. Unfortunately, they lost all these improvements within two months of stopping the exercise programme – so if you are going to embark on these exercises, remember that you have to keep them up to reap long-term benefits.

The exercises should be practised every day. The number of repeats given for each exercise is the number you should try to achieve at first. Once you have been practising these exercises for a few days, you should be able to increase the number of repeats.

If you are the kind of person who always tries very hard and 'pushes yourself', take it gently here. Do not force yourself at any point in these exercises: and if you feel at all unwell, stop and try again later.

Exercise 1: Clearing the nose

Keep your mouth closed throughout. Sit on the floor and close your right nostril with your right thumb. Breathe out via the left nostril.

Close your left nostril with your right index finger and breathe in via the right nostril.

Do this fast with no break between the out-breath and in-breath. Perform ten breaths in all. Rest, then repeat using the left hand and starting with an out-breath via the right nostril.

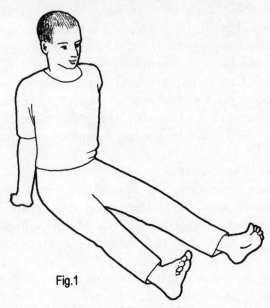

Fig.1

Exercise 2

Sit with your legs slightly apart, back straight, shoulders pulled back, arms held close against the chest, and hands on the floor (Fig. 1).

Look straight ahead and breathe out via the mouth, then in via the nose. The breathing count is fast: 1, 2, 1, 2. Take six to ten breaths, then rest.

Relax the arms, bend over, gently resting the elbows and arms on your legs, and empty your lungs slowly via the mouth. This is the **resting position**.

Exercise 3

Sit with your back straight, looking straight ahead, and pull your shoulders back.

Raise your elbows at the sides, then bring your hands in and place the palms across your chest with the fingers interlocked (Fig. 2).

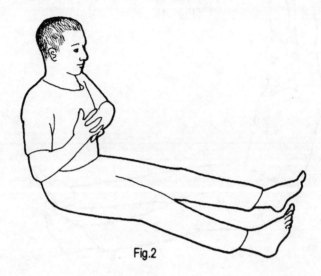

Fig.2

Breathe out via the mouth while extending your arms in front of you and turning your hands so the palms are outwards, with the fingers still interlocked (Fig. 3).

Bring your arms back to the initial position (Fig. 2).

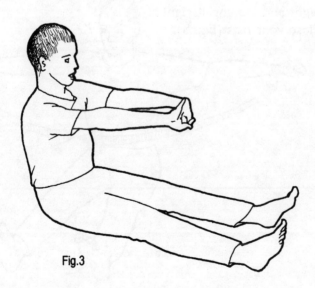

Fig.3

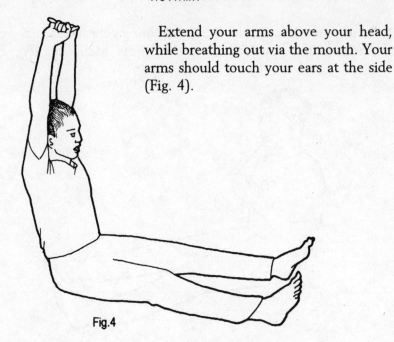

Extend your arms above your head, while breathing out via the mouth. Your arms should touch your ears at the side (Fig. 4).

Fig.4

Return to the initial position (Fig. 2), breathing in via the nose. Repeat the whole exercise five times, to a fast count. Return to the resting position.

Exercise 4

Sit with your arms outstretched, back straight and looking straight ahead. Close your fists (Fig. 5).

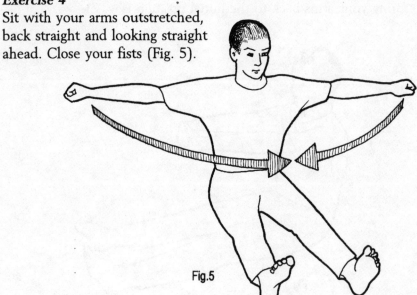

Fig.5

Bring your fists together in front of you, keeping your arms straight while breathing out via the mouth.

Return the arms to the initial position, breathing in via the nose. Repeat five times to a fast count. Return to the resting position and breathe slowly.

Exercise 5

Take up the position shown for Exercise 2 (Fig. 1). Keep your head straight: do not move it during the breathing cycle.

Breathe out via the mouth for five seconds.

Close your mouth, keep completely still but relaxed, and wait for three seconds.

Breathe in through your nose for three seconds.

Do this exercise four or five times at first, then increase later. Return to the resting position and breathe slowly.

Exercise 6

Lie with your head, back and feet in firm contact with the floor. Your knees and feet should be together with both knees bent, your arms straight out at either side with fingers together (Fig. 6).

Bring your arms down to your sides, while breathing out via the mouth.

Return your arms to the initial position, breathing in via the nose. Repeat five times to a rapid count. Aim to gradually increase this to ten times.

Rest with your arms by your sides, breathing slowly through the mouth.

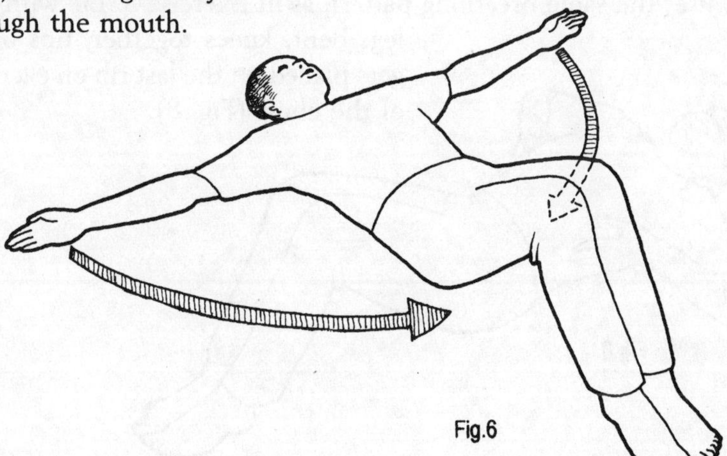

Fig.6

Exercise 7
Lie with the small of your back pressing hard into the floor, legs bent, feet and knees together. Hold your head with your hands at the base of the skull and smile (Fig. 7).

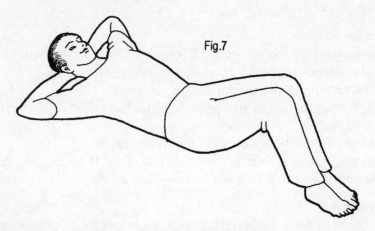

Fig.7

Breathe out rapidly and loudly while raising the head, trying to touch your chin and even your elbows against your chest.

Breathe in via the nose as your head returns to the initial position. Your breath must be noisy and you should try to smile throughout. Check that your back is still pressed into the floor.

Repeat ten times, then rest with your arms beside your body, breathing slowly via the mouth. Repeat the whole exercise.

Exercise 8
This uses the same breathing pattern as in Exercise 5. Lie with your legs bent, knees together, tips of fingers placed on the last rib on each side of the chest (Fig. 8).

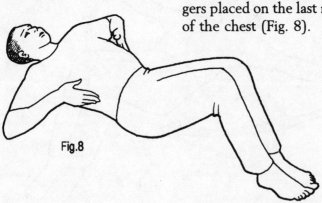

Fig.8

Breathe out via the mouth (five seconds), at the same time raising your head and placing your chin on your chest.

Keep your chin on your chest, your back well in contact with floor, and hold for three seconds, without moving.

With your chin still on your chest, push your legs up towards the ceiling while breathing in via the nose (Fig. 9). The in-breath should take three seconds.

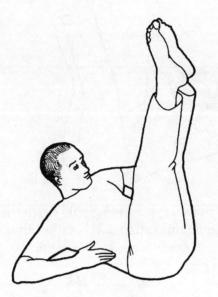

Fig.9

Return to the initial position, breathing out via the mouth for five seconds. Rest and breathe normally.

Repeat the exercise three to five times. Aim to increase to eight times.

Exercise 9

Lie on your back with your legs held vertically. Push your back into the floor. Hold the back of your head with your hands and lift your head so that your chin touches your chest (Fig. 10).

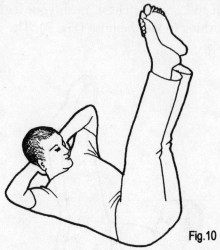

Fig.10

Drop your foot – if possible your heel should touch the back of your thigh (Fig. 11). As you do this you should breathe out noisily via your mouth. Let your leg bounce back to the vertical position while breathing in via the nose.

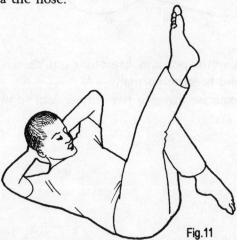

Fig.11

Repeat with the right leg, then the left leg again. Do this 10–12 times.
Relax with your legs down, arms along the side of the body, and breathe slowly.

Exercise 10
Lie with your legs bent, arms by your sides (Fig. 12).

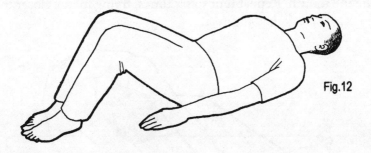

Fig.12

Raise your hips very slowly, breathing out through your mouth for five seconds. You should be supporting yourself on your arms and shoulders (Fig. 13). Your knees and feet are together. Hold this position, and your breath, for three seconds.

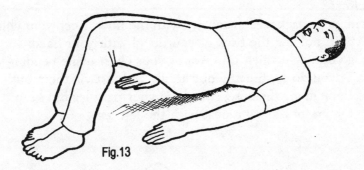

Fig.13

Breathe in through your nose for three seconds as you return to the starting position.

Do the exercise four to five times at first, then relax with your legs and arms down, breathing slowly.

Exercise 11
Sit in the position shown for Exercise 2 (Fig. 1) but raise your arms vertically, interlock your fingers and turn your palms towards the ceiling. Stretch upwards with your hands, so that your upper arms touch your ears.

Breathing out through the mouth, bend over on to one leg (Fig. 14). Now swing your body horizontally so that you are over the other leg, breathing in via the nose. Swing back again to the first leg, breathing out via the mouth. Repeat four to six times, trying to flex closer to the knee each time. Relax and rest.

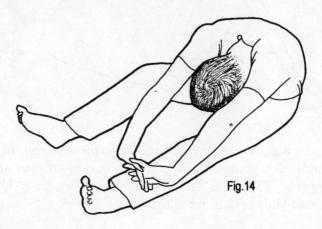

Fig.14

Exercise 12

Lie with your back well in contact with the floor. Keep your chin on your chest, holding the back of your head with your hands.

Bring your right thigh up towards your chest while bending your knee. As you do so, breathe out noisily and fast via the mouth.

Breathing in via the nose, straighten your right leg but keep it just above the ground. Now repeat with the left leg.

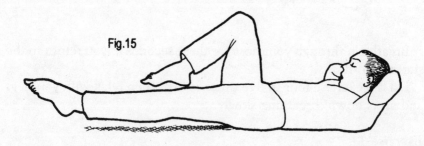

Fig.15

Bend and straighten each leg alternately (Fig. 15), repeating eight to ten times. Keep both legs off the floor throughout, and pull up hard on your head.

Exercise 13

This uses the same breathing pattern as Exercise 5. Lie with your knees bent, and your head, back and feet in firm contact with the floor (Fig. 12).

During the next part of the exercise, breathe out to a count of five seconds. Slowly bring your legs towards your chest, at the same time raising your head from the floor and placing your chin on your chest. Grasp your legs with your hands, getting your chin as close to your knees as possible (Fig. 16)

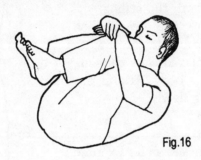

Fig.16

Stay in this position for three seconds while holding your breath. As you return to the starting position, breathe in to a count of three seconds. Repeat the exercise three to five times, then rest.

Exercise 14

Stand with your legs shoulder-width apart, back straight, shoulders pulled back and arms above your head. Interlock your fingers and turn your palms towards the ceiling. Your upper arms should be touching your ears (Fig. 17).

Breathe out for five seconds, hold for three seconds, then breathe in for three seconds. Keep still as you do this, and breathe with your whole body, holding your arms up towards the ceiling.

Repeat three to five times, then gently bend downwards, as low as you can, arms relaxed and dangling on each side of the body. Rest in this position, breathing slowly.

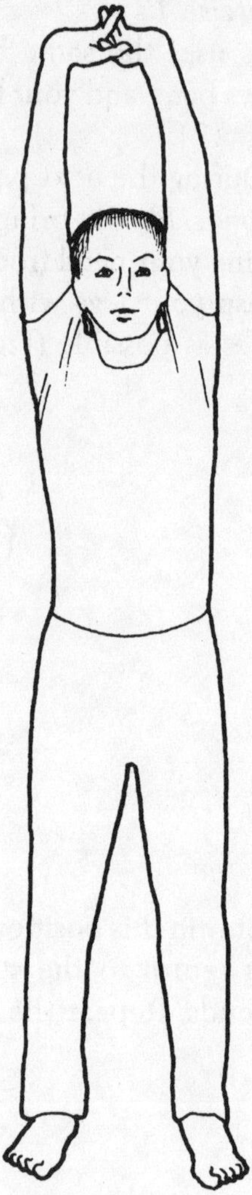

Exercise 15

Start in the position shown for Exercise 14 (Fig. 17). Bend down slowly, breathing out for five seconds. Do not force your back if it feels uncomfortable. If your palms touch the floor, push downwards.

Hold this position, and your breath, for three seconds.

Come back up to the starting position, while breathing in for three seconds.

Repeat three to five times, then rest in the same position as at the end of Exercise 14.

Fig.17

Exercise 16

Start on the floor with your legs bent, knees and feet together, arms close beside your body (Fig. 12).

This exercise follows a different breathing pattern: 3–3–3 (out-hold-in).

Sit up quickly and swing your arms up towards the ceiling, while breathing in (three seconds).

Your arms should stretch up straight and touch your ears at the side (Fig. 18). Hold this position, and your breath, for three seconds.

Return slowly to the starting position, breathing in for three seconds. Repeat three to five times, then rest, either lying on the floor or in the resting position (see p. 432).

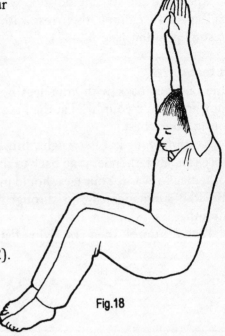

Fig.18

Exercise 17

Lie flat, legs straight, with your head and back in good contact with the floor, arms pointing straight upwards (Fig. 19).

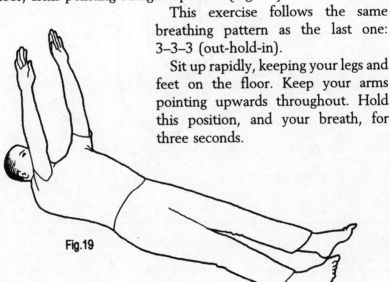

This exercise follows the same breathing pattern as the last one: 3–3–3 (out-hold-in).

Sit up rapidly, keeping your legs and feet on the floor. Keep your arms pointing upwards throughout. Hold this position, and your breath, for three seconds.

Fig.19

Return to the starting position while breathing in (three seconds).

Repeat five times, then rest, either lying on the floor or in the resting position (see p. 432).

Exercise 18

Lie on your back with your legs held vertically and toes stretched upwards. Hold your head at the base of the skull, and push your chin on to your chest.

Keeping your knees straight, bring one leg forward towards your face (Fig. 20), then let it go back to the starting position and bring the other leg forward. Your legs should move with a fast scissoring action. Breathe spontaneously, in through the nose and out through the mouth.

Kick 20 times, then rest, lying flat and breathing slowly.

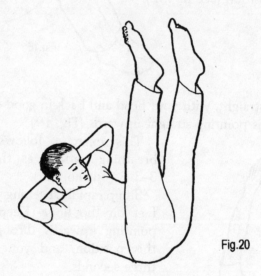

Fig.20

Holidays and asthma

Holidays should be problem-free if you get your asthma under good control in advance, by using your preventer regularly.

Take spare inhalers (kept in a separate bag) in case any get lost or stolen, or you get stranded and have to stay longer. Dry powder inhalers may be affected by very humid climates (see p. 379). If travelling abroad, check with your travel agent that your nebulizer will work on the local voltage. Consider taking a spacer (see p. 380) for emergencies. Choose your holiday insurance carefully (see p. 235).

Flying need not be a problem. The air pressure in the cabin does not fall low enough to trouble most asthmatics. Take your inhalers on board in your hand luggage – the ban on aerosols does not apply to them. If you might need to use a nebulizer during the flight, check in advance that the airline is agreeable, by contacting the airline yourself – don't rely on the travel agent. Some airlines have a more sympathetic attitude than others (a few even carry their own nebulizers) so shop around. If you are affected by perfumes and cigarette smoke, or are ultra-sensitive to peanuts, check whether the airline can provide clean air, free of these hazards. Some countries demand that passengers be sprayed with insecticide on arrival, which might trigger asthma attacks: check in advance with the airline. Anyone with food allergy should inform the airline directly, not the travel agent.

Plan your holiday to avoid allergens, especially pollen (see pp. 177–8) and house dust mite (see p. 116 and p. 154). Some asthmatics with mite allergy take their own bedding or covers with them. A no-smoking hotel is a good idea.

Holiday activities in cold air, such as skiing, can be problematic (see p. 294–5). Some countries ban asthmatics from scuba diving completely, even though they have good qualifications obtained elsewhere (e.g. Britain). Check with your travel agent or holiday company before booking a diving holiday.

As soon as you arrive at your destination, check that the telephone works and find out about the nearest doctor, hospital and ambulance service, just in case you have an attack (see p. 50).

METHODS THAT PROMOTE CALMNESS AND RELAXATION

Feeling calm and in control is extremely valuable during an asthma attack. You can cultivate this calmness in various different ways, so that it comes more easily when you need it. This is valuable for all asthmatics, whether adults or children. The parents of asthmatic children can also benefit from learning to relax and take the anxieties of asthma in their stride. This can make all the difference during asthma attacks, when a calm adult is helpful to a child, but a panicky adult is positively harmful.

In the long term, if asthmatics become more relaxed this may result in their asthma gradually becoming less troublesome anyway, especially if they learn to breathe more slowly and smoothly.

There are many different approaches to cultivating calmness and relaxation. Indeed, some of the techniques described elsewhere in this chapter, such as acupuncture and yoga, will also promote relaxation and calm breathing.

The therapies described here fall into three broad groups, although there are no sharp dividing lines between them, and what you get out of them depends very much on the sort of person you are:

- Some of the methods listed here are self-help relaxation techniques which you are taught, such as relaxation exercises, meditation, biofeedback or autogenic training. With these approaches, you have to do the 'work' (that is, learning to relax) for yourself.
- Others are forms of therapy in which the asthmatic's role is far more passive, as with relaxing massage, reflexology or short courses of hypnotherapy aimed at inducing relaxation. Here the therapist does the work.
- Others take a more fundamental approach to the internal causes of tension – they try to deal with more deep-seated emotional problems that are blocking your attempts to relax and control your asthma. These include the various brands of psychotherapy and psychoanalysis, long-term hypnotherapy with psychotherapeutic aims, and biodynamic massage.

Generally speaking, if you want to learn to relax, the first group of methods are probably going to be more helpful than the second group in the long run, because taking an active role puts you in charge of your asthma symptoms. This will be very good for your self-confidence and sense of control over asthma. However, relaxation treatments in which you have a passive role can be very helpful for managing bursts of short-term stress, or as a 'starter' to calm you down a bit before beginning some other kind of treatment.

The third type of approach may help you a lot, especially if you have tried and failed with relaxation exercises, or if you suspect some strong psychological element in your asthma (see pp. 34–41). By tackling the problems at a deeper level, you are likely to achieve a more profound and long-lasting solution to your difficulties.

Relaxation exercises

There are many different ways of improving your ability to relax. One is to contract and then release muscles methodically in each part of the body, starting with the hands. One trial with asthmatic children found that repeated sessions of this training increased their peak flow by as much as 32 per cent. Some children responded much better than others.

Another relaxation technique uses guided imagery and asks you to lie still and picture the scenes described ('The golden sunlight filters through the leaves of the trees as you slowly float downstream . . .' etc.), in order to induce a more relaxed state of mind. This works for some people, but not others. There are many relaxation tapes available which employ guided imagery. If you cannot find any in local bookshops or other outlets, they can be bought by mail order (see p. 482).

There are also tapes of music that are intended to produce a relaxed or meditative state of mind. Some of these are quite good and, if nothing else, they will probably help you get to sleep.

Autogenic Training

This technique requires you to concentrate on different parts of your body in turn and imagine them growing warm and heavy. Beginning with 'My right arm is heavy and warm . . .' (repeated three times, either out loud or in your head) you work your way through 'My left arm . . .', 'Both my arms . . .', 'My right leg . . .', 'My left leg . . .', 'Both my legs . . .', 'My head-and-neck . . .', and finally 'My torso . . .' At the end you should feel more relaxed, and you stay quietly in this state for several minutes. One of the merits of autogenic training is that you do the exercises in different positions, so it teaches you to relax in a sitting position as well as lying down, which can be useful in everyday life.

By repeating this exercise two or three times a day, most people eventually achieve greater relaxation, and the sense that they can calm down quite quickly whenever they need to. It sounds simple, and you could in theory teach it to yourself, but it is useful to have a class to go to regularly and a teacher to encourage you and help with any problems that arise.

For those with asthma, teachers of autogenic training may add more specific lines at the end of the exercise, such as 'My breathing is calm and regular' or 'My breathing is smooth and easy.'

Autogenic training can be seen as a kind of self-hypnosis technique. It can also incorporate some elements of psychotherapy, for those who have strong emotional reactions during the training, although teachers vary in the extent to which they include this.

One study showed that asthmatics who practised autogenic training for eight months had better lung function, as measured by forced vital capacity and other tests for asthma (see p. 303).

Your local community college, health center, or the Internet can provide information on finding classes.

Meditation

Meditation is a practice that involves stilling the mind – emptying it of thoughts, or focusing it on one simple object, such as a candle flame. This is extremely difficult for most people at first, but with practice it gradually becomes easier. The mind becomes clearer and more focused, and this leads to an increase in calmness and the ability to cope with stress.

There are many different forms of meditation, with different psychological outcomes. Most are part of a spiritual tradition such as Zen Buddhism, Tibetan Buddhism, Hinduism or Daoism. Meditation also forms part of the practice of yoga (when taught in its full form) and some martial arts.

If you want to learn to meditate, there are many books and tapes on this subject (see p. 482), or you could go to classes in a local Buddhist centre – these are now found in most parts of the world.

The only form of meditation that has been scientifically tested in relation to asthma is transcendental meditation (TM), which is expensive to learn, being taught by a rather commercialized international organization using local TM teachers. This study showed some benefits to asthmatics for transcendental meditation.

Biofeedback

The most strictly scientific of all alternative treatments, biofeedback simply uses measuring devices to tell you what state some part of your body is in. With this information shown continuously (by swinging needles on dials, or as flashing lights or bleeping sound signals) you can gradually learn to influence the signal and so alter that bodily state, even though it is supposedly under involuntary control. Biofeedback can teach people to lower their blood pressure, reduce the amount of acid produced by the stomach, increase the flow of blood to their hands or regulate their heart rate. Before the invention of biofeedback, scientists believed that such functions were completely beyond voluntary control, even though yoga practitioners had long claimed to be able to influence them.

Scientific trials with instruments that measure the diameter of the airways have shown that asthmatics can quickly learn to influence the airway muscles and so open up narrowed airways. This exciting discovery has, unfortunately, never been developed for general use by asthmatics. The bulky laboratory apparatus that measures airway diameter would have to be turned into a compact and inexpensive machine that could serve as a widely available training device.

In the meantime, asthmatics can still benefit from the relaxation training that biofeedback offers. Most biofeedback classes use machines that measure the electrical resistance of the skin to teach relaxation, or electronic devices measuring output from the brain. The machines measuring brain output can also be used to teach people to enter a state of mind similar to meditation, which in turn produces profound relaxation.

Massage

Most forms of massage are relaxing to some extent, and if you go for regular massage treatments it could improve your general sense of calmness and ability to cope. Massage may also help with loosening up tensions in the neck, chest and back, which develop as a result of asthma attacks (see p. 400).

Massage is often accompanied by use of aromatherapy oils, and you should bear in mind that some of these can provoke asthma attacks (see p. 232).

Biodynamic massage

Biodynamic massage involves a much gentler touch than other forms of massage and has different objectives, in that it aims to deal with bodily tensions that are a result of blocked emotions. It can be a very powerful way of accessing the source of recurrent emotional difficulties. This approach may be particularly suitable for some asthmatics. It has more in common with psychotherapy than with ordinary forms of massage.

Reflexology

This form of therapy is based on the belief that stimulating specific zones on the soles of the feet can induce healing processes, both physical and emotional. Many claims are made for reflexology, but one of the most convincing is that it induces relaxation. However, a study carried out by Danish reflexologists showed that there was no improvement in asthma symptoms from reflexology – not even, strangely enough, any placebo effect.

Hypnotherapy

Some forms of hypnotherapy are quite brief (one to six sessions) and use hypnotic trances, combined with suggestions from the therapist, to achieve relaxation or a change in personal habits (for example, giving up smoking). Other forms are more long-term and use hypnosis as a means towards achieving personal insight into emotional problems. This approach has much more in common with psychotherapy.

Studies of hypnotherapy suggest that it can help some asthmatics. Those who are easily hypnotized (more suggestible – see pp. 35–6) are more likely to benefit.

Make sure you get a really well-qualified hypnotherapist. There are a great many about who have had very inadequate training. If possible, choose someone who is also a qualified doctor (see p. 463).

Some doctors have expressed concern that hypnotherapy may reduce people's awareness of asthma symptoms without giving them any actual improvement in their airways, which could put them at risk of developing a severe asthma attack. With this in mind, keep up your peak-flow readings while undergoing hypnotherapy, so that you have an early warning of worsening asthma symptoms.

Psychotherapy and counselling

Some people find any kind of relaxation technique or meditation difficult or even upsetting. Slowing down forces them to think about things that they were trying not to think about, and all kinds of negative emotions bubble to the surface.

If this happens to you, you should not lose heart, because you have at least begun to identify the problems which may be making your asthma worse. Rather than giving up completely on relaxation, it makes sense to try something that will actually address these underlying difficulties, such as psychotherapy. Ultimately, it is much more painful and exhausting to keep repressing unpleasant feelings or memories than it is to bring them out into the open, in a safe and supportive situation, where you can deal with them constructively. Sorting out such problems allows you to move on and live life more fully – and it may well improve your asthma symptoms.

There are a million-and-one different brands of therapy to choose from these days, and the range may seem baffling. The good news here is that recent research shows they *all* work, and they all work to about the same extent, despite profound differences in approach. So choose something that appeals to you instinctively, or (better still) choose a therapist who has been recommended by someone you trust. Research also shows that the one factor of overwhelming importance is good rapport between therapist and client. It seems to be that, rather than any specific theory or method, which actually produces the good effects of therapy.

Appendix 1

Useful addresses

ASTHMA AND ALLERGY SUPPORT ORGANIZATIONS

United Kingdom
National Asthma Campaign
Providence House
Providence Place
London N1 0NT
Tel: 0171 226 2260
Fax: 0171 704 0740
Web-site: *www.asthma.org.uk*
Helpline: 0845 7 010203
The helpline is staffed from 9 a.m. to 7 p.m. by trained asthma nurses who can answer queries about asthma. Calls are charged at local rates. There are local NAC groups, free leaflets on various topics, a regular magazine, special publications for teenagers, local swimming clubs, and holiday schemes for children with asthma and/or eczema.

The British Allergy Foundation
Deepdene House
30 Bellgrove Road
Welling
Kent DA16 3PY
The main service offered is a telephone help-line, where callers can obtain immediate advice from an experienced allergy nurse. The help-line is open from 9 a.m.–5 p.m., Monday to Friday, on 0891 516500. Calls cost 50p per minute, including VAT, at all times. Proceeds go to support the work of BAF.

There are also support groups throughout the UK, which organize regular meetings and can give advice.

The National Society for Research into Allergy
PO Box 45
Hinckley
Leics LE10 1JY
Tel: 01455 851546
This organization takes a broader and less conventional view of allergy than the British Allergy Foundation. There is a quarterly magazine, and an advice service which can put you in touch with a suitable medical practitioner in your area.

The Anaphylaxis Campaign
The Ridges
2 Clockhouse Road
Farnborough
Hampshire GU14 7QY
Tel: 01252 542029
Fax: 01252 377140
Web-site: *www.anaphylaxis.org.uk/whom.html*
A truly excellent campaigning organization that has achieved far greater recognition of the problems of, for example, peanut allergy. Many lives must have been saved by their hard work in making caterers and food manufacturers aware of the risks. The newsletter will keep you up to date with potential new hazards.

Republic of Ireland
Asthma Society of Ireland
Eden House
15–17 Eden Quay
Dublin 1
Tel: 1 878 8511

Australia
National Asthma Campaign
Level 1
1 Palmerston Crescent
South Melbourne
Victoria 3205

Tel: 03 9214 1476
Fax: 03 9214 1400
Hotline: 1800 032 495 (for ordering publications)
E-mail: *nac@netlink.com.au*

Asthma Foundation of Western Australia
61 Heytesbury Road
Subiaco
Western Australia 6008
Tel: 08 9382 1666
Fax: 08 9388 1469

Asthma Australia
69 Flemington Road
North Melbourne
Victoria 3051
Tel: 03 9326 7088
Fax: 03 9326 7055

New Zealand

The Asthma and Respiratory Foundation of New Zealand
Rossmore House
123 Moleworth Street
PO Box 1459
Wellington
New Zealand
Tel: 04 499 4592
Fax: 04 499 4594
E-mail: *arf@asthmanz.co.nz*
Web-site: *www.asthmanz.co.nz*
Produces various useful leaflets and a newsletter. There are also local
asthma associations throughout New Zealand, and this central orga-
nization can put you in touch with these.

Canada
Allergy Asthma Information Association
30 Eglinton Avenue West
Suite 750
Mississauga

Ontario L5R 3E7
Tel: 905 712 2242
Fax: 905 712 2245
The central office can put you in touch with the office for your region.

The Asthma Society of Canada
425–130 Bridgeland Avenue
Toronto
Ontario M6A 1Z4
Tel: 416 787 4050
Fax: 416 787 5807
E-mail: *asthma@myna.com*
Asthma Infoline: 1 800 787 3880

USA
Asthma and Allergy Foundation of America
1125 Fifteenth Street, NW
Suite 502
Washington, DC 20005
Tel: 202 466 7643
Fax 202 466 8940
Web-site: *www.aafa.org*

Allergy and Asthma Network – Mothers of Asthmatics
2751 Prosperity Avenue
Suite 150
Fairfax
Virginia 22031
Tel: 703 641 9595
Fax: 703 573 7794
Web-site: *www.aanma.org*
Toll-free helpline: 800 878 4403

Asthma Education and Resource Council
5 Bon Air Road
Suite 110
Larkspur
California 94977
Tel: 415 924 3647
Fax: 415 927 7387

National Jewish Medical and Research Centre
1400 Jackson Street
Denver
Colorado 80206
Toll-free helpline: 1 800 222 LUNG

Food Allergy Network
4744 Holly Avenue
Fairfax
Virginia 22030 5647
Tel: 703 691 3179
Fax: 703 691 2713

ASTHMA INFORMATION ON THE INTERNET

There is a staggering amount of information about asthma on the Internet. Much of it is very basic stuff, however, which is already thoroughly covered by this book. There is also some misleading and incorrect information – anyone can put information on to the Internet, with no medical vetting, or even common-sense vetting. So be wary of any sites that have an amateurish feel to them, or are run by one person only. If you are thinking of following advice from any website, talk to your doctor first.

You may find the Internet useful for keeping up with new developments in asthma treatment. Try the following sites:
www.pslgroup.com/docguide.htm (Select 'Search', then search for 'asthma'.)
www.mediconsult.com

For educating children about asthma (not just those who are asthmatic but also, perhaps, their brothers and sisters) try the asthma information aimed at 8- to 15-year-olds on:
www.med.virginia.edu/cmc/tutorials/asthma

For information about specific drugs, the following site may be helpful, but remember that some information may apply only to the USA:
www.intelihealth.com Select 'Drug Search'

One area in which the Internet can be useful is occupational asthma, especially if you are involved in any kind of dispute about what caused your asthma. A good place to start is the excellent web-site maintained by the Department of Public Health Sciences at Edinburgh University:

www.med.ed.ac.uk

This includes a Directory of Internet Sites in Occupational and Environmental Health, which you can use to pursue your particular query or concern.

Australian readers may also like to try the site maintained by the National Occupational Health and Safety Commission of Australia: *www.worksafe.gov.au*

Our favourite web-site by far is created and maintained by Dr Martin Stern of Leicester, a mine of accurate, up-to-date information for those with allergy, asthma and especially anaphylaxis – this site makes you realize how thin and insubstantial most web-sites are. Medical controversies (e.g. about who should carry injectable adrenaline) are argued through fully, in language anyone can understand. There is more information on anaphylaxis here than we were able to include in the book, and it is updated regularly. You can also send queries to Dr Stern. You can find the site on:

www.users.globalnet.co.uk/~aair/anaphylaxis.htm

STOPPING SMOKING

If you are trying to stop smoking you can get encouragement and advice from:

Nicotine Dependence Center
Mayo Clinic
200 First Street SW
Rochester
Minnesota 55095
Tel: 1 800 344 5984
Fax: 507 266 7236
Web-site: *www.mayo.edu / ndc*

If you feel strongly about passive smoking, you might want to join one of these campaigning organizations:

ASH (Action on Smoking and Health)
2013 H Street NW
Washington, D.C. 20006
Tel: 202 659 4310
Web-site: *www.ash.org*

Americans for Nonsmoker's Rights
2530 San Pablo Ave, Suite J
Berkeley
California 94702
Tel: 510 841 3032
Web-site: *www.no-smoke.org*

SOURCES OF USEFUL INFORMATION ABOUT AIR QUALITY

If you are traveling or moving and wish to check the local levels of air pollution, you can write to:

EMPACT Program
Office of Environmental Information
U.S. EPA (2831)
401 M Street SW
Washington, D.C. 20460
Fax: 202 565 1966
Web-site: *www.epa.gov / empact*

The EPA's website, AIRNOW *(www.epa.gov / airnow)*, provides real-time air pollution data by city as well as information about the health and environmental effects of ozone.

POLLEN AND MOULD-SPORE COUNTS

If you are allergic only to grass pollen, the counts given on television or radio may be sufficient. But if you react to other pollens or to mould spores, you will need more detailed information.
In the USA, you can call a toll-free line: 1 800 9 POLLEN for pollen counts and forecasts.

There is also detailed information available on the Internet at:
www.aaaai.org
This site is valuable because it provides separate counts for trees, grasses, 'weeds' and mould spores, and specifies the predominant allergen at the time for different regions of the USA.

EMERGENCY ALERT BRACELETS

Anyone who suffers from anaphylactic shock (see p. 111), or has very severe and sudden asthma attacks, or is allergic to latex (see p. 282) or penicillin, should wear an emergency alert bracelet or pendant. Key medical information is engraved on the bracelet, and there is also a telephone number which gives medical staff access to a computer database where essential medical data about you is available.

These useful items are sold by a non-profit-making company:

MedicAlert Foundation
2323 Colorado Avenue
Turlock
California 95382-2018
Tel: 1 800 IDALERT (1 800 432 5378)
Fax: 209 669 2495
Web-site: *www.medicalert.org*
(In Canada, telephone 416 696 0142.)

FINDING A WELL-QUALIFIED ALTERNATIVE THERAPIST

Personal recommendation is often the best way to find a really good alternative therapist, so ask around locally. The Yellow Pages can also be a good starting point, but do check credentials. With the commoner therapies, such as osteopathy or acupuncture, it is not difficult to find someone locally. But if you are interested in trying the less common approaches—and some of these are extremely helpful for asthma—you may find it impossible to locate anyone. The following contact adresses may be helpful in this case.

Yoga International (www.yimag.com) and *Yoga Journal* (www.yogajournal.com) magazines both provide on-line directories of yoga associations, teachers, and classes as well as helpful information about getting started in a yoga practice of your own. A print version of *Yoga Journal's Source 2000* can be purchased by calling 1 800 I DO YOGA.
For addresses of Feldenkrais teachers, contact:

The Feldenkrais Guild

PO Box 489
Albany
Oregon 97321 0143
Tel: 541 926 0981
Fax: 541 926 0572
E-mail: *feldenkrais@peak.org*
Web-site: *www.feldenkrais.com*
This organization covers the USA and Canada. Their web-site can be
used to obtain addresses of Feldenkrais Guilds in several European
countries.

FINDING AN ALLERGIST

The Physician Referral Database, available on the Internet on
www.aaaai.org can be helpful in finding a well-qualified allergist in the
USA.

FINDING A PSYCHOTHERAPIST OR COUNSELLOR

There is no substitute for a personal recommendation if you are
searching for a good therapist or counsellor. Your family doctor or
friends may be able to recommend someone suitable in your area. A
directory of qualified psychotherapists as well as useful information
on various aspects of psychological health are available from:

American Psychological Association

750 First Street NW
Washington, D.C. 20002
Tel: 202 336 5500
Web-site: *www.apa.org*

If you have access to the Internet, you can contact the United States
Co-counseling Circle at *http://users.multipro.com/circle*.
   Otherwise, try the following coordinators:
Judy Hartling: 413 747 3924 or *judy_a_hartling@spfdcol.edu*
Bob Sawyer: 860 423 6292 or *bobsawyer7@aol.com*
Jlynn Silvers: 860 523 8665 or *jlynnalive@aol.com*

BREAST-FEEDING SUPPORT ORGANIZATIONS

Many of these are voluntary groups, funded by donations. When writing to them, please enclose a large, stamped self-addressed envelope to save them time and money.

La Leche League International
9616 Minneapolis Avenue
Franklin Park
Illinois 60131
Tel: 312 455 7730
Hotline: 1 800 LALECHE (open 9 a.m.–3 p.m. Central Standard Time, for advice, and so forth)
Web-site: *www.lalecheleague.org/LLLICatMain96.html*

International Lactation Consultant Organization
4101 Lake Boone Trail
Raleigh
North Carolina 27607
Tel: 919 787 5181
Web-site: *www.ilca.org/jhl.html*

MAGAZINES ON BREAST FEEDING

La Leche League's New Beginnings
1400 N. Meacham Road
Schaumburg
Illinois 60173
Tel: 847 519 7730
Web-site: *www.lalecheleague.org*

Mothering
The Magazine of Natural Family Living
PO Box 1690
Sante Fe
New Mexico 87504
Tel: 1 800 984 8116
Web-site: *www.mothering.com*

Nuturing Magazine
Magazine of Natural Parenting
#373, 918 Sixteenth Avenue NW
Calgary, Alberta
Canada T2M OK3
Web-site: *www.nuturing.ca*

Appendix 2

Allergen particles – the range of sizes

(A micron is a thousandth of a millimetre.)

Type of particle	Size (diameter) of particle
Absidia spores	2–4 microns
Alder pollen	22–34 microns
Alternaria spores	4–10 microns, some larger
Amaranth pollen	20–40 microns
Arthrinium spores	4–10 microns
Ash pollen	18–27 microns
Aspergillus spores	2–4 microns, some smaller than 2 microns
Aspergillus tereus	less than 2 microns
Aureobasidium spores	2–10 microns
Australian white cypress-pine	20–24 microns
Bacteria	0.1 micron–5 microns
Bald 'cypress' pollen	28–36 microns
Birch pollen	18–28 microns
Bird allergens	see 'Feather allergens'
Cat allergen	less than 2.5 microns (perhaps as low as 0.05 micron) up to 20 microns or more
Cladosporium spores	4–10 microns
Coal dust	1–100 microns
Coniophora cerebella spores	14 microns × 9 microns
Cryptostroma spores	2–4 microns
Cypress pollen	19–38 microns
Diesel exhaust particulates	1–10 microns, most are 2.5 microns or less
Dock pollen	21–27 microns
Dog allergen	no figures available

Dry rot spores	4–10 microns
Epicoccum spores	over 10 microns
Feather allergens	most are 1 micron
Flour	1–90 microns
Fog and mist	2–100 microns
Goosefoot pollen	20–30 microns
Graphium spores	2–10 microns
Grass pollen	25–37 microns
Greasy particles found in domestic air	0.01 micron–5 microns
Hazel pollen	18–23 microns
Horsetail (*Equisetum*) spores	38–56 microns
House dust mites	200–300 microns
House-dust mite droppings	4–20 microns
House-dust mite droppings – fragmented	0.5 micron–3 microns
Japanese red cedar pollen	24–32 microns
Micropolyspora faeni spores	less than 2 microns
Mould spores	less than 2 microns to over 10 microns (*see individual entries if you know which mould is your allergen*)
Mucor spores	2–10 microns
Nocardia asteroides spores	less than 2 microns
Mugwort pollen	18–24 microns
Olive pollen	17–28 microns
Paxillus panuoides spores	4–5 microns
Pellitory pollen	14–19 microns
Penicillium spores	mostly 2–4 microns, some larger
Pine pollen	60–85 microns, but air bladders keep it airborne despite its large size
Plane pollen	18–25 microns
Plantain pollen	16–36 microns
Pollen	5–200 microns although the main allergenic pollens fall in the range 10–40 microns, with the majority between 20 and 35 microns (*see individual entries if you know*

	which pollen is your allergen)
Pollen fragments* (see below)	0.5 micron upwards
Privet pollen	28–38 microns
Puccinia spores	over 10 microns
Ragweed pollen	19–20 microns
Rat urinary proteins	associated with particles of 5–10 microns
Redwood pollen	22–25 microns
Smog	0.01 micron–2 microns
Smoke from cigarettes	see 'Tobacco smoke particles'
Smoke from coal fires and boilers	0.01 micron–4 microns
Smoke from oil-burning boilers, etc.	0.04 micron–1 micron
Sporobolomyces spores	2–10 microns
Thermoactionmyces spores	less than 2 microns
Tobacco smoke particles	0.01 micron–1 micron
Ustilago spores	4–10 microns
Viruses	0.02–0.3 micron
Wet rot spores	see *Coniophora cerebella* spores and *Paxillus panuoides* spores

* Covers all smaller-than-pollen-grain particles carrying pollen allergens. This includes both fragmented pollen grains, and very small particles containing pollen-type allergens that are released by the plant at the same time as the pollen. These are known to exist for ragweed, some grasses, Japanese red cedar and Australian white cypress-pine. They may exist for other plants, but this has not been widely investigated.

Appendix 3

Products for those with asthma

Spacers for use with aerosol inhalers

Collapsible spacers
A collapsible spacer that you can carry in your pocket may be very useful, especially for small children.

Suppliers include:
Allergy Control Products, WE Pharmaceuticals Inc

Dose-counters for inhalers
For use with aerosol inhalers, the dose-counter displays the number of inhalations taken in the current day, and announces when the inhaler is almost empty.

Suppliers include:
Allergy Control Products, National Allergy Supply, Newmed Corp.

Inspiratory Muscle Trainers
These devices strengthen the diaphragm and other muscles that power the in-breath (see p. 430). The Powerbreathe device, designed

by university-based research scientists studying respiration, is one of the best.

Suppliers include:
Allergy Supply Company

Buteyko Technique videos
Classes in Buteyko are very expensive, so you may want to try learning it at home. Basic instructions are given on pp. 425–8. There are also training videos, which you may find helpful. If you have access to the Internet, you can check *www.wt.com.au/~pkolb/diy.htm* for local suppliers. Some offer on-line support as part of the video package, which may be the most useful element.

Suppliers include:
Buteyko Asthma Education

Reducing indoor pollution

Water-based paints, stains, and finishes
These can be bought in many large DIY stores now, but there are also specialist suppliers. They pioneered the move to produce products that would not irritate the airways, and all the ingredients in their products are vetted very carefully to make the finishes as problem-free as possible. These products may be the best choice for many asthmatics.

Suppliers include:
Livos Phytochemistry, The Healthy House

Mite-proof bedding and covers
First, don't be taken in by vague terms such as 'anti-allergenic'. This may just mean that the pillows contain polyester fibre or foam filling rather than feathers, and new research shows that these actually harbour *more* house dust mites.

Covers need to form a barrier against dust-mite *droppings*, including fragments of droppings, which can be extremely small. The mites themselves are considerably larger.

A summary of points to check before you buy:

1. Ask how large the pores are: they should be less than one micron (often written as 1 μm; it equals one thousandth of a millimetre).
2. Stitch-holes along the seams of covers can provide entry holes for mites, and exit holes for droppings. Check how the seams are constructed. Ideally, they should be welded or sealed in some way.
3. Mattress covers for long-term use should enclose the *whole* mattress, not just the top and sides.
4. Check how the covers are fastened once in place. The fastening needs to be good, because the covers should form a *complete seal* around the mattress, pillow or duvet, so that mites cannot enter and dropping particles cannot leave.
5. Covers that just fold around a mattress and do not fasten together are unlikely to work. If the covers have a zipper, check that this does not provide an access route for mites. Some manufacturers supply a roll of special adhesive tape to block the tiny holes between the teeth of the zip: this helps considerably in keeping mites out and allergen in. Where this is not supplied, you can seal the zip with any strong fabric tape – hardware shops usually sell various kinds for repairing tents, etc. This tape seal should be renewed every three months.
6. Ask for a sample of the fabric used, so that you can check how soft and pliable it is. Some of the fabrics are quite stiff, and you may notice them rustling when you roll over, or feel them. If you are a light sleeper, this might bother you.
7. Also check the sample to see how strong the fabric is – will it tear easily?
8. Ask how long the covers are guaranteed for.
9. Ask what type of material it is. Generally speaking, the synthetics known as 'polyolefins' are less durable and more papery than other types of fabric.
10. Ask how the covers should be cleaned: can they be washed if necessary? At what temperature? (Only 55°C (135°F) and above will kill mites.)
11. Are the covers safe for babies and young children? The ones made from a synthetic fabric, or with a plastic membrane, carry a risk of suffocation. The Egyptian cotton covers should be risk-free in this respect, but check with the manufacturer.

There are five basic types of cover:

1. Covers made of a plastic such as polythene or PVC, which are completely impermeable. Nothing can get through them, but that, unfortunately, includes water vapour. Moisture may collect on the inner surface, next to the mattress or pillow, and this can produce a growth of mould. In addition, plastic covers can feel cold, hard and uncomfortable, the sheets tend to slip off them, and the perspiration that you produce can accumulate in between you and the mattress. However, such covers are cheap and effective as far as mite-control is concerned. (And unlike the other kinds, they protect the mattress against bed-wetting, which may be necessary for a small child.) You can buy plastic sheeting and use strong packing tape to turn it into a cover. To make it more comfortable, put a thick blanket between the sheet and the mattress cover (This blanket will, of course, need to be washed every two weeks at 60°C (140°F) and dried thoroughly afterwards.) A long strip of double-sided sellotape between the plastic mattress cover and the blanket should prevent slippage. Plastic covers should not be used on pillows for young children, as there is a risk of suffocation. With mattress covers, there should be a thick blanket between the cover and the sheet to prevent suffocation. Be sure that the cover cannot become loosened in the night.

Suppliers include:
Any hardware shop for plastic sheeting 'by the yard'.

2. Covers of the 'micro-porous' or 'semi-permeable' kind. These are *either* made of a fairly soft synthetic fabric with tiny pores to let water vapour through, *or* made of cotton with a plastic membrane added, the membrane having tiny pores. (The latter may be referred to as a 'laminated natural fabric'.) Most modern covers are of this kind. The crucial question to ask is: how big are the pores? A cover with relatively large pores will act as a barrier to the mites themselves, but not to their droppings – or the fragments of droppings, which are very much smaller. Such a cover is probably of little use, because, if there are any dust mites at all in the mattress or pillow already, they will remain there, multiplying happily, and their allergenic droppings will be able to escape. So if covers merely claim to 'keep out dust mites' as some brands do, be aware that they may be of little value.

Before you buy, ask *how big the pores are* in the cover. To form a barrier to fragments of droppings, they should be *less than 0.5 micron in diameter.* (A micron is a thousandth of a millimetre.) These covers, fitted to duvets, can make the sleeper feel warmer than before, so if you are buying a new duvet, it may be advisable to go for one with a lower tog rating. There may be a risk of suffocation if these covers are used for young children – check with the manufacturer.

Suppliers include:
Allergy Control Products, American Allergy Supply, The Allergy Store, Allergy Supply Company, National Allergy Supply

3. A few covers are made from a material with a plastic membrane added, but without any pores. The membrane used is of a special kind which can absorb moisture and transmit it to the other side of the fabric by a chemical process. These covers are very strong, and while they are more expensive, they do come with a guarantee. There may be a risk of suffocation if these covers are used for young children – check with the manufacturer. It is possible that they will make the duvet feel warmer, as the microporous covers do.

Suppliers include:
Allergy Control Products

4. A new type of anti-mite cover is made from very high-quality Egyptian cotton, and the pores in this are small enough to exclude dust mite droppings. They can be washed at very high temperatures and come with a lifetime guarantee. They can also withstand dry heat, which means you can use an electric blanket to dry out the bed thoroughly during the day (see pp. 134–5). Because they are made of pure cotton, they are also suitable for people who are sensitive to synthetic fabrics, and plastics. Be sure that you are buying covers designed specifically for anti-mite purposes: not all Egyptian cotton is made to this high standard.

Suppliers include:
Medivac Healthcare

5. Some covers work on a completely different principle, being treated with a pesticide that kills the mites. We cannot recommend that you buy this type of cover.

Pillows with built-in covers

If you are going to buy a new pillow anyway, these are an attractive option. Most of the questions listed above are relevant to these products as well. Talk to the manufacturer about how you should go about controlling the dust mite levels on the outer surface (since you cannot take the covers off and wash them).

Suppliers include:
National Allergy Supply

Partial mattress covers for travelling

If you travel a lot, and are badly affected by mattresses when away from home, you could also buy a cover that just fits over the top and sides of the mattress (with an elasticized edge, like a shower cap). These are cheaper than full mattress covers, widely available at department stores, and can be fitted very quickly. They do decrease the amounts of allergen breathed in, but mite allergens will still fall out underneath and eventually get into the sleeper's airways, so they are not recommended for long-term use at home. While removing the bedding and fitting the mattress cover, wear a mask to keep allergens out of your airways.

Washable bedding

Washable pillows and duvets

If you have a large washing machine and a tumble-dryer, these may be a good alternative to anti-mite covers. They should be able to withstand repeated washing at 60° C (140° F) or more. One advantage of these products is that there is no risk of suffocation for young children, whereas some of the covers may carry this risk.

Suppliers include:
Allergy Control Products

Washable blankets

If they can be washed at 60° C (140° F) or more, these are very useful as under-blankets, or as an alternative to a duvet.

Suppliers include:
Allergy Control Products, National Allergy Supply

Anti-mite washing solution

This can be useful for items that cannot be washed at 60° C (140° F). You can add it to the wash in the washing machine, or you can soak clothes in it before washing. The pesticide used is benzyl benzoate.

It seems likely that this all washes out of the clothing during the rinse cycle. Note that this chemical can (in much larger doses — used for treating scabies) cause skin irritation. Whether trace amounts left in clothing by the washing procedure would irritate the skin is unknown at present.

You can also use eucalyptus oil to kill mites in cooler washes.

Suppliers include:
Allergy Control Products, National Allergy Supply

Sprays for house dust mite

Take care to distinguish between sprays that kill mites and those that inactivate mite allergen. A few sprays (e.g., Acarosan) contain two different ingredients and can do both these jobs.

Sprays that kill mites

These sprays usually contain benzyl benzoate or a pyrethroid (pyrethrum) compound. The latter is derived from a plant and is therefore sold as 'natural', but remember that hemlock and belladonna are 'natural' too and that any pesticide is potentially toxic to people as well as pests. Pyrethrum, in particular, can provoke allergic reactions in those susceptible to allergy. Never use mite-killing spray on bedding, or on carpets where babies crawl or children play. Consider all the alternatives before resorting to long-term use of sprays.

Suppliers include:
Allergy Control Products, National Allergy Supply

Sprays that inactivate allergen

There are two kinds of spray that inactivate allergen, and both should work against a variety of allergens, not just dust mite:

1. Some sprays contain tannic acid, which changes the allergen chemically and makes it inactive as an allergen. The spray works on dust-mite and cat allergens, and may well work on others. Tannic acid is found in tea and is assumed to be harmless, but the tannic acid sprays commonly sold are very variable in composition and contain many impurities, so it is hard to be sure about their long-term safety. We would not recommend these sprays for use on bedding which is next to your skin or near your face. Tannic acid may stain some fabrics, so test on a small hidden area first.

Suppliers include:
Allergy Control Products, The Allergy Store, National Allergy Supply

2. Those containing polysaccharides, which stick the allergen particles together, so that they become heavy and do not float about and get inhaled.

Suppliers include:
The Healthy House

Dehumidifiers
A dehumidifier will only be effective if you reduce the sources of moisture entering the air – if you dry clothes indoors and boil food with no lids on the saucepans, the dehumidifier will be fighting a losing battle.

Dehumidifiers to combat moulds
Any dehumidifier will be of some help in combating moulds, but the more powerful it is the better. Before buying one, ask yourself if opening windows and improving ventilation in other ways would not help just as much. Remember that you will have to keep windows closed for the dehumidifier to be effective.

Suppliers include:
Allergy Control Products, National Allergy Supply

Dehumidifiers to combat house dust mites
Any dehumidifier will help to make life more difficult for house dust mites, but to reduce the humidity drastically, and so *kill* mites, you need a really powerful dehumidifier especially designed for this job. Ask what level of humidity the machine can achieve: it should be less than 50 per cent for prolonged periods of time to kill significant numbers of mites. The lower the humidity achieved by the machine, the more impact it will have on the mites.

Suppliers include:
Medivac Healthcare

Humidity meter
You might find one of these useful if you want to check how your dehumidifier is performing, find out which rooms need treatment most urgently, or see how well various anti-humidity measures are doing in reducing the moisture in your home.

Suppliers include:
Allergy Control Products, National Allergy Supply

Vacuum cleaners
Ordinary vacuum cleaners break up dust-mite faeces and spray tiny allergen particles into the air. This increases the amount of allergen inhaled.

Many different vacuum cleaners are now claimed by their manufacturers to be useful for those with mite allergy. For most of these machines, the claims about how much dust is extracted from the emitted air are based on the effectiveness of the HEPA filters used to filter the exhaust. The problem is that there is often no airtight seal around the filter, so a lot of dusty air goes round the edges, rather than through the filter. Unfiltered air can also escape from the joints of the vacuum cleaner, if these become distorted very slightly while the cleaner is in use, as often happens with the plastic casing of ordinary vacuum cleaners when subjected to heat and high working pressures from the machine's motor.

When manufacturers quote the filtration rate for their vacuum cleaner, they are often simply quoting the effectiveness of the filter itself, tested in isolation. This gives no real indication of the amount of dust escaping from the machine. A slightly better test is to assess the amount of dust in the exhaust stream from the vacuum cleaner (as done in published tests of vacuum cleaners), but this does not measure the amount of *allergen* emitted, nor take account of leakage from the joints of the machine when the motor gets hot. The best testing method is to look at the level of allergen in the air after vacuuming a room: this tests the emissions from the machine as a whole, and by looking at the allergen, rather than at dust particles, it measures what actually causes asthma attacks.

Only one type of anti-allergy vacuum cleaner, the Medivac, has been tested in this way. A scientific trial conducted at Wythenshawe Hospital in Manchester, England, has shown that there is no increase in the amount of mite allergen in the air after using this machine, whereas there is three times as much allergen in the air after using a standard vacuum cleaner.

The Medivac has a metal body, which prevents the joints from becoming distorted and leaky. It relies on a very high-quality filter, which is protected from clogging by dust, and never needs changing. This is not the cheapest vacuum cleaner, but it is the only one that has been properly tested and shown to keep mite allergen out of the air.

Suppliers include:
Medivac Healthcare

Central vacuum systems (built-in vacuum systems)
This is a good option if you can afford it. The system can be installed in new houses, or in existing houses as long as they have cavity walls. A high-power vacuum unit is installed in the garage, basement or other storage area, and concealed pipes lead to each room in the house. There is an inlet hole (fairly inconspicuous) in each room, and you plug your flexible vacuum hose into one of these. The dust is sucked up efficiently, and taken directly out of the room, through the pipes and into the central vacuum unit. Your local Yellow Pages or the Internet can direct you to a supplier.

Filters for fitting to ordinary vacuum cleaners
These fit over the exhaust of a conventional vacuum cleaner. They will reduce the amount of dust allergen thrown out, but certainly won't eliminate it. You need to take other anti-dust measures if using these filters (see pp. 140–1).

Suppliers include:
Allergy Control Products, National Allergy Supply

Anti-mite steam cleaners
There is one steam cleaner currently on sale, called the Medivap, which has been specifically designed to combat house-dust mite. By means of high pressures, it produces steam at a temperature *above* boiling point which inactivates the main dust-mite allergen as well as

killing the mites. Independent scientific trials have shown that *all* the mites in a carpet are killed by the process, and the primary allergen, Der p1, is inactivated.

Suppliers include:
Medivac Healthcare

Dusters which hold dust electrostatically

Dusters which hold the dust electrostatically, so that it does not become airborne when you dust, are useful as an alternative to wet-dusting for those allergic to house dust mite.

Suppliers include:
Allergy Control Products, American Allergy Supply, Allergy Supply Company, National Allergy Supply

Carpets and bedding covers with built-in pesticide

There are various anti-mite products on sale which are impregnated with acaricides (pesticides that kill mites).

Although the chemical used will have been tested for safety, the long-term effects of daily close contact simply cannot be predicted. Many doctors feel uneasy about anyone having such prolonged and constant exposure to pesticide-treated items. In the case of bedding covers, sleeping next to pesticide-treated cloth night after night seems particularly worrying. Carpets treated with pesticides are also a cause for concern in houses with babies and young children, who tend to have a lot of direct contact with carpets.

We would advise against buying such products, especially as there are viable alternatives that do not rely on pesticides.

Masks

To work properly, a mask must fit tightly against the nose and face, forming a seal at all edges. Beards and moustaches tend to prevent this.

There are two basic types of mask: those that have a dust filter only, and those that combine a dust filter with an activated carbon filter to take out gases and chemical vapours.

Summary of questions to ask:
   1. Does the mask take out particles, or gases, or both?

2. What is the smallest size of particle that it will filter out?
   Check this against the size of airborne allergen particles
   shown in Appendix 2.
3. Does it conform to any standards?
4. How long is it expected to last? Can the filters be replaced?

Dust masks

A claim that a mask removes '95 per cent of particulates' is meaning-
less unless the size of those particulates is given.

Dust masks that are manufactured and sold for the protection of
workers (see pp. 277–9) have to meet certain standards based on the
smallest particle size they will filter out efficiently. (These are known
as **dust respirators**.)

Masks sold *only* for protection from traffic pollutants are not
governed by any compulsory standards in Britain at the time this
book went to press.

Standards for dust masks

The standards applied in Britain to industrial dust masks (respirators)
are as follows. (In all cases, particles smaller than 0.5 micron will also
be removed, but with less efficiency.)
Health and Safety Executive Standards
EN 149 FFP 3SL Filters out particles of 0.5 micron and above with an
efficiency of 98 per cent.
EN 149 FFP2S Filters out particles of 0.5 micron and above with an
efficiency of 92 per cent.
EN 149 FFP1 Filters out particles of 0.5 micron and above with an
efficiency of 78 per cent.

Nuisance dust masks

Nuisance dust masks only filter out particles larger than 5 microns.
There are no compulsory standards set for the efficiency with which
they remove these particles. The manufacturers are allowed to state
that such masks filter out pollen, but fragments of pollen grains can be
smaller than 5 microns.

The dust masks sold in chemists' shops are designed only for
nuisance dusts. Thus, they will not give full protection against pollen
fragments or particles of dust-mite allergens made airborne during
vacuum cleaning, despite the claim on the packet that they are 'suitable
for those sensitive to dust.'

You should check the size of the particles that you need protection from, using Appendix 2.

Masks to protect against dust-mite allergens

If you are sensitive to house dust mite, and need a mask for times of high exposure, such as housework, the best buy is a 3M mask which conforms to standard EN 149 FFP2S (see above). This is used by researchers working with house-dust mites to prevent allergic reactions.

Suppliers include:
3M, National Allergy Supply

Masks to protect against pollutants

These contain activated carbon. There should also be a dust filter between the activated carbon layer and the nose/mouth, so that granules of activated carbon are not inhaled — avoid any mask that contains activated carbon alone.

Activated carbon acts like a 'molecular magnet', holding a variety of airborne chemicals. (It does not hold nitrogen dioxide, but can be specially treated to give it this ability.)

The capacity of activated carbon to hold chemicals declines with use, because the surface of the carbon becomes coated with chemicals already filtered from the air. So it is important to replace the filter regularly. There are, at present, no standards for the removal of gas or chemical vapours (unlike dust particles) so the effectiveness of these masks has to be taken on trust. However, one mask sold for cyclists did well in testing by *Health Which?* (see below).

As well as being useful against most traffic and industrial pollution, these masks will filter out solvent vapour from paint or other DIY activities, irritant volatile substances from oil-seed rape plants, and other chemical substances, such as petrol fumes.

Cycle shops now sell masks that may be of use to some asthmatics. In a survey conducted by *Health Which?* (June 1998 issue) the best performing masks were the Techno Gold which is a combined mask (although only dust filtration was tested) and Urban Survival Sports, which filters dusts only. Both conform to standard EN 149.

Suppliers include:
Allergy Control Products, The Allergy Store — or any cycle shop

Relaxation and meditation tapes

Relaxation tapes include those that have music only, those that combine music with natural sounds such as waves breaking or birdsong, and those that combine music with speech — instructions on how to relax, or visualizations of peaceful scenery that are intended to induce relaxation. There are also music tapes which are intended to induce a meditative state, rather than simply helping you relax, and tapes that have specific instructions on how to meditate. You may need to try out several different tapes before you find one that is just right for you.

Suppliers include:
Inner Traditions International, Sounds True

Bacterial (gut flora) replacers

Following a course of antibiotics, it is advisable to replace the natural health-giving bacteria in the gut (called the gut flora) some of which may have been killed by the antibiotic. Bacterial replacers can also be helpful as part of the treatment for 'candidiasis'. You will find replacers in any healthfood shop, but often these have been stored at too high a temperature and the bacteria are no longer viable. It is best to buy replacers mail-order, from a company that ensures fast delivery and guarantees the number of live organisms in the product.

Suppliers include:
CAG Functional Foods

ADDRESSES OF SUPPLIERS

Allergy Control Products
96 Danbury Road, Ridgefield, Connecticut, 06877 USA
Tel: 1 800 422 DUST
Fax: 203 431 8963
E-mail: *info@allergycontrol.com*
Web-site: *www.allergycontrol.com*

The Allergy Store
8567 Coral Way, Suite 108, Miami, Florida, 33155 USA
Tel: 305 223 2847 (local)
1 888 337 5665 (toll-free)
Fax: 305 220 3334
Web-site: *www.allergystore-2.com*

This company sells boxspring casings, as well as other anti-mite bedding covers.

Allergy Supply Company
11994 Star Court, Herndon, Virginia, 20171 USA
Tel: 1 800 323 6744. Within Washington, DC, tel: 703 391 2011
Fax: 1 800 681 5454
E-mail: *allergy@allergysupply.com*
Web-site: *www.allergysupply.com*

American Allergy Supply
PO Box 722022, Houston, Texas, 77272–2022 USA
Tel: 1 800 321 1096 or 1 800 221 6483
E-mail: *American@neosoft.com*
Web-site: *www.neosoft.com*
This company offers covers for box-spring bed bases, as well as mattress and pillow covers.

Buteyko Asthma Education (USA)
Tel: 1 877 ASTHMA 3
Web-site: *www.buteyko-usa.com*
Offers training courses in the USA as well as home training products.

CAG Functional Foods
222 South Fifteenth Street, Suite 770, Omaha, Nebraska, 68102-7315 USA
Tel: 402 595 7315 or 1 888 828 4242
Fax: 402 595 4498
Web-site: *www.culturelle.com*

The Healthy House
Cold Harbour, Ruscombe, Stroud, Gloucestershire GL6 6DA
Tel: 01453 752216
Fax: 01453 753533
Note that much of the bedding in their catalogue is designed for those with chemical sensitivity, rather than mite allergy: make sure you are buying the right products.

Inner Traditions International
One Park Street, Rochester, Vermont, 05767 USA
Tel: 1 800 2 GO TO IT
Fax: 802 767 3726
E-mail: *orders@InnerTraditions.com*
Web-site: *www.InnerTraditions.com*
This publishing company offers cassettes and CDs for meditation and relaxation.

Livos Phytochemistry of America
P O Box 1740, Mashpee, Massachusetts, 02649 USA
Tel: 508 477 7955
Fax: 508 477 7988
Web-site: *www.livos.com*

3M
3M Product Information Center
3M Center, Bldg 304-1-01, St. Paul, Minnesota, 55144-1000 USA
Tel: 1 800 3M HELPS
Fax: 1 800 713 6329
Web-site: *www.3M.com*

Medivac Healthcare Ltd
Wilmslow House, Grove Way, Wilmslow, Cheshire SK9 5AG
Tel: 01625 539401
Fax: 01625 539507
Web-site: *www.medivac.co.uk*
This company produces the Medivac vacuum cleaner, designed specifically to combat dust mites. An electronic dust monitor comes free with the machine to assess the dustiness of the air.

Newmed Corporation
76 Treble Cove Rd, Bldg 2, Billerica, Massachusetts 01862 USA
Tel: 1 800 863 9633
Fax: 978 439 5170
E-mail: *info@doser.com*
Web-site: *www.doser.com*

National Allergy Supply
1620 Satellite Blvd., Suite D, PO Box 1658, Duluth, Georgia 30096-8440
USA
Tel: 1 800 522 1448
Fax: 770 623 5568
Web-site: *www.nationalallergysupply.com*

Sounds True
PO Box 8010, Boulder, Colorado 80306-8010 USA
Tel: 303 665 3151
Fax: 303 665 5292
Toll-free line: 1 800 333 9185
E-mail: *info@soundstrue.com*
This company sells excellent tapes, CDs and videos, covering a very
wide range of musical and spiritual traditions. A good place to start if
you want to learn to meditate, to practise yoga, to understand yourself
better, or just to relax. A free catalogue is available, and can be sent
anywhere in the world, as can orders.

WE Pharmaceuticals
PO Box 1142, Ramona, California 92065 USA
Tel: 1 800 262 9555
Web page (includes mail-order facility): *www.weez.com*

Index

Abnormal heart rhythm, 419
Accuhaler, 379
Aching, in the chest, 419
Aching muscles, 182
Activated carbon, 481–2
Acupuncture, 410–13
Acute, 31, 241
Adrenaline, 38, 75, 342, **347–8**, 418
  emergency use, 55–7
  for anaphylaxis, 55–7
  for aspirin sensitivity, 54
  inhalers, 55–6, 62, 347–8, 469
  injections, 17, 62, **348**
  maximum dose, 55–6
Adult-onset asthma, 43
  possible causes, 29
Aeroplanes, 445
Aerosols, 222–3
  see also Inhalers, aerosol
Aftershave, 226
Age at which asthma begins, 29–30,
  43–4
Aikido, 429–30
Air,
  food in, 179
  particles in, *158–9, 162–3*
Air conditioning, 90, 152–3, 175
Air filters, 152, 161, 165, 169
  for cars, 482
Air fresheners, 17, 222, 233
'Air hunger', 312, 419
Air pollution, 78, 80, 203, **204–15**
  coping with, 213–15, 482

finding information on, 459
from cars, 206–12, 213–15
indoor, 166, **221–6, 234–5**
industrial, 207, 211, 212–3
Air sacs, *20, 21*
Airway muscles, *21*, 22, 23
  control over, 417–8, 449
Airway narrowing, 20–21, 22–3,
  417–19, 449
  awareness of, 49, 61
Airway resistance, **31**
Airways, 20–23, *21*
  damage to, 327
  'twitchy', 23
Alcoholic drinks, 180, 265–6, 332
  and sinusitis, 244
Alexander Technique, 403
Allergens, 31, 109, **110**
  airborne, 111, *158–9, 162–3*
  and nocturnal asthma, 76–7
  at work, 268–9, **280–3**
  delayed reactions to, 29, 114, 119,
    121, 174
  desensitization for, 197–202
  dust mite, 131
  how to avoid, 127–178
  identifying, **115–25**, 301–2
  in schools, 17
  size of particles, 158–9, 162–3,
    466–8
Allergic bronchopulmonary
  aspergillosis, 246
Allergic diseases, 31

Allergies, 31, **110–12**
  blocking with drugs, 106, 338
  development of, 26–8, 29
  identifying, 113–26, 301–2
  inheritance of, 25–8
  link with asthma, 110
  tests for, 113, 301–2, 304–5, 395
  to infectious fungi, 246–9
  see also Food allergy
Allergists, 321, 300, 301–2, 462
Allerpet-C, 164
Alternaria, 165
Alternative medicine, 394–451
  types most useful for asthma, 394–5
Alternative therapists, 125, 252,
    395–6, 460–1
Altitude sickness, 295
Alveoli, 20, *21*
Ambulance service, 50–2, 55–7
Ammonia, 270
Anaphylactic shock *see* Anaphylaxis
Anaphylaxis, 31, 48–9, 111–12
  causes of, 111–2
  coping with 55–7, 452, 456
  food and exercise, 70
  in children, 17
  symptoms of, 48–9, 57
  treatment of, 55–7, 62–3, 301
Animals, allergy to, 119–20, 156–65,
    283
Anti-allergic drugs, 335
Antibiotics, 92–3, 237–8
  allergy to, 124
  and risk of asthma, 92–3
  bacterial resistance to, 241–3
  for chest infections, 93, 237–8
  for sinusitis, 241–5
Anti-cholinergics, 235, **345**
  and exercise, 72
  and night-time asthma, 76
  safety of, 328
  side-effects of, 365–6
Anti-fungal drugs, 247–8, 252

Anti-histamines, 266, 339
  and skin-prick tests, 125
  see also Ketotifen
Anti-inflammatory drugs, 341, 363
  see also Preventers
Antioxidants, 98–9, 103, 104
Anti-muscarinic bronchodilators, 335
Anti-venom, 111
Anxiety, 37, 39–40, 182, 419
  in parents, 11, 38
Aromatherapy, 234, 409
Arthritis, 377
Aspergillus, 246
Aspirin-like drugs, 257–61
  effect on exercise-induced asthma,
    73
  in cold remedies, 238
Aspirin sensitivity, 257–61
  and sinusitis, 244
  coping with attacks, 55
  recognizing attacks, 47–8
Asthma,
  causes of epidemic, 81–3
  diagnosis of, 79, 270–1, 275, 306–14
  effect on airways, 327
  effect on posture, 400, 415
  fear of, 43, 309
  growing out of, 42
  inheritance of, 25–6
  over-treatment of, 390
  prevention of, 87–95, 96–104
  return of, 43
  'stigma' of, 34, 306
  support groups, 452–6
  symptoms of, 23–4, 307–9
  treatment variations, 331–3, 389
  triggers for, 2–3
  under-treatment of, 390–91
  why it begins, 28–30, 81–4, 230,
    263, 295–6
  work-related, 268–86
  worldwide variations in, 79–81
Asthmagens, 268–9

Asthma nurses, 298, 321
Athletes, 68, 69, 293–6
Athlete's foot, 247–8
Atopic, 25, 32
Atropine-type drugs, 335
Attacks, 45–58
  averting, 49, 60–1, 70–3
  best positions during, 54
  breathing during, 415, 417
  calmness during, 446
  cause of, 20–23, 58, **60**, 98
  coping with, **50–58**, 70, 348, 379,
    383–4
  during pregnancy, 290
  exercise-induced, 68–73
  rapid onset, 46
  recognizing, 45–9
  slow onset, 46
  what to do afterwards, 59–63
  see also Fatal asthma attacks
Autogenic Training, 447–8, 462
Autohaler, 378–9
Automobiles see Cars
Autonomic nervous system, 417–18
Autumn (fall),
  asthma worse in, 65–6, 117–18

B-2 agonists, 335
B-2 bronchodilators, 335
B-2 relievers, **342–5**
  and exercise, 71–2
  brand names of, 371–2
  British guidelines on, 343
  during an attack, 51–2
  in tablets or syrup, 344, 365
  international guidelines on, 343
  long-acting, 76, 344–5
  over-use of, 36, 322–6, **323**, 333, 343
  parenteral, 344, 365
  risks of, 322–6, 350
  short-acting, 322–6, 342–4
  side effects, 76, 363–5
  US guidelines on, 333, 343

Babies, reducing asthma risk for, 89–93
Bacteria, 26,
Bacterial replacers, 243, 483
Bad breath, 240
Balloons, 125
Bathrooms, 141
Bean dust, 124, 212, 281
Becotide see Steroids
Bedrooms, 139–41, 143–7
Beds, 130, 132–7, 148, 160, 470–5
Beer, 180
'Belly breathers', 422
Beta-2 agonists, 335
Beta-blockers, 62–3, 236, 262
Beta-carotene, 99, 104, 213
Biodynamic Massage, 450
Biofeedback, 70, 449
Birch, 122, *159*, 171, 175, 232
Blankets, 134, 475
Bleach, 223
Blood samples, 305
Blood tests, 305, 346–7
'Blue one', 370
  see also Relievers
Blurred vision, 419
Breast-feeding, 91, 92, 292, 464–5
Breathing, 20–22, 53, 414–19
  control of, 417–19
  'correct', 404–6, 414–16, 421–3
  patterns, 404–6, 414–16
  stops while asleep, 256
Breathing apparatus, 277
Breathing exercises, 397, 421–45
  for clearing mucus, 59
  to improve out-breath, 429–30
  to strengthen muscles, 430–45, 469
Breathlessness, 23, 36, 46, 51–2, 68,
  74, 311, 313, 419
Bricanyl see B-2 relievers
Brittle asthma, **32**, 35, 112, 182, 216,
  256
  treatment of, 346, 384
Bronchi and bronchioles, 20, *21*

Bronchiectasis, 313
Bronchiolitis, 311
Bronchitis, 32, 308, 309
  chronic, 216, 313
Bronchoconstriction, paradoxical, 364
Bronchodilators, 32, 334
  see also Relievers
Bronchospasm, 22
'Brown one', 370
  see also Preventers
Bunk beds, 137
Burping, 254
Buteyko Method, 423–8, 470

Cafés, 181
Caffeine, 265
Cancer, 314
Candida, 249–52
  in the throat, 352
Cannabis, 407
Carbon dioxide, 21, 419–20
Carbon monoxide, 313
Cars, 84, 214
  filters for, 482
  paints for, 225
  pollution from, 206–12, 213–15
Carpet beetles, 115
Carpets, 116, 145, 149, 480
  shampooing, 140
Cats, 119–20, 156–165
  eliminating allergens of, 156–60
  size of allergen, 157, 162–3, 466
  ubiquity of allergens, 165
Causes of asthma, 26–7, 28–9
Celery, 70
Cemfuel, 213
Central heating, 66, 118, 166
Chemical sensitivity, 225–6, 465, 486
Chemicals, household, 221–35
Chemical spills, 270
Chest infections, 237–9
  see also Bronchitis
Chest pain, 24, 254

Chest physicians, 300
Chickenpox, 360
Childbirth, 289–90
Children with asthma,
  and dust mites, 89–90, 137–8, 149
  and elimination diets, 193
  and exercise, 69
  dealing with attacks, 11, 39, 44, **50–8**
  diagnosis, 307–8, 310–14
  growing out of it, 42
  learning difficulties, 74
  night-time attacks, 74
  preventing asthma in, 87–95
  psychological factors, 38–9, 69, 74,
    446–7
  recognizing attacks, 47
  self-esteem, 14
  sleepiness, 74
  using spacers, 382
  why it begins, 29
Chiropractors, 400–2
Chlamydia pneumoniae, 256
Chlorine, 70, 223, 270, 295
Choking, 254, 256
Christmas trees, 118
Chronic, 32, 241
Chronic obstructive pulmonary disease
    (COPD, CORD or COAD), 32,
    216, 309
Cigarettes see Smoking
Cilia, 245, 314
Cladosporium, 122
Cleaning products, 223
Cleanliness, and asthma risk, 27, 93
Clickhaler, 379
Clothes and allergens, 120, 138, 276
Coal smoke, 211–12, 222
Cockroaches, 123, 178, 206
Coffee, 265
Coking plants, 207
Cold air, **227**, 295–6, 317
Colds and chest infections, 71, 106,
    237–9

and sinusitis, 241
and steroid use, 238–9
remedies for, 238
Comfort blankets, 138
Comforters *see* Duvets
Conditioning, 35–6, 233
Condoms, 125, 131, 282
Confusion, 419
Constipation, 182
Consultants, 299–301
Contact dermatitis, 305
Cookers, 221
COPD, 32, 216, 309
Corticosteroids, 335
Cortisol, 75, 335
Cotton, 124
Coughing,
  and misdiagnosis, 308, 313
  as symptom of asthma, 23, 308
  as symptom of sinusitis, 240
  first sign of asthma, 275
  habitual, 312
Cough medicines, 349
Cough-variant asthma, 308
Counselling, 451, 463
Covers *see* Mattresses
Crohn's disease, 182
Cromoglycate, 328, **338**, 407
  and exercise, 71
  brand-names of, 371
  side-effects of, 361
Crying and asthma attacks, 34
Curtains (drapes), 143–4, 151
Cushing's syndrome, 356
Cyclosporin, 329, 341, 363
Cystic fibrosis, 245, 246, 313

Damp, 114, 116, 117–8, 139–140,
  154, **166–8**, 170
  weather, 227
Death, fear of, 419
Deaths *see* Fatal asthma attacks
Decongestants, 242, 243

Dehumidifiers, 145, 148–9, 151–2,
  169, 476–7
Dehydration, 53, 59
  and exercise, 71
Denial, 39
Depression, 40–1, 182, 419
Desensitization, 107, **197–202**, 226
Deserts, 116, 118
Diabetics, 264, 355
Diagnosis of asthma, 79, 270–1, 275,
  306–14
Diaphragm, 414–17, *416*, 421–2
  breathing with, 421–3
Diarrhoea, 48, 182
Diesel exhaust, *159*, 204, **210–11**, *210*
  reducing, 458–9
Diet and asthma, 96–104, 179–82
Digoxin, 263
Diskhaler, 379
DIY, 223
Dizziness, 48, 419
Doctors, 298–302, 388
Dogs, 119–20, 165
Dose counters, 379, 469
Drapes *see* Curtains
Dried fruit, 180
Drugs, 319–75
  abuse of, 14
  'addiction to', 36, 330–1
  and children, 11–14
  and sport, 296
  brand-names of, **370–5**
  controversies about, 319–33
  decisions about, 388–92
  differing policies on, 331–3, 343,
    389–90
  do they work?, 319–20
  during pregnancy, 287–8
  for exercise induced asthma, 71–2
  for night-time asthma, 75–6
  getting information on, 456
  mixtures of, 348
  new, 105–7, 329, 346, 363

obsolete, 347
psychological addiction to, 36
reducing dose, 390
safety of, 321–33
side-effects of, 350–69
'stepping up', 389
stopping, 64, 395–6
what they do, 334–49
Dry cleaning, 131, 138, 157
Dry-powder inhalers, 369, 379
Duodenal ulcers, 182
Dust, 125–6, 212
Dusting, 140, 145, 479
Dust mites, 84, 115–16, 127–55, *132*
    allergens of, 125, 131, *158, 162*
    and babies, 29, 89–90
    and cleanliness, 115, 127–8
    and humidity, 116, 130, 145
    and semen, 131
    effects of washing on, 130–1, 475
    identifying allergy to, 115–16
    in clothing, 138
    in food, 154
    in hair, 138
    in schools, 17
    in toys, 137–8
    likes and dislikes of, 115–16, 130–1,
        145–6
    masks for, 481
    outside the home, 154–5
    products for combatting, 470–81
    reducing exposure to, 127–55
    sprays for, 149, *150*, 475–6
Duvets (comforters), 133, 470–3

Earache, 240
Eczema, 25, 29, 42, 155, 299
Edema, 182
Elastic bands, 125
Electric blankets, 134–5
Elemental diets, 192
Elimination diet, 181–93
    for children, 193

Emergency treatment, 50–8
Emotional factors, 34–41, 67
    in children, 14–16
Emphysema, 32, 216, 309
Enzyme Potentiated Desensitization
    (EPD), 200–1
Enzymes, 124, 282
Eosinophils, 106
Ephedrine, 372
Epidemic, 26, 79–85
    causes of, 81–3
    in New Zealand, 205–6, 322–3
Epinephrine *see* Adrenaline
Epi-pen *see* Adrenaline
Estrogen *see* Oestrogen
Excitement and asthma attacks, 34
Exercise-induced asthma, 68–73, 182,
    293–4
    and food, 182
    and refractory effect, 73
    and warming up. 72–3
Exercise test, 304
Exhaust fumes, 206–12, 213–15
Exhaustion, 24, 59, 74, 313, 314
Expectorants, 59, 349
Extrinsic asthma, 34
Eye drops, 236, 262, 354
Eyes, symptoms in, 275

Factories, 207
Fainting, 56–7
Families, 15, 37, 38–9, 67
    effects of asthma on, 13, 15
    inheritance of asthma in, 25–6, 87
Farms, 223, 281
Fat in diet, 100
Fat (obesity), 6, 69, 248, 255
Fatal asthma attacks,
    at work, 277
    causes of, 8–10, 58, 165, 322–3,
        343, 390
    during exercise, 70
    epidemic of, 322–3

from desensitization, 198–9
in children, 11, 16, 17, 47
signs of, 46–7, 315,
speed of, 7
timing of, 7, 74
Feldenkrais Technique, 404–6
Felt-tip pens, 17
Feverishness, 240, 247, 275, 311
Fibre in diet, 99
Fires, bonfires, 225
    coal or wood, 211, 221–2
First aid, 56, 63
Fish, 103, 180
Fish oil, 103
Fitness, 68–9
Flour, 124, 268–9, 280–1
Flowers, 120, 232–4
Flu, 237
Flute, 429
Food additives, 180–1, 260
Food allergy, 17–18, 63, 111, 179
    and exercise, 70
    see also Anaphylaxis, Food
        intolerance
Food and asthma attacks, 70, 98,
    179–82, 281, 282, 312
Food intolerance, 112, 181–96
    symptoms of, 182
Food labelling, 194–6
Foods, packaged, 181
    tinned, 185
Forced expiratory volume, 303
Forced vital capacity, 303
Formaldehyde, 223–4, 285
Freezer treatment, 137
Fruit, 98–9, 180
Fungal infections, 246–52
    in sinusitis, 241
Fungi, 118–19
    see also Moulds

Ganoderma, 118–19
Garages, 225

Gardens, 117, 126, 177, 225, 234
Gas fires, 313
Gas stoves, 207–8, 221
Gastro-oesophageal reflux, 254–5, 310,
    312
Genes for asthma, 25
GER, 254–5, 310, 312
Ginkgo, 407
Glue, 17
Glue ear, 182
Gold salts, 341, 363
Grass, 121–3, 159, 171, 176, 177,
    228–9
Growth suppression, 353, 355–6
Guilt, 29
Gut flora, 483

Hairdressers, 234, 285
Hair-sample tests, 181, 395
Hallucinations, 419
Hamsters, 120
Haptens, 269
Harvesting, 117
Hayfever, 25, 120, 253
Headache, 182, 240, 313, 419
Heartburn, 254–5
    as side-effect of steroids, 352
    mimicking asthma, 310, 312
Heart disease, 314
Heart rhythm, abnormal, 419
Heating, 140, 169, 211, 221–2, 313
Heat recovery units, 153
Heimlich manoeuvre, 59–60
Heiner's Syndrome, 311
Henna, 124
Herbal remedies, 407–8
Histamine, 179–80, 420
Holidays, 445
Homeopathy, 408–9
Hormones, female, 66, 263
Horses, 119–20
Hospitals, 11, 56–7, 116, 282, 285
Hot air ducts, 221

Hot weather, 227
House dust mite *see* Dust mite
House plants, 95, 117, 168
Houses, age of, 225
Housework, 116, 222
HRT, 263
Hydrolysate formula, 91
Hyperactivity, 182
Hyperinflated lungs, 33, 400
Hypersensitivity, 33
Hyperventilation, 22, 36–7, 184,
    311–12, **419–21**
  and Buteyko method, 420, 428
  and panic, 219, 312, 419
  and psychological factors, 36–7
  causes of, 36–7, 397–8, 420–1
  mistaken for asthma, 311–12
  symptoms of, 312, **419–20**
  tests for, 421
  treatments for, 422–8
Hypnotherapy, 36, 73, 450–1
Hyposensitization, 197–200

IgE, 27, 106
IIA, 270
Immune system, 32, 211
Immunoglobulin, 341
Immunotherapy, 197
Indigestion, 182, 254–5
Industrial pollution, 207, 211, 212–13
Infections, 28, 93, 211–12, 257
  see also Fungal infections
Inflammation, 22, **33**, 105–6
  and allergies, 111
Influenza, 237
Inhalations, steam, 349
Inhaled milk, 310
Inhalers, **376–80**
  'addiction to', 1, 36, 330–1
  adrenaline/epinephrine *see*
    Adrenaline
  aerosol, 331, 368, 377–8, 380
  and exercise, 70–72

  at school, 16
  breath-operated, 378
  carrying, 61
  different kinds, 334–5
  dose-counters for, 379, 469
  dry-powder, 369, 379
  identifying, 370–5
  new types of, 107, 368
  non-CFC, 368
  non-drug ingredients, 331, 368–9,
    378, 380
  not working, 46, 51, 335, 343, 378
  propellants in, 331, 368, 378, 380
  side-effects from, 368–9
  use during attacks, 51–2, 379
  see also Drugs
Inheritance and asthma, 25–6, 87
Injectors (adrenaline/epinephrine) *see*
    Adrenaline
Insecticides, 223, 224, 233
  see also Pesticides
Insects, allergy to, 123–4, 283
Insect stings, 17, 111
Insurance, 235
Intal *see* Cromoglycate
Internet, asthma information on,
    456–7
Intertrigo, 246, 248–9
Intrinsic asthma, 34
Inversions, 177, 229
Involuntary muscle, 22
Ionizers, 152
Irritant-induced asthma, 270
Irritants, 3
  and sinusitis, 244
  at home, 221–6
  at work, 269, 283–5
  in schools, 17
  in traffic exhaust fumes, 207–11
Isocyanates, 224, 284–5
Itching, 48–9
  of anus, 250
  of eyes, 275

Jobs, choosing, 273–4, 280–5
Joint pain, 182
Judo, 428–9

Kerosene, 225
Ketotifen, 332, **340**
  side effects of, 361–2
Lactose, in inhalers, 369
Larynx, 21
Late reactions to allergens, 114, 119,
  174
Latex allergy, 124–5, 179, 212, **282**, 283
Laughing, 34
Leukotriene antagonists, 259, 329,
  340–1
  and exercise, 72
  side-effects of, 329, 362–3
Leukotrienes, 105
Lips, swollen, 49
Loss of strength, 419
Low-allergen gardens, 177
Lung-function tests, 303
Lungs, *21*
  damage to, 309, 327
  effect of inhalers on, 380
  how they work, 20–2, 417–19
  over-inflated, 33, 400
  transplants, 34

Magnesium, 99
Management plan, 391–2
Manganese, 101–2
Martial arts, 428–9
Masks, 129, 277–9, 480–2
Massage, 449–50
Mast-cell blockers, 335
Mast cells, 420
Mattresses, 130, 133–6
  covers for, 130, 133–6, 148, 160,
    470–4
Maximum dose of reliever, 51
ME, 412
Measles, 360

Meat, 101
Medic-Alert, 459
Medihaler-Epi, 347
Meditation, 448–9
Menstruation, 66
Menthol, 234, 238
Methotrexate, 329, 363
Methylxanthines, 335
Mice, 119–20
Migraine, 182, 419
Milk, 91, 311, 369
Minerals, 99, 101–2, 103
Mint, 234
Montelukast, 340–1
  side-effects of, 362–3
Mood swings, 419
Mornings, asthma worse in, 74
Moulds, 17, 117–18, 126, 165–70
  identifying allergy to, 117–19, 122,
    126
  infection by, 246–9
  reducing exposure to, 165–70
  spores of, *158–9*, *162–3*, 246, 466–8
Mountains, 116, 294, 295, 317
Mouth,
  breathing through, 418
  swelling of, 56–7
  tingling or itching, 49, **57**
Mouth ulcers, 182
Moving house, 29, 94, 139
Mucus, 22, 23, 33, 298, 345
  colour of, 22, 247, 390
  from the nose, 313
  hard, 106–7
  treatments for, **59–60**, 298–9, 345,
    349
Muscles, aching, 182, 419
Muscle cramps, 419

Nausea, 182, 313
Nebulizers, 384–7
  not working, 386–7
  risks of, 387

Nettle-rash, 48

Neutralization Technique, 201–2

Newspaper ink, 225

Nicotine gum, 218

Night-time asthma, 7, 46–7, 52, **74–7**, 254

  with no symptoms by day, 309

Nitrogen dioxide, **207–8**, 221

  from science lessons, 17

Nocturnal asthma *see* Night-time asthma

Non-specific urethritis *see* NSU

Non-steroidal anti-inflammatory drugs, **258**, 264

Nose.

  blocked, 240, 253, 275, 314

  breathing through, 174, 213, 418, 430

  drops, 242, *260*, 354

  operations on, 8

  polyps in, 257–9

  runny, 253, 275, 313

  unblocking, 425, 432

Nozovent, 430

NSAIDs, 258, 264

NSU, and risk of asthma, 88

Numbness, 419

Nuvance, 105–6

Obesity, 6, 69, 248, 255

Occupational asthma, 268–86, **269**

  advance warning of, 275

  diagnosis of, 270–1, 275–6

  getting information on, 456–7

  prevention of, 272–9

Oedema, 182

Oestrogen, 66, 263

Offices, 285

Oil-seed rape, 123, 482

Omega-3 oils, 103

Onychomycosis, 248–9

Open fires, 222

Operatic exercises, 431–45

Operations, 7, 260–1

Oral steroids *see* Steroid tablets

Oral tolerance, 155

Osteopaths, 243, 400–2

Over-treatment, 390

Overbreathing *see* Hyperventilation

Oxygen, 21–2

  effects of shortage, 23, 24

  in nebulizers, 384

Ozone, 204, 205, **208–9**

Paediatricians, 299–300

Pain,

  around teeth, 240

  in abdomen, 49

  in chest, 24, 254

  in face, 240

Paint, 17, 224, 470

Palpitations, 48

Panic, 219, 312

Panic attacks, 419

Paracetamol, 259

Paradoxical bronchoconstriction, 364

Paraffin, 225

Parasitic worms, 27, 83

Parasympathetic, 75, 345, 418

Parents and children, 37, 38–9, 44

Particles, size of, 466–8

Patch tests, 305

Pavlov's dog, 35

Peak flow, 303

Peak flow meters, 45, 49, **315–17**

  and exercise, 71

Peat burning, 222

Pediatricians *see* Paediatricians

Perfume, 226, 232–5

Periods, 66

Personality and asthma, 35

Pesticides, 223, 224, 226, 270

  for dust mites, 149, **150**, 160, 475–6

Petrol, 225, 226

Pets, 119–120

  allergens from, *158*, 162

  in schools, 17

Phlegm, 247
  see also Mucus
Phobias, 419
Photocopiers, 285
Physiotherapists, 59, 298
Pill (contraceptive), 184, 249, 263, 338
Pillows, 133–4, 470–3
Placebo effect, 36
Plastics, 226
Pneumonia, 256, 311
Pollen, 158–9
  and time of day, 171, 172
  at night, 172
  avoiding, 170–8, 459–60
  counts and forecasts, 172–3, 459–60
  identifying allergy to, 120–3, 126
  sensitization to, 88
  'shower', 172
  size of, 158–9, 162–3, 466–8
Pollution see Air pollution
Polyps, 257–9
Polyurethane foam, 224
Powerbreathe device, 430–1, 469–70
Power stations, 207
Post-nasal drip, 33, 240, 313
Posture, typical asthmatic, 400, 415
Pregnancy, 28, 287–92
  and asthma prevention, 28, 88–9, 91
Preventers, 334–41
  after an attack, 59
  benefits of, 327–8
Prevention of asthma, 87–95, 96–104
Propellants see Inhalers
Propolis, 237
Prostaglandins, 257
Provocation tests, 305
Psychological effects of drugs, 356
Psychological factors, 34–41, 412–13, 451
  and inhaler use, 36
  and smells, 233
  in children, 14–5
  outdated beliefs about, 16, 34
Psychotherapy, 451, 463

Puffers, 377
Pulse, 47, 48
Pyrethroids, 224

RADS, 270
Ragweed, 121, 159, 171
Rape, oil-seed, 123
Rash, 47–8, 248, 275
RAST, 305
Rats, 119–20
Reactive Airways Dysfunction
    Syndrome, 270
Rebound congestion, 242
Reflexology, 450
Regurgitation of food, 254
Relaxation, 446–50, 482–3
Relievers, 334–5, 341–7
  and exercise, 71–2, 296
  for night-time asthma, 76
  not working, 46, 51
  older types, 347
  use during attacks, 51–2
Residual volume, 303
Respirators, 277
Respiratory sensitizers, 268–9
Respiratory synctial virus, 93, 311
Restaurants, 181
Reversibility test, 304
Rhinitis 33, 182, 257, 313
  see also Hayfever
Rheumatoid arthritis, 182
Rib-cage, 400, 414–17
Ringing in the ears, 419
Roaches, 123, 178
Rotohaler, 379
RSV infections, 93, 311
Rubber (latex), 125, 282, 283

Salicylates, 259–60
Salt, 100, 264
Sawdust, 124, 212
Schools, 15–17
Scuba diving, 295, 445

Seasonal symptoms, 65–6
Selective B-2 adrenoceptor stimulants, 335
Selenium, 101–2
Shiatsu, 411
Shingles, 360
Shortness of breath, 23
Showers, en suite, 139
Sickness *see* Vomiting
Side-effects, 350–69
Silent chest, 47
Singing, 292, 429
Sinuses, 242
Sinusitis, 240–5, 257, 314
Skin-prick tests, **125–6**, 300, 301–2, **304–5**, 304–5
Sky-diving, 295
Sleep,
  apnoea, 77, 256
  disturbed, 36–7, 256
  loss of, 36–7
Sleeping pills, 53
'Small particles', 215
Smell, loss of, 240, 257, 260–1
Smells triggering asthma, 98, 232–5
Smoke, 211–12, 225
Smoking, 43, 203, 216–20, 256
  passive, 217–8, 308
  stopping, 216–20, 457–8
  while pregnant, 89
Snake bites, 111
Sneezing, 275
Snoring, 256, 289
Soft toys, 137
Soil bacteria, 27
Soldering, 30, 284
Sore throat, 240
Soya milk, 91
Soybean dust, 124, 212, 281
Spacers, 380–4
  collapsible, 469
  in emergency, *383–4*
  priming, 382–3

Specialists, 275, 299–301
Spiders, allergy to, 283
Spinhaler, 379
Spirometer, 303
Spores, size of, *158–9, 162–3*, 466–8
  see also Moulds
Sport, 23, 68–73, 267, 293–6
  and children, 16, 69
  causing asthma, 295–6
Sprays, for dust mites, 149, **150**, 160, 475–6
Steam-cleaning, 140, **143**, 149, 151–2, 160, **479**
Steam inhalations, 349
Steroid card, 359
Steroids, 326–8, **335–8**, 389–90
  and exercise, 71–2
  and growth, 353, 355–6
  and infections, 238–9, 360
  and sport, 296
  as tablets, 12, 52, 59, 239, 330, 337–8
  benefits of, 327–8
  brand-names of, 370–1, 373
  dose of, 351–2
  earlier use of, 327–8
  increasing dose, 52, 238–9, 247
  in drops, 253, 354
  inhaled, 42, 76, 326–8, 333, **336–7**
  oral, 354, 373
  safety of, 326–8, 351–2
  side-effects of, 350, 351–60
  Swedish policy on, 327–8
Stomach ulcers, 182
Strangulation, feeling of, 24
Stress,
  caused by asthma, 14–15
  effects on asthma, 34–5, 37–8, 67, 418
  improving asthma, 37–8, 418
  treatment of, 447–51
  triggering asthma, 29
Suggestion, 35

Sulphur dioxide, 204, **207**, 270
  from cleaning products, 223
  from food and drink, 180–1
  from science lessons, 17
Summer, symptoms worse in, 65–6,
  121–3
Swallowing difficulties, 254, 419
Swaing coolers, 116
Sweating, 275
Swelling of lips and tongue, 49, **56–7**
Swimming, 73, 295
Swimming pools, 223
Sympathetic nervous system, 418
Symptoms,
  diary of, 65
  of a severe asthma attack, 46–7
  of aspirin sensitivity, 47–8
  of asthma, 23–5, 307–9
  seasonal, 65–6, 126
  variations in, 65–7
  when lying down, 310

TB, 27, 246
T helper cells, 27, 106, 107
T'ai chi, 428–9
Taste,
  loss of, 240
  unpleasant, 254
Teddy bears, 137
Teenagers with asthma, 13–14, 18
Terfenadine, 72, 332
Tests, 113–14, 181, **303–5**, 306–7
  for allergy, 113, 301–2, 304–5, 395
  lung function, 303
Theophylline, 76, 332–3, **346–7**
  brand-names of, 374–5
  risks of, 266, 350, **367**
  side-effects of, 12, 255, 350, 366–8
  US policy on, 332–3
Throat, sore, 240
Thrush, 249, 352
Thunderstorms, 229–31
Tightness in chest, 23

Tingling, of hands, feet, tongue, lips,
  419
Tiredness, 24, 59, 74, 182, 313, 314
Toddlers, 29
Tomatoes, 100
Tonsilitis, 94
Trachea (windpipe), 20, **21**
  narrowing of, 24–5
Traffic pollution, 207–15
Tremors, 419
Trichophyton, 247
Triggers for asthma, **2–3**
  in schools, 17
  interaction with allergies, 114
Tuberculosis, 27, 246
Turbohaler, 379–80
Twitches, 419

Under-treatment, 390
Ureaplasma urealyticum, 88
Urethritis, 88

Vaccinations, 94–5
  against asthma, 107
  for TB, 27
Vacuum cleaners, 115–16, 140–41,
  169, **477–9**
  emptying, 138
Vegetables, 99
Vegetarians, 101, 103
Ventilation, 120, 140, 146, 153,
  167–8
Ventolin *see* B-2 relievers
Virus infections, 26–8
  see also Colds and chest infections,
  RSV infections
Vital capacity, 303
Vitamin C, 98–9, **103**, 237
  and air pollution, 213
Vitamin E, 100
  and air pollution, 213
Vitamin supplements, 102–4, 213
Vocal chord dysfunction, 69–70, 311

Volatiles, 175, 482
Vomiting, 24, 48, 49, 310
  in anaphylaxis, 56–7

Waivers, 18
Washable bedding, 474–5
Washing, and the risk of asthma, 93
Washing powder, 124
Weather, 227–31
Weight loss, 314
Weight (obesity), 6, 69, 248, **255**
Wheezing, **24**, 308
  coming on suddenly, 310
  in babies, 307–8
  non-asthmatic, 310, 313
Wheezy bronchitis, 79, 308
Wind, 250
Wind instruments, 429
Wine, 180

Winter, symptoms worse in, 65–6, 118
Wood dust, 124, 212, 281
Wood smoke, 211–12, 222
Wool, allergy to, 115, 124
Work-aggravated asthma, 269–70
Work-related asthma, 268–86
  advance warning of, 275
  getting information on, 456–7

Xanthines, 335
X-rays, 305

Yeast, 194, 250
Yoga, 397–9, 431

Zafirlukast, 340, 362
Zileuton, 341, 363
Zinc, 101–2

A note on the authors

Professor Jonathan Brostoff is Professor of Allergy and Environmental Health and Director of the Centre for Allergy Research at University College London, and Director of the Diagnostic Immunology Laboratory at University College London Hospitals.

Currently Physician in charge of the Allergy Clinic at the Middlesex Hospital, he sees a wide range of allergic patients with both inhalant and food allergies. He is editor (with Professors Ivan Roitt and David Male) of a standard Immunology textbook and co-author with Professor Stephen Challacombe of the principal textbook of Food Allergy and Intolerance. He is recognised as a leading international authority in his field.

He is founder of the charity, the Allergy Research Foundation, whose aim is the better education of doctors and health-care professionals in allergy and allied diseases.

Linda Gamlin trained as a biochemist and worked in scientific research for several years. She now specialises in writing about allergic diseases, the immune system, alternative medicine and the effects of diet and environment on health. In 1994 she won the Rhône-Poulenc Science Book Prize, junior category. She writes for medical journals, newspapers and a range of magazines, including *New Scientist*, *Positive Health* and *Healthy Eating*.

Food Allergies and Food Intolerance

The Complete Guide to Their Identification and Treatment

Jonathan Brostoff, M.D., and Linda Gamlin
ISBN 0-89281-875-1 • Paper, $19.95
480 pages, 6 x 9

An international authority on food allergy and intolerance shows how sensitivity to foods is responsible for many chronic and misdiagnosed ailments including migraines, sinus problems, and persistent fatigue.

"Should be compulsory reading."

New Scientist

Genetically Engineered Food: Changing the Nature of Nature

What You Need to Know to Protect Yourself, Your Family, and Our Planet

Martin Teitel, Ph.D., and Kimberly Wilson
FOREWORD BY RALPH NADER
ISBN 0-89281-888-3 • Paper, $12.95
192 pages, 6 x 9

Corn plants that kill monarch butterflies, tomatoes with fish genes, french fries registered as pesticides, soybeans that thrive on herbicide—these are foods whose genetic structures are altered in ways that could never occur in nature, and they are already in many of the products you buy in supermarkets— unlabeled, unwanted, and largely untested. This is the first book to take a comprehensive look at genetic engineering in food and its many disturbing ramifications.

The Estrogen Alternative

Natural Hormone Therapy with Botanical Progesterone

THIRD EDITION
Raquel Martin with Judi Gerstung, D.C.
ISBN 0-89281-893-X • Paper, $14.95
288 pages, 6 x 9

"Any woman who is considering synthetic hormone therapy or who wishes to get off of it owes herself the reading of this densely informative book. The simplicity and safety of the solution is almost shocking. One might ask why every suffering woman is not using botanical progesterone."

World Health News

The Arthritis Bible

A Comprehensive Guide to Alternative Therapies and Conventional Treatments for Arthritic Diseases Including Osteoarthrosis, Rheumatoid Arthritis, Gout, Fibromyalgia, and More

Craig Weatherby and Leonid Gordin, M.D.
ISBN 0-89281-825-5 • Paper, $14.95
272 pages, 6 x 9

A specialist in functional medicine provides the most up-to-date information on a variety of treatments, including drugs, exercise, physical therapy, diet, vitamins, herbs, nutraceuticals, and homeopathy.

"The Arthritis Bible is an outstanding resource to anyone with arthritic symptoms, as it blends the best of conventional and complementary medicine to help alleviate the pain and suffering in these patients."

Stephen T. Sinatra, M.D.
Author of *Optimum Health*

The Encyclopedia of Aromatherapy

Chrissie Wildwood
ISBN 0-89281-638-4 • Paper, $24.95
320 pages, 7⅛ x 9⅝
75 color and 19 black-and-white illustrations

The Encyclopedia of Aromatherapy explores the many aspects of this healing art in a single illustrated volume. The author discusses all things aromatic, from essential oils and fragrant gardens to therapeutic massage and beauty products.

"The most elegantly comprehensive package on the whole art and science of aromatherapy written to date…an indispensable reference."
Aromatherapy Quarterly

Aromatherapy and Massage for Mother and Baby

Allison England, R.N.
ISBN 0-89281-898-0 • Paper, $14.95
160 pages, 6 x 9
15 black-and-white illustrations

This newly revised edition of the definitive guide provides expert advice on using essential oils in massage, baths, compresses, lotions, and inhalations. Special sections on massage for pregnant women and newborns give complete instructions for using massage to ease discomforts of pregnancy and relieve the pain of labor and birth, as well as soothe and comfort restless babies and facilitate the bonding of mother and child.

"One of the best books on aromatherapy. Basic advice on purchasing, storing, and using essential oils is applicable for anyone interested in aromatherapy for better physical and emotional health."
The Herb Companion

Black Cumin
The Magical Egyptian Herb for Allergies, Asthma, and Immune Disorders

Peter Schleicher, M.D., and Mohamed Saleh, M.D.
ISBN 0-89281-843-3 • Paper, $9.95
96 pages, 5 x 7¾
10 black-and-white photographs

The extraordinary healing powers of black cumin have been known for centuries in the Middle East, and now its importance is revealed to the rest of the world. Because of its complex chemical structure—it has over one hundred active ingredients—black cumin has positive effects on the respiratory, immune, circulatory, digestive, and urinary systems. Includes specific recipes for infections and allergies, and precise directions for their preparation.

Magnet Therapy
The Gentle and Effective Way to Balance Body Systems

Ghanshyam Singh Birla and Colette Hemlin
ISBN 0-89281-841-7 • Paper, $12.95
160 pages, 6 x 9
37 black-and-white illustrations

Used successfully by more than 100 million people worldwide, magnet therapy has helped relieve pain, reduce blood pressure, enhance cellular regeneration, and even reduce tumor growth. Based on their years of work using magnets within the ancient Ayurvedic healing tradition, the authors present the history and science of this increasingly popular treatment. Complete with case studies and resource listings, *Magnet Therapy* is the comprehensive guide to one of the world's oldest proven healing systems.

Parenting Begins Before Conception

A Guide to Preparing Body, Mind, and Spirit
For You and Your Future Child

Carista Luminare-Rosen, Ph.D.
ISBN 0-89281-827-1 • Paper, $16.95
352 pages, 6 x 9
9 black-and-white illustrations

*"Parenting Begins Before Conception is a guide that every potential
parent will want to read. Nothing is more empowering than working
consciously with your baby's soul—even before that child is conceived.
I highly recommend Dr. Luminare-Rosen's work."*

Christiane Northrup, M.D., F.A.C.O.G.
Author of *Women's Bodies, Women's Wisdom*

Child Astrology

A Guide to Nurturing Your Child's Natural Gifts

M. J. Abadie
0-89281-722-4 • Paper, $14.95
272 pages, 6 x 9
11 astrological tables

A professional astrologer and psychotherapist offers a comprehensive look at the planets and their influence on your child's
emotional, intellectual, physical, and spiritual development in
this hands-on guide. With its planetary tables and clear instructions, even parents with no previous knowledge of astrology
can assist their child's development with an approach tailored
expressly to the child's individual gifts.

Chinese Massage for Infants and Children

Traditional Techniques for Alleviating Colic, Colds, Earaches, and Other Common Childhood Conditions

Kyle Cline, L.M.T.
ISBN 0-89281-797-6 • $19.95 pb
160 pages, 8 x 10
180 black-and-white line drawings

A leading practitioner of Chinese medicine provides a parents' handbook of simple massage techniques that can alleviate most common childhood ailments. *Chinese Massage for Infants and Children* first grounds parents in the basics of Chinese medicine, then illustrates 9 massage techniques, 63 massage points, and 22 complete massage plans. With additional information on a general health plan for all children and on using Chinese herbal remedies, this book can substantially reduce visits to the pediatrician and use of prescription medicines, while improving the bond between parent and child that is at the heart of good health.

Bach Flower Remedies for Children

A Parent's Guide

Barbara Mazzarella
ISBN 0-89281-649-X • $14.95
192 pages, 6 x 9

The first easy-to-use guide to safe and gentle Bach Flower remedies especially for children's well-being. Includes profiles of the 38 remedies along with practical applications for common childhood compaints. Each chapter incorporates a short story demonstrating the positive aspects of each flower type. Combined with the energies of the flowers themselves, these meditations and stories will help children overcome distress and grow into healthy, well-adjusted adults.